W9-CBG-502

ADDITIONAL PRAISE FOR *INSANE CONSEQUENCES*

"*Insane Consequences* does an amazing job explaining the impact of the failed mental health system on the criminal justice system. Every advocate, police chief, sheriff, district attorney, and mayor should read it."
—Chief (ret.) Michael Biasotti, author of the
International Association Chiefs of Police resolution on
Assisted Outpatient Treatment in the care of the severely mentally ill,
and a past Distinguished Fellow, US Department of Homeland Security

"DJ Jaffe has written a readily accessible and up-to-date book on serious mental disorders that should be a must-read for laypersons interested in mental disorders, family members of mentally ill persons, and patients themselves. A wide variety of mental disorders are described with clarity and graphic case examples. Moreover, the author points out clearly that lack of treatment facilities for the seriously mentally ill has led to their criminalization, with many more of these individuals now in jails than in psychiatric hospitals."
—Robert Paul Liberman, MD,
Distinguished Professor of Psychiatry, UCLA School of Medicine,
and director of the UCLA Psychiatric Rehabilitation Program

"In this important, thoroughly researched book, Jaffe exposes what is probably the largest, most audacious bait and switch operation in US history: unbeknownst to the public, what Jaffe calls 'the mental health industry' siphons off billions of taxpayer dollars each year, designed to serve the seriously mentally ill, to scientifically baseless or irrelevant programs (like prevention, when no one has the faintest idea of how to prevent major mental illness). Worse still, the small proportion of funds that go to the seriously ill are used to prevent treatment (under the false flag of civil rights) rather than to provide it."
—Rael Jean Isaac, coauthor of *Madness in the Streets:
How Psychiatry and the Law Abandoned the Mentally Ill*

"Jaffe's book is to the mental health industry what Al Gore's *An Inconvenient Truth* was to climate change. We can no longer afford to ignore the most seriously ill. My son and all people living with mental illness have a right to treatment. This book provides real solutions that will save money and lives."

—Liza Long, author of *The Price of Silence:*
A Mom's Perspective on Mental Illness,
a 2015 Books for a Better Life award winner

"Jaffe gives us vital answers. There is no other book that so completely identifies, specifically, how the United States is condemning tens of millions of seriously mentally ill citizens to tragic lives of extreme isolation, homelessness, incarceration, violence, suicide, and the lost chance of recovery. Much more than a screed against the mental health industry, lawmakers, the justice system, and an apathetic public, this book provides science-based commonsense answers that work. It should be mandatory reading for all involved in mental illness treatment, public safety, healthcare legislation, the justice system, and helping family caregivers."

—Xavier Amador, PhD, author of the international bestseller
I Am Not Sick, I Don't Need Help! How to Help Persons with
Mental Illness Accept Treatment;
former director of Psychology and professor in the
Department of Psychiatry, Columbia University;
and past member of the board of directors,
the National Alliance on Mental Illness

"I am proud that Jaffe, a constituent and member of the Harlem chapter of National Alliance on Mental Illness, has been tirelessly advocating to help the seriously mentally ill. Through increased awareness and improved public policy as outlined in this book, we can combat the challenges we face to ameliorate mental health."

—Charles Rangel, former representative from New York

"In the complicated and often crazy world of mental illness, Jaffe provides important guidance to journalists seeking a sound bite while he conveys controversial information."

—Eleanor Clift, Washington correspondent, *Daily Beast*

"*Insane Consequences* is a thorough accounting of the innumerable tragedies and lost opportunities brought about by America's broken mental health system. This book is the culmination of Jaffe's long history of speaking truth to power and provides a compelling counterargument to those who would attempt to maintain the current status quo."

—John Snook, executive director of the Treatment Advocacy Center

"In *Insane Consequences*, Jaffe marshals compelling case accounts and empirical data to show how America's mental health system—such as it is—grossly misallocates resources by focusing on the 'worried well' at the expense of those with serious brain disorders. One result is that our nation's jails have become de facto psychiatric institutions. This is a serious ethical transgression that Jaffe's hard-hitting account makes impossible to ignore."

—Dominic Sisti, PhD, director of the Scattergood Program
for Applied Ethics of Behavioral Health Care
and assistant professor of medical ethics and health policy at the
Perelman School of Medicine at the University of Pennsylvania

"Want to know what's wrong with America's disastrous mental health system? Look no further than Jaffe's thoughtful, clear, and insightful presentation on the shortfalls in a system that tolerates abuse, neglect, and suffering as a matter of official policy. Want to fix the system? Jaffe discusses this in the same straightforward, head-on manner. *Insane Consequences* is a must for any mental health library. It is a how-to manual for mental health advocates, and a road map for legislators implementing much-needed changes. Well done, Mr. Jaffe."

—Stephen B. Seager, MD, producer/director of the
award-winning documentary *Shattered Families:
The Collapse of America's Mental Health System,*
and author of *Behind the Gates of Gomorrah:
A Year with the Criminally Insane*

"*Insane Consequences* is the first candid book about mental illness that I have read. It really pulls no punches. It speaks the truth about our system, instead of the usual sugar-coated version. You should read this book, even if you are not affected by mental health issues. It's time to start educating the public about mental illness."

—Mia St. John, five-time World Boxing Council champion

insane consequences

insane

consequences

How the Mental Health Industry
Fails the Mentally Ill

DJ Jaffe

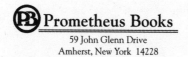 Prometheus Books

59 John Glenn Drive
Amherst, New York 14228

Inquiries should be addressed to
Prometheus Books
59 John Glenn Drive
Amherst, New York 14228
VOICE: 716–691–0133
FAX: 716–691–0137
WWW.PROMETHEUSBOOKS.COM

21 20 19 18 17   5 4 3 2 1

Library of Congress Cataloging-in-Publication Data

Names: Jaffe, D. J., 1954- author.
Title: Insane consequences : how the mental health industry fails the mentally ill /
    by DJ Jaffe ; foreword by E. Fuller Torrey, MD.
Description: Amherst, New York : Prometheus Books, 2017. | Includes index.
Identifiers: LCCN 2016050213 (print) | LCCN 2016051482 (ebook) |
    ISBN 9781633882911 (hardback) | ISBN 9781633882928 (ebook)
Subjects: LCSH: Mental health services. | Mentally ill—Care. | BISAC: MEDICAL /
    Public Health. | PSYCHOLOGY / Mental Health.
Classification: LCC RC455 .J28 2017 (print) | LCC RC455 (ebook) |
    DDC 362.2—dc23
LC record available at https://lccn.loc.gov/2016050213

*To Lynn, whose minute-to-minute battle against schizophrenia
demonstrates a heroic mental and physical fortitude
that makes me realize how weak I am.*

*To Dr. E. Fuller Torrey who took the time to teach me and thousands of others
what we need to know to rage successfully against the machine.*

*And to my wife, Rose, who stuck by my side for thirty-five years
in spite of everything I did to make walking out the saner choice.*

CONTENTS

SECTION 3: THE MENTAL HEALTH INDUSTRY

SECTION 4: THE INDUSTRY IS IN DENIAL

SECTION 5: DIVERTING FUNDS TO WHAT DOESN'T WORK

SECTION 6: FAILING THE SERIOUSLY MENTALLY ILL

SECTION 7: WHERE DO WE GO?

"What is remarkable about recent history is how the traditional advocates of the downtrodden played a major although unwitting role in putting the mentally ill into conditions that would have shocked previous generations of Americans."
—Clayton E. Cramer, author of
*My Brother Ron: A Personal and Social History
of the Deinstitutionalization of the Mentally Ill*

FOREWORD

by E. Fuller Torrey, MD

Episodes of violent behavior, including homicides, committed by individuals with serious mental illness who are not being treated are a growing problem and have become a national disgrace. It has been widely claimed that the public mental illness treatment system is failing because of a lack of funding. But as is true in the American medical care system in general, the United States spends more on public mental illness services than most other countries, yet this funding results in significantly poorer services. The United States excels in putting people with serious mental illness in jails and prisons or leaving them on the streets to fend for themselves. The problem is not a lack of funding, but rather how the funds are spent. We say that many of our sickest patients have a thinking disorder, yet the thinking that created the current mental illness treatment funding system is much more disordered than the thinking of our patients.

Imagine having a $3.7 billion federal agency that is supposed to be coordinating federal policies for individuals with serious mental illness, but among its 575 employees it does not have a single psychiatrist; this was the situation with the federal Substance Abuse and Mental Health Services Administration (SAMHSA). And at the state level things are not much better; currently only three states employ psychiatrists to oversee the state mental illness treatment system. A leadership void created the current mental illness mess.

Insane Consequences is one of the most important books written on how to reform the system. DJ Jaffe is the consummate public advocate. I know of nobody in the mental illness/mental health field who works as hard as he does, or is as effective. When the Government Accountability Office (GAO) issues a relevant report, DJ reads all 128 pages, plus the appendix while the rest of us read only the executive summary. When the US Senate introduces relevant legislation, DJ reads the entire bill, most of which is written in federal legalese; the rest of us wait for someone else to summarize it. He is an expert in exploring government websites to fish out those small but damaging facts that the government agency retrospectively wishes it had not released. Many of us who advocate for improved mental illness services for individuals with serious mental illness have used DJ's findings and ideas many times. He is invariably generous and selfless in sharing what he has found, never asking to be publicly credited.

Because DJ has studied the mental illness/mental health field so thoroughly, his ideas for reforming it deserve careful attention. DJ Jaffe represents the very best principles of democracy—one man really can make a difference. It has been a great pleasure to have worked with him for over twenty years, and it is an honor to contribute a foreword to this fine book.

E. Fuller Torrey, MD
Bethesda, Maryland
January 2017

AUTHOR'S NOTES

DEFINITIONS

Where possible, this book differentiates between "serious mental illness" (SMI) and "any mental illness." Briefly, "mental illness" encompasses the over three hundred diagnoses listed in the *Diagnostic and Statistical Manual* (*DSM*). "Serious mental illnesses" are the subset that *substantially* interfere with or limit the ability for someone to engage in major life activities. See chapters 4 and 5. The book also differentiates between "mental health" advocates who don't advocate for the most seriously ill and "mental illness" advocates who do. In the mental health industry, "peers" and "consumers" refer to people who have a mental illness, used mental health services or received a diagnosis. "Antipsychiatry" refers to groups and individuals who generally deny that mental illness exists or that treatment is useful. They believe both treatment and psychiatry are damage or torture.

STUDIES AND INTERVIEWS

Because single studies can be found to support any position, we examined multiple studies, often relying on collections created by the Treatment Advocacy Center (TAC) or Mental Illness Policy Org. (MIPO). Where possible, we quoted studies appertaining to *serious* mental illness, not *any* mental illness. We tried to provide URLs for the studies when they were available or to the abstract when they were not. However, authors often sanitize abstracts to downplay unpleasant or politically incorrect findings, so we have relied on the actual study rather than the abstract. Most studies are peer-reviewed, but we did include some non-peer-reviewed information from reputable sources like Dr. Thomas Insel, former director of the National Institute of Mental Health (NIMH).

During years of advocacy, the author has spoken with and corresponded with thousands of individuals with mental illness and their families, and quoted some in this book. Real names were used when permission was granted. Names and some identifying information were changed in the few cases where individuals preferred to remain anonymous or could not be located.

PROCEEDS

One hundred percent of the author's net proceeds will be donated to organizations working to improve care for people with serious mental illnesses, including the Treatment Advocacy Center in Arlington, Virginia, and Mental Illness Policy Org. in New York City.

UPDATES

To keep up to date on mental illness policy, visit Mental Illness Policy Org. at http://mentalillnesspolicy.org/, follow us on twitter at @MentalIll Policy, and like our Facebook page at https://www.facebook.com/Mental -Illness-Policy-Org-323404203517/.

Also visit the Treatment Advocacy Center at http://www.treatment advocacycenter.org/, follow it on twitter, @TreatmentAdvCtr, or like it on Facebook at https://www.facebook.com/TreatmentAdvocacyCtr/.

To support efforts to improve care, make a tax deductible donation to either organization.

DISCLAIMER

This book does not contain medical advice or legal advice. Do not rely on it. Contact a doctor or lawyer if you need medical or legal advice.

HOW I GOT INVOLVED

On September 2, 1985, my wife, Rose, and I picked up her eighteen-year-old sister, Lynn, at LaGuardia Airport. Lynn had been one of the best-liked, highest-performing students in her Wisconsin high school. She was attending community college and living at home with her lovable, babushka-wearing, Hungarian-immigrant mom, a hard-working, church-going widow who cleaned houses to support herself and Lynn. But recently their relationship soured. They started having bitter fights. One day, in an unprovoked, psychotic rage, Lynn slapped the mom she loved. She was hospitalized for "being mental," then came home, and after several weeks, when her medications wore off, she repeated the behavior.

My wife and I thought the problem was due to an American teen living with an old-world mom and that moving Lynn to New York City to live with us aging hippies would solve all her problems. We were that stupid.

At first, Lynn was the perfect New Yorker, taking long walks in Central Park, people-watching in our Chelsea neighborhood, and shopping in the East Village. But slowly, as the weeks went by, her concentration became scattered and her speech became rushed, breathless, and pressured. Delusional thoughts would come cascading out of her mouth in an uncontrollable barrage of disconnected ideas that made no sense, even to her. She started becoming paranoid, convinced that conversations taking place across the street involved plots to kill her.

One afternoon, after she spent hours screaming at the voices in her head, we took her to the emergency room. She was admitted, diagnosed, medicated, and provided rehabilitative therapy. But to "protect her privacy," her doctor wouldn't tell us her diagnosis, what medications he'd given Lynn, or what would happen when her hospitalization ended. Lynn returned home to us and stopped taking the antipsychotic medications we didn't even know she'd been prescribed. She deteriorated again, started screaming at voices only she could hear, and engaged in pitched arguments with herself about Jesus, God, and the devil.

We tried to get her to go back to the hospital, but she refused. She didn't think the problem was with her; she knew it was with us. She "knew" we were plotting to kill her. Her illness told her so. "I know you're trying to poison me. I'm going to kill you first," she said more than once. We called the police, hoping they could get her to the hospital, but when they arrived, Lynn went mute, so they didn't see evidence of her being a "danger to self or others." "We can only help after she becomes violent, not before," the displeased officer informed us.

Eventually, she slipped into catatonia, was rehospitalized, and the pattern repeated: hospitalize, stabilize on medications, go off medication, rehospitalize. After Lynn underwent several ins and outs, a nurse remarked, "Well, people with schizophrenia often feel that . . ." "Schizophrenia? Is that what she has?" my wife asked. "Didn't your doctor discuss that with you?" the nurse innocently inquired. Nope. Never did.

I started researching schizophrenia and was astounded by the depth of my ignorance. I thought schizophrenia meant a split personality. That it was psychological, not medical, and people with it were just plain "nuts."

It's a real *physical* disorder, but because it affects the brain, people who suffer from it sometimes don't even know they are ill and therefore can't regulate their thoughts or behavior. They become victims of their hallucinations and delusions and often can't think straight.

The next time the hospital released Lynn, we got her into a day treatment program that was supposed to offer the structure people with schizophrenia often find comforting and help her reintegrate and regain skills she had lost. But a few weeks later, the program director called and said he didn't want Lynn in the program anymore because she wouldn't attend group therapy. We asked Lynn why, and she told us that in group therapy everyone talked about suicide and she found it depressing and against her Catholic religion, which proscribes suicide. In other words, she had two very good reasons for not attending group therapy, and because of that, they were going to end her treatment. That was the moment when I realized how dysfunctional and disconnected the mental health system had become from the needs of the seriously mentally ill.

I started raising money for the New York City chapter of the National Alliance on Mental Illness (NAMI) and eventually joined the board. The NAMI chapter was staffed by exceedingly dedicated volunteers, primarily aging mothers of persons with serious mental illness. These heroic moms answered helpline calls from other moms and gave out fact sheets. The most frequent calls were what one would expect: How do I find the right doctor? How do I find the right medicine? Is there a housing program for my relative? How do I plan my estate?

But one common call was "My seriously mentally ill son/daughter/ mother/father/sister/brother is locked in his room. He 'knows' the FBI planted a transmitter in his head and won't come out. He won't eat because he 'knows' the food is poisoned, won't shower because he doesn't want to wash away his protective field, and can't sleep for fear of attack. What can I do?" There was no answer to this question, no fact sheet we could write. The law prevents parents from helping psychotic or delusional loved ones who refuse treatment until *after* they become a danger. As ludicrous as it sounds, rather than preventing violence, the law requires it.

That realization led me on a thirty-year journey to try to find out what is wrong with the mental health system and what can be done to fix it. This book is the product of that search.

OVERVIEW OF EVERYTHING

"It's hard to determine which is more delusional: the mental health system or the people it's intended to treat."
—Dr. E. Fuller Torrey

America's mental health system is insane, expensive, and ineffective. Under the guise of protecting civil rights, it is killing people. Under the guise of increasing freedom, it is increasing incarceration. Under the guise of facilitating recovery, it ensures that fewer recover. In the name of protecting privacy, it causes suicide. America treats the least seriously ill ("the worried well") and forces the most seriously ill to fend for themselves. The ability to get help has become inversely related to need. We move sick people from hospitals to jails and label it progress. Government funds those who created the problems rather than those with solutions. The more dysfunctional the system becomes, the more money we throw at it. Our mental health system is not based on science and has nothing to do with compassion. As a result, there are ten times more people with mental illness incarcerated as hospitalized. "Being Mentally Ill" has essentially become a crime.

Our system forces people with serious mental illness to suffer. Your happy, smart, popular child enters his late teens or early twenties, and then slowly schizophrenia strikes. First, he becomes withdrawn, scared, and noncommunicative. Then he becomes imprisoned in a straitjacket of paranoid psychotic thinking that spews forth whenever he talks. My own sister-in-law told me in a single sentence:

> The FBI planted a transmitter in my head God is the Messiah did you see *Jeopardy!* maybe I'm too smart they're after me trying to kill me why

19

is everyone around here so crazy I like the Beatles Johnny is gay Kathy you know what she did I'm gonna be an astronaut that way the beams won't get me. Hahaha.

You attempt to use reason to convince your child that something is wrong and to get help, but he's too sick to know he's sick. He refuses to go to a doctor because "I'm not crazy, and I know you're beaming thoughts into my head."

You find a social worker who tries to win your son over. He refuses her help too. And because he is over the age of eighteen, or as young as twelve in California, Illinois, and West Virginia, he has the right to refuse all treatment.[1] Federally funded lawyers will defend his right to be psychotic. You call the mental health department, so your son starts threatening you: "You want to get rid of me I'm gonna kill you I'm not crazy you're crazy get out of my room! Stop poisoning my food!"

Out of options, you call the police. But they can't help either because he's not dangerous enough yet. Even if you manage to get your son into a hospital, privacy laws will prevent you from learning what's wrong or what's next. He will be discharged to your care without your knowing what the diagnosis is, what medications he should be taking, when the next doctor appointment is, or what to do. Will your son stay on the medications? Will he go off them and become violent to himself, toward you, or maybe toward a bystander? Will that make him a headline? Will you become the headline when the public blames you for being the mom of the next "Psychotic Killer Goes on Rampage"?

There are forty-three million Americans over eighteen affected with "any mental illness" and ten million with "serious mental illness."[2] At least 140,000 of these seriously mentally ill are homeless and often can be seen foraging in Dumpsters, engaged in pitched battles with demons only they can see.[3] Some 392,037 are in jails and prisons.[4] An additional 755,360 are on probation or parole, and many of them will return to jail or prison multiple times.[5] At least 95,000 who need hospitalization can't get a bed because of the deadly shortage.[6] More than 5,000 kill themselves every year.[7] Their untreated mental illnesses make them more likely to be murdered and more likely to be victims of violent crime than the mentally healthy.[8] They die up to twenty-five years earlier than others. While most people with mental illness do not become violent, those with *untreated serious mental illness* are more likely than others to become violent. Their victims are most likely to be members of their own families. The public becomes aware of the issue only when strangers are killed en masse:

- Aaron Alexis had untreated mental illness when he shot and killed twelve people in September 2013, thereby becoming the "DC Navy Yard Shooter."[9]
- One L. Goh shot and killed seven and injured three at Oikos University in California in April 2012. He had schizophrenia.[10]
- Seung-Hui Cho had untreated mental illness when he killed thirty-two and wounded seventeen in April 2007 at Virginia Tech.[11]

Maintaining our failed mental health system is expensive. In 2014, the federal government spent $147 billion in taxpayer funds on mental health.[12] And that doesn't include state spending. The New York State Office of Mental Health alone spends $3.5 billion annually.[13] Since 2005, California has been investing in excess of $1 billion in public funds annually on mental health and has little to show for it.[14] We are spending more, yet the problems are getting worse.

WE HAVE TO STOP IGNORING THE SERIOUSLY ILL

Mental "health" advocates blame the problem on lack of funding. They are wrong. The mental health advocates themselves are the problem.[15] One hundred percent of adults feel sad at some point and can have their mental health improved. Eighteen percent had some sort of mental illness in the past year. But only four percent had a "serious" mental illness like schizophrenia, bipolar disorder, or severe, major depression.[16] As documented in section seven, the mental health industry persuaded the government to ignore the four percent with a serious mental illness and invest the funds on improving the mental health of all others.

The mental health industry cherry-picks the most compliant and least symptomatic. It labels all other patients "high-needs" and claims it is not set up to help them. A psychiatric social worker admitted to me, "A rampant problem with not only the mental health system but the entire healthcare system is it discriminates against potential clients it perceives as being too difficult to handle."

While ignoring those with serious illnesses, the mental health industry expands the number of people entitled to services by inventing new illnesses like bullying and cyberbullying. It declares poverty, bad grades, divorce, sexual dysfunction, and unemployment to be mental illnesses and diverts mental health funding to them. It even persuaded the Substance Abuse and Mental Health Services Administration (SAMHSA), which develops the nation's mental health policy, and state mental health authorities to ignore science and fund politically correct pop psychology that improves nothing but the industry's own coffers. The industry convinced the states to shutter psychiatric hospitals that serve the seriously ill and enact laws that prevent the seriously ill from being helped until after they become "a danger to self or others."

Until the 1940s, public funds were used to treat the "insane." Then we moved to helping the "mentally ill," then to the even broader mission of "improving mental health," then to the broader mission of addressing "behavioral health," and today we've arrived at denying that the seriously ill exist and divert the funds to "wellness services" for everyone.

The industry is "medicalizing ever larger swaths of human experience."[17] The American Psychiatric Association fuels this trend with each new edition of the *Diagnostic and Statistical Manual* (*DSM*), which defines ever greater numbers of normal emotional reactions, such as grief over losing a parent, as mental disorders.[18] Outreach workers pour into elementary schools looking for barely symptomatic children to engorge the mental health system.

Meanwhile, everyone ignores the seriously mentally ill in plain sight. No one stands outside homeless shelters or prison doors to help those who really have serious mental illnesses stay in treatment. It's become harder to get into Bellevue than Harvard. And if the most seriously ill can find a hospital to admit them, they will be discharged "sicker and quicker." They wind up in jails, prisons, shelters, and nursing homes, moving from an institution that was appropriate to others that are not.

The solution is to replace mission creep with mission control. We have to stop ignoring the most seriously ill. We have to spend less on mental

health and more on serious mental illness. And we have to base our policies on science.

Insane Consequences will show how the mental health industry wrested
control of mental illness policy and spending from the government. The
industry focuses on improving the mental health of everyone rather than
delivering treatment to the 4 percent with serious mental illness. Their "three
main strategies when discussing schizophrenia and other forms of psychotic
illness *is to deny it, romanticize it, or trivialize it.*"[19] This book argues that the
government has to recognize certain unpleasant truths about the most seriously mentally ill that the mental health industry convinced it to ignore:
not everyone recovers, sometimes hospitals are necessary, involuntary treatment is preferable to incarceration, and there is a group of the most seriously
ill who—*left untreated*—become suicidal, homeless, criminal, incarcerated,
and, yes, sometimes violent. To solve these problems, we should focus our
resources on science-based treatments for those who need help the most
rather than on those who need help the least. We should move away from
a system that requires tragedy before treatment to one that offers treatment
before tragedy. Pretending the seriously mentally ill don't exist is no solution.

Section 1 describes the *Insane Consequences* of ignoring the most
seriously ill: increased homelessness, suicide, victimization, perpetration,
arrest, violence, imprisonment, and suffering. It documents the drain on
the criminal justice system, the danger to the public and patients, and the
cost to taxpayers.

Section 2 details the difference between poor mental health and serious
mental illness for those new to the subject. While the boundary between
the two is debatable, the extremities are clear. It describes the science of
serious mental illness because policy should be driven by that science.

Section 3 introduces the major mental health organizations that fail
the most seriously ill, with particular attention to the Substance Abuse
and Mental Health Services Administration (SAMHSA), the Center for
Mental Health Services (CMHS), and the nonprofits they fund. It also
identifies the good guys who are trying to convince the government to treat
the most seriously ill.

Sections 4 and 5 document exactly how SAMHSA and the mental health industry prevent help from reaching the seriously mentally ill and encourage the government to waste money on programs that don't help.

Section 6 identifies the major federal actions and US Supreme Court decisions that fail the seriously ill.

Section 7 lays out a road map for reform. It proposes ways to eliminate wasteful mental health spending and increase the efficacy of existing spending.

After reading this book, I hope you will conclude that lack of money is not as big a problem as lack of leadership. We have to narrowly focus our resources on delivering actual treatment to those known to be the most seriously mentally ill rather than on all the softer sideshows that receive funding now. We have to adopt policies grounded in science. That path will improve the lives of people with the most serious mental illnesses, save money, keep the public, police, and patients safer, and make us a better country.

INFAMOUS MENTALLY ILL ADULTS WHO WENT OFF TREATMENT

Adults with untreated serious mental illness can cause devastating consequences for the public, police, and the ill individuals and their families.

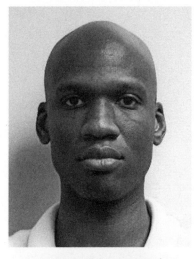

Washington, DC, Naval Yard Shooting

Mentally ill Aaron Alexis was not in treatment when he shot and killed twelve people in the Washington, DC, Navy Yard.[1] (Photo: US Navy)

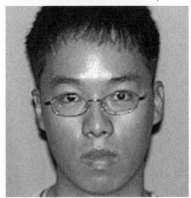

Virginia Tech Shooting

Mentally ill Seung-Hui Cho was not in treatment when he killed thirty-two and wounded seventeen at Virginia Tech.[2] (Photo: Virginia State Police)

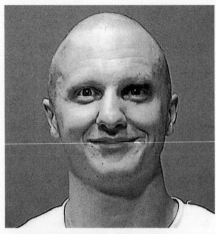

Gabrielle Giffords's Shooting

Mentally ill Jared Loughner was not in treatment when he killed six and wounded US Representative Gabrielle Giffords.[3] (Photo: US Marshals Service)

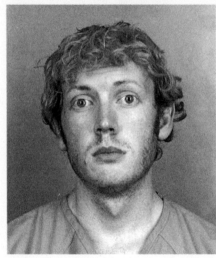

Aurora, Colorado, Theater Shooting

Mentally ill James Holmes was not in treatment when he shot and killed twelve in an Aurora, Colorado, theater.[4] (Photo: Arapahoe County Detention Center)

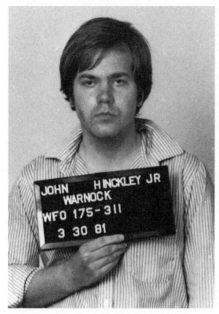

Ronald Reagan Shooting

Mentally ill John Hinckley was not in treatment when he shot President Reagan.[5] (Photo: FBI)

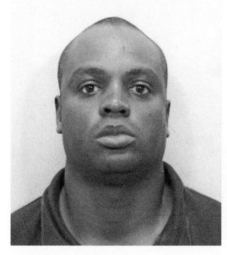

Texas Chevron Station Police Shooting

Mentally ill Shannon J. Miles was not in treatment when he shot and killed Harris County Deputy Sheriff Darren Goforth at a Chevron station north of Houston.[6] (Photo: Harris County Sheriff)

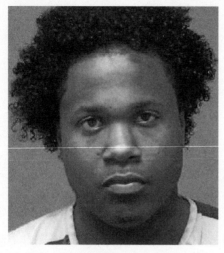

New York City Police Shooting

Mentally ill Ismaaiyl Brinsley was not in treatment when he ambushed and killed two police officers sitting in their patrol car in Brooklyn, New York.[7] (Photo: Springfield, OH, Police)

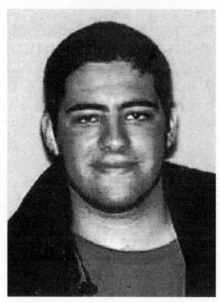

Santa Monica College Shooting

Mentally ill John Zawahri wasn't known to be in treatment when he killed five and wounded more in a mass shooting at Santa Monica College.[8] (Photo: Santa Monica Police Department)

Section 1

THE INSANE CONSEQUENCES

Chapter 1

HUMAN CONSEQUENCES OF IGNORING THE SERIOUSLY MENTALLY ILL

"We have a Humpty Dumpty mental health system."
—Unknown

INTRODUCTION

When the mental "illness" system disappeared and the mental "health" system replaced it, homelessness, hospitalization, crime, arrest, violence, incarceration, shootings of and by police, and expenditures for mental illness all went up. The only metrics going down are the number of psychiatric beds available to treat the seriously mentally ill and the number of nonprofits, government agencies, advocates, and politicians that care. We're in this mess because the mental health industry convinced the government to abandon treating the most seriously mentally ill in favor of serving the highest functioning. This focus on improving mental health over treating serious mental illness has *Insane Consequences*.

High-profile tragedies are so common that the National Association of State Mental Health Program Directors (NASMHPD) created a "toolkit" to deflect media criticism away from state mental health directors when they are appropriately "put on the hot seat" after someone with untreated serious mental illness goes on a rampage.[1] Their "toolkit" includes fact sheets to convince the media that mental illness is not associated with violence, violence by the mentally ill cannot be predicted, and the public has nothing to fear. All this is false.

INCREASED VIOLENCE IN THE COMMUNITY

Mass murders by people with untreated serious mental illness are exceedingly rare, but seem increasingly common. James Holmes gained celebrity status when he shot and killed twelve people in an Aurora, Colorado, movie theater. He was previously identified by a school psychologist as being mentally ill and potentially dangerous, but he was not required to be in treatment.[2] Jared Loughner shot Representative Gabrielle Giffords and killed six people in Arizona in January 2011. He, too, was known to be mentally ill and potentially dangerous but was not required to be in treatment.[3] Mentally ill John Zawahri wasn't known to be in treatment when he killed five and wounded more in a mass shooting at Santa Monica College. The siblings of John Hinckley knew he was mentally ill and tried to have him hospitalized for mental illness, before he shot President Reagan, but were unsuccessful.[4]

Mother Jones found 63 percent of mass shooters between 1982 and 2012 had mental illness.[5] Getting mentally ill shooters into treatment might have saved the lives of others, and prevented them from being buried alive behind bars. According to psychiatrist E. Fuller Torrey, author of nine books on serious mental illness and scores of studies, up to 10 percent of all US homicides are likely due to untreated serious mental illness.[6] A 2008 study found that more than twenty-six thousand Americans with a mental illness were incarcerated for murder.[7]

Parents and family members, not the public, are the most likely victims of violence by people with untreated serious mental illness. Of the four thousand homicides in the United States in 2013, where someone killed his own family member, 29 percent were by someone with serious mental illness.[8]

- Palm Beach, FL: On January 9, 2013, twenty-three-year-old Alan Farajian fatally stabbed his mother, Gloria Farajian, because of an argument over a TV show. Farajian suffered from bipolar disorder and schizophrenia and had stopped taking medication for those illnesses.[9]
- Ocoee, FL: On February 18, 2013, twenty-one-year-old Meagan Jones fatally stabbed her mother, sixty-five-year-old Linda Jones.

Linda told authorities that Meagan had bipolar disorder and was off her medication.[10]
- Cresson, TX: On January 9, 2013, thirty-year-old Jacob Dwight Farren attacked his mother, fifty-four-year-old Beverly Farren, with a hammer. She said her son was diagnosed with bipolar disorder and wouldn't take medication for that illness.[11]

As shown in appendix B, overwhelming evidence from the United States and other countries shows a clear connection between *untreated* serious mental illness and violence. Dr. Thomas Insel, immediate past director of the National Institute on Mental Health (NIMH), cited the extensiveness of the evidence:

> I'd like to say something which I think is unpopular with many people in the mental health community. But the data I believe are fairly unambiguous. . . . An active psychotic illness is associated with irrational behavior and violence can be part of that. The numbers are stunning. . . . There is a fifteen fold reduction in risk of homicide, with and without treatment.[12]

After looking at all the research over multiple years, violence researcher John Monahan declared:

> The data that have recently become available, fairly read, suggest the one conclusion I did not want to reach: whether the sample is people who are selected for treatment as inmates or patients in institutions or people randomly chosen from the open community, and no matter how many social or demographic factors are statistically taken into account, there appears to be a relationship between mental disorder and violent behavior.[13]

Violence is not associated with poor mental health, mental illness, or serious mental illness. It is clearly associated with serious mental illness *that is allowed to go untreated.*

INCREASED VIOLENCE IN PSYCHIATRIC WORKPLACES

So many mentally ill are going without treatment that psychiatric work-places are becoming increasingly dangerous. According to the American Psychiatric Nurses Association (APNA), 75–100 percent of the nursing staff on acute psychiatric units had been assaulted during their careers.[14] It wasn't always like that. Historically, violent patients would remain hospitalized while orderlies controlled them and doctors medicated them; then the danger passed and the patient could be safely released. No longer. As a result of lawsuits brought by mental health industry lawyers, patients, even those involuntarily committed because they are dangerous, maintain the right to refuse treatment.[15] On top of making medicating more difficult, SAMHSA and mental health industry advocates are working to ban the use of restraints and seclusion.[16] When a patient lashes out, the hospital now has little choice but to call the police and have the individual jailed. Mental health advocates are turning patients into prisoners and making hospitals more dangerous for everyone.

As will be seen in chapter 9, treatment could reduce the violence, but advocates and the industry refuse to admit that a connection between untreated serious mental illness and violence exists.

INCREASED HOMELESSNESS

In January 2015, the most extensive survey ever undertaken found 564,708 people were homeless on a given night in the United States.[17] Depending on the age group in question, and how homelessness is defined, the consensus estimate as of 2014 was that, at minimum, 25 percent of the American homeless—140,000 individuals—were *seriously* mentally ill at any given point in time. Forty-five percent of the homeless—250,000 individuals—had *any* mental illness. More would be labeled homeless if these were annual counts rather than point-in-time counts.

It is not surprising so many seriously ill are homeless. Leaving serious mental illness untreated can cause bizarre behavior that makes living with families untenable and homelessness inevitable. Jennifer Hoff's son became seriously mentally ill at the age of twelve. She spoke at a 2014 rally held to protest California's neglect of the seriously mentally ill:

My son was so sick he was kept in residential treatment from age twelve to eighteen for safety. He has "crazy boy" tattooed across his face. But when he turned eighteen, he was discharged to live homeless on the streets in front of the Civic Center in Santa Ana. When we tried to get him housing and help . . . his case manager said I'd be a better mother if I supported his "choice of housing." I still have that text. I have them all. So we watched—and they watched. They stood by and watched him go off his medications. Today my son is incarcerated.[18]

Being homeless is a terrible way to live. Many shelters won't accept unmedicated seriously mentally ill adults because their intense delusions and sometimes aggressive behavior make it impossible to maintain order. Even so-called "good" shelters often won't accept families with seriously ill children, by claiming they are full. During the day homeless untreated mentally ill cower down streets, scream at voices only they can hear, and forage Dumpsters for food. At night, they search for a street grate that might provide some heat. The seriously mentally ill commit quality-of-life crimes such as trespassing to find a place to sleep or stealing food to eat. Mentally ill who are homeless are more likely to be raped, assaulted, and injured.[19]

INCREASED SUBSTANCE ABUSE

People with serious mental illness often use pot, alcohol, or harder drugs to quell the delusions infesting their heads, leading to higher arrest rates and greater crime. According to a 2006 study, 74 percent of state prisoners, 76 percent of local jail inmates, and 63 percent of state prisoners who had mental health problems used drugs in the month before their arrest.[20] Of adults without mental illness, 6 percent have a substance use disorder. But among those with any mental illness, the percentage is three times higher (18 percent), and for those with serious mental illness, it is almost four times higher (23 percent).[21]

INCREASED SUICIDE

Suicide is always horrible but thankfully rare. Forty-two thousand suicides are completed each year, representing .012 percent of the population.[22] But a disproportionate number, 13 percent, or about five thousand suicides, are likely committed by people with serious mental illness.[23] The lifetime risk to those with schizophrenia is 5 percent and to those with bipolar disorder is 10–15 percent.[24] Suicide rates are up to fifteen times higher for people with serious mental illness in the ninety days following discharge from a psychiatric hospitalization than they are for the general population.[25]

Mental health advocates claim up to 90 percent of suicides are mental illness related. That may be untrue. Whenever anyone takes his life after having lost a spouse or job, received a bad grade in school or a disturbing medical diagnosis, the industry puts the suicide in the mental illness column, even though losing a job, getting a bad grade, and receiving a new medical diagnosis are not mental illnesses. As documented in chapter 12, instead of treatment, the mental health industry uses suicide prevention funds for unproven "awareness" programs featuring their logos and targeted to those least likely to commit suicide. Suicide funds have become a cash cow for mental health nonprofit organizations.

INCREASED VICTIMIZATION

People with untreated serious mental illness are more often victimized than the general public. In their psychotic and delusional state, they are often robbed and raped in shelters, randomly beaten in the street, stuck up by drug dealers, and forced to live a hellish existence. One study found "more than one quarter of persons with serious mental illness (over three million persons) had been victims of a violent crime in the past year, a rate more than 11 times higher than the general population. ... Depending on the type of violent crime (rape/sexual assault, robbery, assault, and their subcategories), victimization was 6 to 23 times greater among persons with serious mental illness than among the general population."[26] Another study found "compared to community controls, patients with schizophrenia-spectrum disorders were significantly more likely to have a record of violent ... and sexually violent victimization."[27] Latifah, the mother of one seriously ill young man, told me,

My son was living at a group home. But he went off his medication and started walking around pounding his bare chest like Tarzan. He would do it for hours so the group home "disappeared" him.[28] We called the police who told us, "He has a right to leave." The only way we could get the police to take our report was to say he didn't have his medications, and ask how it would look if they didn't even take our report and something bad happened. A week later, we got a call saying he was in a hospital in Philadelphia. We drove down, walked into his room, and my stomach turned. Ali's nose was mangled. Teeth were missing. He had a gash in his cheek and bruises that hadn't healed yet. He says, "Hi mom" like nothing happened. He wouldn't tell us what did happen but we think some of the homeless people beat him up to steal his winter coat.

Studies show that some of the increased victimization of persons with mental illness is the result of living in homeless shelters. Other studies attribute the higher than average incidence of victimization of persons with mental illness to their increased use of substances.[29] But while "co-morbid substance misuse and criminality both heighten the chances of victimization, they cannot fully account for the increased rates."[30] The higher incidence of victimization can result from the illness itself.[31] The same treatments and policies that can restore sanity and reduce homelessness, incarceration, arrest, and suicide can also reduce victimization. But as will be seen in sections four and five, the mental health system stands in the way of implementing them.

THE DESTRUCTION OF FAMILIES

Leaving people with serious mental illness untreated takes a devastating and invisible toll on families. A delusional, hallucinating loved one who is constantly yelling at the voices in her head, causes all members of the family to walk on eggshells, forced to stand back for fear of creating a scene or worse. Parents and siblings who are unable to force ill relatives into treatment are instead forced to take out orders of protection. The needs of the ill prevent parents from addressing the needs of other children. Families have to cope with drugs and strangers brought into the house. Few can withstand the strain:

- "My husband left me. Neither one of us can live with the tension in the house caused by our daughter. He can walk out. I won't abandon her."—Rose
- "My son can't take me anymore. That's part of his angst—being 'dependent' on his mom. I don't blame him. I wish he didn't need me and could live independently, drive again. Hopefully someday."—Mary Palafox, after years of providing care to her mentally ill son.
- "My daughter is extremely bright, earned an advanced degree and had a promising career in human resource management. About nine years ago, however, she spiraled out of control. She suffers from a psychotic illness but does not believe she is seriously ill and so cannot be in the vicinity of her 9-year-old son as a result of the disturbing behaviors she has exhibited, including kidnapping. As a result, she is now homeless."—Kathleen Branch[32]

If the mental health industry is the villain, moms and dads are the heroes, with siblings and children of the ill not far behind. Moms do everything they can to keep their families together and prevent loved ones from becoming the next "psychotic killer" headline. But they are looked on as pariahs by the mental health industry. Too many doctors, social workers, and mental health administrators will spout platitudes about the importance of family involvement until the family disagrees with their decision to deny their loved ones needed care. Then all bets are off. "The family doesn't understand" or "We have to empower the patient," they are told.

Families are thwarted by hospitals that have shut their doors, community programs that declare their family members "high-needs patients," doctors who are forced by administrators to hide behind patient privacy laws and prevent parents from getting the information they need to help, and industry-supported laws that require their loved ones to become dangerous before they can be treated. Those who work in the system may be well-meaning, but they've acquiesced to bean counting, box-checking "quality improvement" plans that lower quality, prevent improvement, and cause mayhem for families. In one year, an estimated 1,149 persons were killed by a relative with serious mental illness.[33] Rael Jean Isaac, coauthor of *Madness in the Streets*, put it succinctly: "The family is the new mental institution."[34] Aging parents try to provide case management, housing, and treatment to psychotic and delusional loved ones without the information they need or the authority to enforce compliance. Renee, whose son suffers from schizophrenia, told me,

> I try to get my son to see a doctor, but he doesn't believe he is ill, and thinks I'm the ill one. I try to convince him, but that only makes the tension escalate. One day he told me he wants to be a nuclear engineer, and yet he can't even understand his cousin is not Osama-bin Laden.

Trying to get treatment for an ill family member takes countless hours, scores of daily calls, callbacks, hours on hold, and visits to facilities, and success is not guaranteed. Researchers at Harvard investigated how difficult it is to get an appointment with a psychiatrist.

"Posing as patients, investigators called 360 psychiatrists listed in a major insurer's database. . . . In round one of calling, investigators were able to reach 119 of the 360 psychiatrists (33%). Of 216 unanswered calls, 35 were returned. After two calling rounds, appointments were made with 93 psychiatrists (26%)."[35]

It's not necessarily the fault of the psychiatrists; that's the system they work in. Chirlane McCray, the powerful First Lady of New York City, wrote about her experience when she tried to get help for her daughter, Chiara:

> "I'm sorry, but the doctor isn't taking new patients right now." It took me a moment to grasp what the receptionist was telling me. After hours of internet research, innumerable phone calls, and frustrating discussions with some well-meaning but distant professionals, the psychiatrist we had identified as a good fit for Chiara wouldn't be able to help us. I hung up the phone and put my head down on the table. My first impulse was to leave it there until the world started making sense again, but there was no time for that. My daughter needed help.[36]

Laura Pogliano is a middle-class, single, educated mom and an informed and unstoppable advocate who lives in the suburbs of Baltimore. She described the effort she went through to get one single hospitalization (he had thirteen) for her son, Zac:

We had four hearings. The first was for the emergency petition to remove him from the house to care at the nearest ER and then transfer to Hopkins [hospital]. Next week, there was mental health court inside Hopkins (miracle) to remove competency so he could be treated. In the third week, there was a hearing for a medical panel who decided if he was bad off enough to force meds and what meds to prescribe. Finally, there was a 48-hour appeal process. From EP [emergency petition] to injection, fifteen days passed, all while in care and racking up a huge bill, without so much as an aspirin.

In spite of her heroic ongoing efforts, on January 18, 2015, Zac was found dead in his room.

These hours of phone calls take parents away from their other children and often cause them to lose hours of pay or even their jobs. Whole families can become homeless. The burden on low-income families is almost unfathomable. One sweet, elderly church lady I met at a Harlem NAMI chapter meeting told me why she couldn't appeal the state's decision not to provide her daughter housing: "I don't have enough minutes." It never occurred to me that something as simple as cell phone minutes could be a barrier to care. She went on to tell me that even if he had enough minutes, her boss—she makes beds at a hospital—would never let her take a break long enough to make the innumerable calls.

In spite of their efforts, parents are inevitably blamed when something goes wrong. Loretta Bodtmann, the mom of a mentally ill son, spoke for all families when she wrote in a Facebook group,

> When a family can no longer deal with an SMI (seriously mentally ill) family member who has become violent and the family can't get help, the families are blamed for being negligent and not caring. When a family cannot physically or emotionally deal with an SMI family member, they are blamed for their weakness. Their years long efforts with trying to care for them are ignored. It's like people expect families of the SMI to be perfect, and if they are not, everything is their fault. Even if they've taken care of their SMI family member with heroic virtue and much sacrifice, it's still the family's fault. We've all been blamed in some way somehow by others for the actions of our ill children.

Susan Schick was the mother of mentally ill John Schick, who shot six people on March 8, 2012, at the Western Psychiatric Institute in Pittsburgh before being shot by responding officers.[37] Susan tried to get John help for years before the incident. As if losing a son wasn't enough, she had to hire lawyers because she herself was sued by his victims who said the shootings were her fault for "abandoning" her son. She told the attorneys who forced her into giving a gut-wrenching deposition what every mom of someone with serious mental illness knows. "I think the overwhelming issue here was not that he was feeling abandoned by us, but that he needed to get the psychiatric care he needed. And I couldn't compel that, my husband couldn't compel that, nor could the doctors."[38]

The most frequent question I hear from parents is, "Who will take care of my mentally ill loved one after I die?"

In the following chapter, we discuss the impact that abandoning the most seriously mentally ill has had on the criminal justice system.

Chapter 2

CRIMINAL JUSTICE CONSEQUENCES OF IGNORING THE SERIOUSLY MENTALLY ILL

> *"We have two mental health systems today, serving two mutually exclusive populations: Community programs serve those who seek and accept treatment. Those who refuse, or are too sick to seek treatment voluntarily, become a law enforcement responsibility. . . . [M]ental health officials seem unwilling to recognize or take responsibility for this second more symptomatic group."*
>
> —Chief of Police (ret.) Michael Biasotti[1]

INCREASED DRAIN ON POLICE

The failure of the mental health system is forcing police to fill the gap. Lompoc, California, police chief Pat Walsh told a Santa Barbara committee that "30–40 percent of all calls for service in Lompoc involved the mentally ill."[2] According to a March 17, 2016, report in the *Green Bay Press Gazette*, "Green Bay, Wisconsin police respond to 20,000 to 32,000 mental illness–related incidents every year . . . amounting to 25 to 40 percent of the 80,000 calls for service the department receives annually." These numbers are typical of police departments throughout the country.

Leaving serious mental illness untreated forces people with mental illness into the criminal justice system. It causes homelessness, violence, suicide, and victimization. Without treatment, many mentally ill homeless camp in public, loiter, panhandle, store their belongings in public, and engage in other activities classified as crimes.[3] Failing to find a bathroom you can use and urinating in public three times can also lead to arrest under "three strikes and you're out" laws. Persons with untreated serious mental illness may develop psychosis and believe a celebrity is in love with them, forcing police to arrest them to stop the stalking.[4]

Michael Biasotti is the former chief of police in New Windsor, New York, past president of the New York State Association of Chiefs of Police, has a daughter with serious mental illness, and is a recognized expert on policing the mentally ill. He conducted a nationwide survey of 2,406 senior law enforcement officials that found that local law enforcement authorities are overwhelmed "dealing with the unintended consequences of a policy change that in effect removed the daily care of our nation's severely mentally ill population from the medical community and placed it with the criminal justice system."[5] Officers blame the mental health system for failing to provide hospitalization or treatment even after officers identify someone as needing them. In an op-ed Chief Biasotti explained what happens when officers try to take someone with mental illness to a hospital:

> We wait hours for psychiatrists to evaluate them, only to find the doctor overrules us and refuses to admit the patient. If the individual is admitted, they will generally be discharged before being fully stabilized or having effective community services put in place. The easier solution for our officers is to take people with serious mental illness to jail, something we are loath to do to sick people who need help, not incarceration. But the mental health system gives us little choice.[6]

One officer described the mental health system as having a "catch and release attitude."

DANGER TO POLICE AND FROM POLICE

Getting treatment from the mental health system is so difficult that parents sometimes try to have a loved one arrested in the hopes that police will arrange shelter or care. Parents call this a "mercy booking." When Heather Jacobson couldn't get treatment for her son, she arranged a mercy booking:

> My mentally ill son went missing and was off his medication. The psychiatrist's nurse would not even take info from me about him, much less

help me find him. Two weeks later he called and asked me to pick him up. He had been living in the woods at a drug fest. I got him home and didn't know what to do, since he didn't know he was ill and therefore wouldn't accept voluntary treatment. My only hope to save him was to call the police. They came and picked him up on a warrant. Since then whenever he disappears I file a missing persons' report and have been "lucky" because going missing was a probation violation that enabled police to pick him up.[7]

Other times family members have to call police because they feel in danger. When police are called the situation is usually peacefully resolved, but sometimes it ends in tragedy for the police. Mental Illness Policy Org. has a collection of over one hundred names of officers killed by persons with untreated serious mental illness over multiple years, and a joint 2013 study by the Treatment Advocacy Center (TAC) and National Sheriffs' Association (NSA) found that at least half the attacks on officers are by people with mental illness, many of whom were apparently not taking their medications at the time of the shooting.[8] The Department of Justice (DOJ) conducted a study on deaths among law enforcement officers who were responding to calls and discovered "at least 20 percent of the cases involved officers responding to a call that involved a subject with a reported mental illness. Close to half of those reportedly mentally ill suspects were either known to be armed or had previously made threats."[9]

- On January 3, 2013, thirty-seven-year-old Peter Jourdan opened fire on two police officers on a Manhattan-bound N train. Officers Michael Levay and Lukasz Kozicki were shot multiple times during the incident. Jourdan died in the shootout. His family complained that despite numerous trips to jails and hospitals, Jourdan, diagnosed with schizophrenia, had been routinely sent back to the streets instead of taken someplace for treatment.[10]
- Mentally ill Shannon J. Miles was not in treatment when he shot and killed Harris County Deputy Sheriff Darren Goforth at a Chevron station north of Houston.[11]
- Mentally ill Ismaaiyl Brinsley was not in treatment when he ambushed and killed two police officers sitting in their patrol car in Brooklyn, New York.[12]

But the danger also goes the other way. "Nationally, about half the 375–500 people shot and killed by police each year are mentally ill."[13] Tom Moroney of *Bloomberg News* documented sixty-four people with mental illness who died at the hands of police in 2012.[14] Seventy-six percent (forty-nine people) were armed or appeared to be armed. When the Department of Justice investigated use of force by the Baltimore police department in the wake of concerns raised by the Black Lives Matter movement, it found 20 percent of the incidents were directed at people with mental illness.[15]

> Thirty-one-year-old Juan Antonio Gonzalez of Tulsa, Oklahoma, had bipolar disorder and was refusing treatment. On February 16, 2013, he was fatally shot after a standoff with police. Officers were called to the apartment complex after Gonzalez chased his roommate out of their apartment with a knife.[16]

As Rosanna Esposito, an advocate for the seriously mentally ill, told me, "If someone is untreated, psychosis can render them unpredictable and/or unable to follow an officer's instructions. Paranoia can fuel distrust and suspicion and lead to behavior that causes the officer to fear for his own safety." Most of the shootings of mentally ill by police were classified as "justifiable homicides" in that force was used to protect the officer or the public.[17] Many of those shot by law enforcement officers were people attempting to commit "suicide-by-cop."[18]

When Moshe Pergament aimed a gun that turned out to be a toy at Officer Anthony Sica, Sica shot and killed him. During the investigation, officers found a note on the front seat of Pergament's car addressed "To the officer who shot me" that read, "Officer, It was a plan. I'm sorry to get you involved. I just needed to die. Please remember that this was all my doing. You had no way of knowing. Moe Pergament."[19]

Advocates are quick to criticize police when someone with mental illness is injured or killed by them. What is surprising is that it doesn't happen more often. When laws prevent people with serious mental illness from being treated until *after* they become "a danger to self or others," some will become dangerous. Police *have* to step in. Unlike the mental health system, the police cannot simply pretend the seriously mentally ill don't exist. After police interactions end up harming someone with mental illness, the industry lobbies for contracts to "educate the police," while failing to recognize its own culpability.

Chief Biasotti wrote that he understood the public outrage when persons with mental illness die because of a police action, but he wasn't sure the public understood that "the last thing any police officer wants to do is pull out a gun. It's a sign that something has gone terribly wrong. But increasingly officers are being forced to pull out their guns, and often it's to protect the public from someone with untreated mental illness."[20] Police step in when one condition has been met: the mental health system failed. As a result of the frequency of the failure, police have become major proponents of better treatment for the most seriously ill. As Cheektowaga, New York, police chief David J. Zack told the *Buffalo News*, "You cannot arrest your way out of this problem."[21]

INCREASED DRAIN ON THE COURTS

Letting people with serious mental illness go untreated is gridlocking and bankrupting the court system. One rough estimate, arrived at by extrapolating a 2001 Brooklyn study, pegs the number of excess court bookings at a staggering twelve million a year, each requiring a judge, defense lawyer, prosecutor, court facility, and often an officer to provide transportation between the jail and the court. In the years since, the problem has likely grown worse.

The failure of the mental health system to provide the seriously mentally ill treatment is forcing courts to set up shadow mental health systems called mental health courts. In lieu of sentencing, judges order judicially supervised, community treatment for the mentally ill who come before them.[22] Put another way, after individuals the mental health system refused to treat commit a crime, they are sent to mental health courts where judges order the mental health system to provide treatment. It's a long, unnecessary round-trip that's expensive to taxpayers.

OVERCROWDED JAILS AND PRISONS

As a result of the mental health system's failure to focus on the most seriously ill, in 2014, there were about 265,455 seriously mentally ill in prisons and 125,582 in jails, or 392,037 adults with serious mental illness in jails or prisons.[23] An additional 755,360 seriously mentally ill are on probation or parole.[24] There are now more than ten times more seriously mentally ill persons in jails and prisons than in state hospitals.[25] The incarcerated mentally ill tend to have very severe disorders.[26] If they are untreated, they often rack up new charges while on parole or in prison, and serve longer terms than the non–mentally ill.[27]

Sheriff Tom Dart, who runs the Cook County Jail in Illinois, the largest psychiatric facility in the country, compassionately and rhetorically asked, "What are they here in jail for? They're hungry. Retail theft is enormous. They steal something to feed themselves. Loads of them criminal trespass on land. What is that? They're breaking in to find some place to sleep."[28] Mary Beth Pfeiffer documented in *Crazy in America* how many "climbed a ladder of petty, illness-driven crimes into prison."[29] Treatment for the seriously ill could prevent the ladder from being climbed.

Those incarcerated are often repeat offenders—known to the mental health system and police as "frequent flyers" or "round-trippers."

- Sheriff Dart told *60 Minutes*, "I've got 2500–2800 people with mental illness in my jail today. Many have been in here 50, 60, 100 times. We've got some people in here 400 times."[30]
- According to a study cited by Miami-Dade County, Florida, judge Steve Leifman, over a five-year period ninety-seven people in Miami-Dade County diagnosed with serious mental illness experienced 2,200 arrests, 27,000 days in jail, and 13,000 days in hospitals and emergency rooms. "The cost of all this to Florida taxpayers is conservatively estimated at $13 million, with no demonstrable return on investment."[31]
- In the Los Angeles County Jail, 90 percent of mentally ill inmates are repeat offenders, with 31 percent having been incarcerated ten or more times.[32]
- One frequent flyer in Memphis, Tennessee, Gloria Rodgers, had 259 arrests before she was finally committed to a state psychiatric hospital. "Linda Kraige, diagnosed with bipolar disorder, has been in

Virginia's Roanoke County Jail so many times that, when asked to name her best friend, she named the deputy at the jail."[33]

Off-loading the mentally ill to jails is often encouraged by politicians. Former New York City mayor Rudy Giuliani ordered the arrest of anyone who habitually used an unlicensed squeegee to earn a living, an occupation that included many mentally ill.[34] He was credited with cleaning up the streets, and no one knew or cared that he crammed the jails.

SUFFERING WHILE INCARCERATED

Behind bars, the seriously mentally ill are rarely treated and disproportionately victimized. They are preyed upon by other inmates who know they are too meek to defend themselves or are offended by their symptoms.[35] According to a 2006 study by the Department of Justice's Bureau of Justice Statistics, mentally ill state prisoners are twice as likely as other prisoners to have been injured in a prison fight.[36] As a result of their psychotic behavior or inability to follow instructions, they are routinely thrown into solitary confinement.

New York Times reporters Michael Winerip and Michael Schwirtz wrote a heartbreaking series throughout 2014 that brought attention to constant beatings and abuse of mentally ill prisoners at New York's Riker's Island jail that eventually led to a federal investigation. In *Crazy: A Father's Search Through America's Mental Health Madness*, former *Washington Post* reporter, now mental illness advocate and writer, Pete Earley, described visiting Miami's notorious Dade County Jail and finding unwashed, psychotic, reeking, and often nude prisoners living for months in dangerously overcrowded cells, sometimes lacking even mattresses.[37] In a 2013 follow-up, CBS Miami found nothing had changed. Judge Steve Leifman, who is credited with bringing the conditions to light, said, "It's hard to believe it's been seven years. I mean when Abu Ghraib came out, there was such international outrage. It was shut down in months. But here it has gone on seven more years."[38] In *Brown v. Plata*, the US Supreme Court affirmed a lower court decision classifying the California prison system as "cruel and unusual punishment." The decision included a photograph of the telephone booth–sized cages California used to hold the mentally ill, sometimes for days at a time.

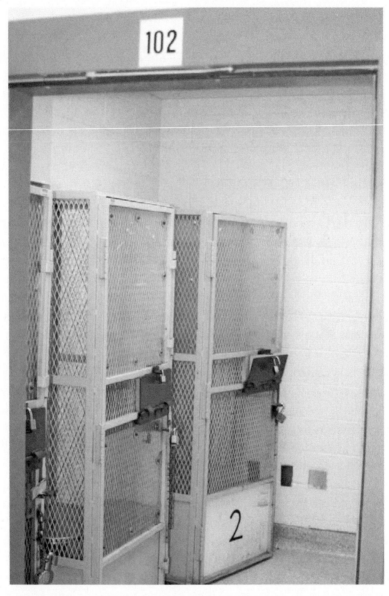

Telephone booth–sized cages used at Salinas Valley State Prison in California to hold mentally ill. (Photo: *Brown v. Plata*, US Supreme Court, Slip Opinion 09-1233 (May 23, 2011)

Even those who get treated in hospitals while incarcerated don't fare much better. In *Behind the Gates of Gomorrah*, about life inside California's Napa State forensic hospital, Dr. Stephen Seager documented an unending stream of daily beatings, rapes, and shakedowns of patients and by patients.[39] He blames so-called mental health advocates for virtually eliminating the doctor's ability to use medications, restraints, or seclusion to guarantee safety and facilitate recovery.

For many incarcerated mentally ill, it is too much. Suicide rates among prisoners are higher than for any other group, and 38 percent of those suicides are people with mental illness.[40] Many a mom has lost a mentally ill child to suicide in jail. In an ultimate act of cant, the American Civil Liberties Union (ACLU), disability rights organizations, and mental health industry advocates are suing to improve the treatment of the seriously ill behind bars while continuing to support policies that lead to incarceration.

In the next chapter, we examine the financial cost of maintaining these failures.

Chapter 3

FINANCIAL CONSEQUENCES

"Our health care system squanders money because it is designed to react to emergencies. Homeless shelters, hospital emergency rooms, jails, prisons—these are expensive and ineffective ways to intervene and there are people who clearly profit from this cycle of continued suffering."

—Pete Earley, author of
*Crazy: A Father's Search Through
America's Mental Health Madness*

INTRODUCTION

The dollars spent on America's mental *health* system is crazy. The Office of Management and Budget (OMB) reported actual federal mental health spending for treatment and income support in 2012 totaled $130 billion, with $147 billion budgeted for 2014. By 2020, the combined federal, state, local, and private funds spent on treatment alone are expected to total $238 billion.[1] That does not include state and local expenditures. Much of the funding is used to support the highest functioning and treatments that lack evidence and is therefore wasted.

The failure to focus funds on the seriously mentally ill causes the most seriously ill to cycle in and out of the most expensive settings: jails, prisons, and hospitals. The former president of the American Psychiatric Association found in Maryland just five hundred "high utilizer" patients accounted for 20 percent of the state's inpatient psychiatric costs and they have been treated in emergency rooms six or more times a year.[2] Their average annual hospital bill was $72,000, or $36.9 million, not including the cost of medications.[3] According to a New York City criminal justice task force, eighty-four seriously mentally ill people were admitted to New York City jails more than eighteen times in 2014.[4] If community treatments were funded to keep the seriously mentally ill in treatment, much of that spending for hospitalization and incarceration could have been saved.

Federal Mental Health Expenditures

(2014 budgeted amounts in billions)

Income Support

	Entitlements	Discretionary	Total
Disability (SSDI)	53		53
Supplemental Security Income (SSI)	31		31
Other	1		1
Subtotals	**85**	**0**	**85**

Surveillance Research & Treatment

	Entitlements	Discretionary	Total
Medicaid	30		30
Medicare	17		17
Other	1	1	2
Veterans Administration		7	7
Department of Defense		3	3
National Institute of Health		2	2
SAMHSA		1	1
Subtotals	**48**	**14**	**62**
Grand Totals	**133**	**14**	**147**

Fig. 3.1.

Data Source: Letter from Office of Management and Budget (OMB) director Sylvia M. Burwell to Congressman Tim Murphy, Subcommittee on Oversight and Investigations of the House Energy and Commerce Committee, November 7, 2013, http://mentalillnesspolicy.org/national-studies/mentalhealthexpenditurenational. pdf (accessed July 19, 2016). These costs do not include programs that primarily address substance abuse, but also benefit individuals with co-occurring mental illness or federal programs that benefit people with mental illness, but do not track them separately. These costs do not include state and local costs like the local share of Medicaid. They do include the federal Mental Health Block Grants, which are distributed locally by states.

The National Alliance on Mental Illness (NAMI), Mental Health America (MHA), and others in the mental health industry only argue for spending more. But incremental funding rarely goes to the seriously mentally ill, while cutbacks always do. Hospitals are closed while bullying, cyberbullying, and stigma programs are expanded. Before investing more, we should ensure that a greater percentage of the existing mega mental health budget goes to serving the most seriously ill. Following is a description of existing funding streams and expenses.

SUMMARY OF MAJOR MENTAL HEALTH SPENDING

Of the $147 billion the federal government budgeted for mental health in 2014, $85 billion was spent on income supports and $62 billion was spent on treatment and research. (See Fig. 3.1.) One hundred thirty-three billion dollars went to mandatory spending primarily for four programs.[5] Two were income support programs: Social Security Disability Income (SSDI), $53 billion, and Supplemental Security Income (SSI), $31 billion.[6] The other two were treatment programs: Medicaid, $30 billion, and Medicare, $17 billion. Fourteen billion dollars were used for discretionary spending, half of which went to the Veterans Health Administration (VHA) and US Department of Veterans Affairs (VA). As will be seen in chapter 7, the discretionary spending that went to the Substance Abuse and Mental Health Services Administration (SAMHSA) was often used to discourage states from using evidence-based programs to serve the seriously ill. Eliminating SAMHSA would allow states to improve treatment received by the seriously ill.

Social Security Disability Income (SSDI) and Supplemental Security Income (SSI)

Social Security Disability Income (SSDI) provides income to people who work and then become disabled. Thirty-one percent of the ten million people who received SSDI in 2014 claimed mental disability.[7] As will be seen in chapter 13, it is likely that many of them are not seriously mentally ill. The definition of mental illness has been dumbed down, and fraud in the program is rampant.

Supplemental Security Income (SSI) is for the poor, disabled, and those without assets. "By 2009, 41% of SSI recipients under age 65 (and about half of children) qualified for SSI on the basis of a mental illness."[8]

Medicare and Medicaid

Medicare provides healthcare to the elderly, and Medicaid provides it to the poor and disabled. According to an analysis of data from the Health-care Cost and Utilization Project (HCUP) by the Treatment Advocacy Center, in 2013, hospitalization for 1.2 million people with mood disorders and schizophrenia cost about $28 billion.[9] Mood disorders accounted for the lion's share of the absolute cost, $17 billion. "But with roughly half as many people diagnosed, schizophrenia was more costly per capita at $11.5 billion. . . . Through Medicare and Medicaid, the public paid 75 percent of the national bill for hospitalization related to schizophrenia [$9 billion] and 50 percent of the bill for mood disorders [also $9 billion]."

As will be seen in chapter 14, Medicaid and Medicare provide important care to people with serious mental illness, but both contain provisions that limit reimbursement for long-term hospital care for the most seriously mentally ill, fund useless services for people with mental illnesses, and—due to the medicalization of normality—cover mental health services for people without mental illness.

STATE AND LOCAL COSTS

According to the National Association of State Mental Health Program Directors, in 2012 states controlled $41 billion in federal and state funds spent on mental health services.[10] States are lowering expenditures by getting out of the business of treating the seriously ill. Between 2009 and 2012, state mental health and substance abuse budgets were cut by $4.35 billion.[11] Nearly 4,500 psychiatric beds that served the most seriously ill—9 percent of state psychiatric bed capacity—were eliminated. While fewer of the seriously ill were served, between 2007 and 2010 the total number of people served grew from 5.5 million to 6.5 million—a 10 percent overall increase. Clearly, state funding is drifting away from the seriously ill.

CRIMINAL JUSTICE COSTS

Our failure to focus funding streams on the seriously ill is causing county criminal justice costs to skyrocket.[12] These costs do not show up in state and federal spending estimates. One study estimated that the cost of schizophrenia alone in the United States included $2.6 billion in direct, non-healthcare costs for law enforcement.[13] For example: "In Florida, there are roughly 17,000 state prison inmates, 9,000 local jail detainees and 1,500 people in forensic hospitals who experience serious mental illnesses. The cost to taxpayers to house them is nearly $1 billion annually."[14] Illinois taxpayers laid out more than $17.8 million to convert existing prison space into facilities to treat and house seriously mentally ill prisoners.[15] A study in Connecticut revealed that individuals with mental illness involved with the justice system during a two-year period incurred costs approximately double the mentally ill with no criminal justice involvement—$48,980 compared with $24,728 per person.[16]

COST SHIFTING ALSO CAUSES MANY PROBLEMS

The failure to treat the seriously ill is also driven by cost shifting. Most of the financial decisions made by county, state, and federal mental health officials are not even intended to improve care for people with serious mental illness or reduce costs to taxpayers. They are intended to shift costs out of their departments and onto other departments or other levels of government. County mental health directors shift mental health department costs to the county criminal justice departments when they fail to provide housing or treatment and people get arrested. State mental health directors shift costs to the federal government by eliminating psychiatric hospital beds and forcing people into the community, where Medicaid pays half. But many of those kicked out of hospitals wind up incarcerated, which shifts costs to localities. In almost all cases, the shift increases total costs to taxpayers. Stated another way, when a person with mental illness gets arrested that is a "success" for the mental health system: one less person it has to treat.

LOST WAGES

Many mental health advocates argue that the cost of mental illness includes lost wages and use a 2008 study that calculated lost wages from serious mental illness at $193.2 billion a year, or a 2016 study that calculated lost wages from schizophrenia alone at $60 billion.[17] But those are misleading. If everyone with untreated serious mental illness could be put back to work, those wages wouldn't be lost. But while politically incorrect to say, with the exception of bipolar disorder, existing treatments are not yet effective enough to return many of the most seriously ill to nonsubsidized employment. The treatments are barely good enough to prevent them from becoming homeless and psychotic. "Approximately 90% of people with serious mental illnesses are unemployed."[18] Many of the seriously ill who do go back to work, and are held up as poster children, work in peer-counselor positions, which are government-funded positions put aside exclusively to those who have intersected with the mental health system.[19] Until there are more effective treatments, lost wages are not a justification for spending more on treatment for the most seriously ill, although it is a reason to spend more on research. Finally, there are also high-functioning people who game the system, claim they have mental disability, often PTSD, so they don't have to work.[20] Spending more on treatment would not return them to work.

The cost of the mental health system and the failure to focus spending on the most seriously ill has become monumental, unsustainable, and often counterproductive. At the same time that we are spending more, the mental illness disaster is getting worse. We need to eliminate programs that don't work and use the savings for programs that do. We also need to replace mission creep with mission control. Rather than trying to help ever-increasing numbers of barely symptomatic people, we should focus on the sickest and spend the money on preventing them from deteriorating to the point where they have to be hospitalized or incarcerated. We can start to address the crisis without spending more. We simply have to spend smarter.

The following section explains the difference between poor mental health, which is well-funded, and serious mental illness, which is not.

MENTAL HEALTH VS. MENTAL ILLNESS: WHAT'S THE DIFFERENCE AND WHY DOES IT MATTER?

Chapter 4

WHAT SERIOUS MENTAL ILLNESS IS NOT

"There is no real epidemic of mental illness, just a much looser definition of sickness."

—Allen Frances, MD, in *Saving Normal*

Poor mental health is not the same as mental illness or "serious" mental illness. One hundred percent of the US population has at some point felt sad, anxious, or nervous and therefore could be considered as having poor *mental health*. But only 18 percent of the population over eighteen (forty-three million adults) had a *mental illness* in the past year, and only 4 percent (ten million adults) had a *serious* mental illness.[1] Our community programs largely help the 100 percent who can have their mental health improved, or the 18 percent with any mental illness, but rarely focus on the 4 percent with serious mental illness. And that is the problem. The ability to get help is inversely related to need. This chapter describes mental health and mental illness. The next chapter discusses serious mental illness.

POOR MENTAL HEALTH

The World Health Organization (WHO) claims anyone who hasn't realized her own potential has poor mental health.[2] The surgeon general ruled that anyone who doesn't have a fulfilling relationship or has difficulty coping with adversity has a mental health problem.[3] The American Psychiatric Association (APA) suggests a "mental health checkup," i.e., a visit to one of its members, for anyone who experiences a problem concentrating, balancing home life with work, or has a change in appetite or sleeping patterns.[4] What WHO, the surgeon general, and the APA are calling mental health issues are really states of normality that everyone experiences at some point.

61

The mental health industry is "'psychologizing' daily existence," trying to convince the public that normal feelings and behaviors are actually mental health issues that it can treat.[5] Anyone who is too sad or too happy, who wants a new job or a new spouse is now deemed to be exhibiting signs of poor mental health, requiring publicly funded intervention. New York's governor Andrew Cuomo boasted that he spent an $8.2 million FEMA mental health grant "to help victims of Hurricane Sandy recognize that, in most cases, their emotional reactions are normal."[6] When New York had a snowstorm in 2015, the Substance Abuse and Mental Health Services Administration (SAMHSA) set up a "distress line" for those who wanted counseling.[7] No illness required.

The mental health industry has succeeded in getting the media to run articles positioning all of the following as "risk factors" for poor mental health: poverty, bad grades, stigma, experiencing global warming, spanking, owing money, perceiving racism, the Internet, illiteracy, wanting a nose job, having back problems or a sexual dysfunction, wanting to be rich, wanting a tan, exercise, religion, and using Facebook.

Because feeling sad is now poor mental health; anything that makes you happier is now a mental health "treatment." Just add the word "therapy." An Internet search found there's dog therapy, horse therapy, art therapy, group therapy, shopping therapy, yoga therapy, laughter yoga therapy, dance therapy, and its subset, tango therapy. There's tai-chi therapy, surfing therapy, meatloaf and mashed potato therapy, cleaning therapy, remarriage therapy, induced after death communication therapy, paintball therapy, and every kind of talk, meditation, massage, acupressure, counseling, and introspection. Holistic treatment has become a euphemism for useless treatment. If it feels good, it must be therapy, and chances are it's receiving government funding. Pop psychology has taken over.

Clearly, something is wrong.

MENTAL ILLNESS

Mental illness is one step down from poor mental health. It is everything the APA puts in its *Diagnostic and Statistical Manual* (*DSM*)—over three hundred conditions.[8] Eighteen percent of adults have some sort of condition that is defined in *DSM*. Half of those people (9 percent) have anxiety and nothing else.[9]

Dr. Allen Frances, lead editor of *DSM-IV* who has become *DSM-5*'s leading critic, noted that *DSM* "sets the crucial boundary between normality and mental illness."[10] They have moved the boundary so far to the right that normality is now an illness. The *DSM* groups constellations of symptoms that occur together as indicating the presence of a mental illness. That works well when extreme symptoms are grouped together. The extreme symptoms of schizophrenia and severe bipolar disorder—hallucinations, delusions, and cognitive impairments—are enough to tell us something is wrong. But with each iteration, the APA has gathered less extreme symptoms together and decided they too indicate the presence of illness.

Dr. Frances calls this "diagnostic inflation" and says it is "running rampant." The latest edition of *DSM* includes "normal grief," "temper tantrums," "everyday forgetting," and eating four meals a day instead of three as symptoms of mental illness.[11] Using the APA definition, the Centers for Disease Control and Prevention (CDC) claims that "nearly 50% of U.S. adults will develop at least one mental illness during their lifetime."[12] The more mental illnesses the APA can describe, the more services its members can bill for. While it is common for someone to go to a medical doctor with a physical complaint and be told nothing is wrong, the same is not true for those who visit psychiatrists. If you walk in the door, you will get a diagnosis and likely a prescription. They're available to anyone with insurance. Normality now has a billing code.

Overdiagnosing is particularly common in children. Dr. Frances wrote in *Psychiatric Times* that partially as a result of his own work, there was a forty fold increase in the diagnosis of childhood bipolar disorder from 2001 to 2010 and that he feared efforts to correct it in *DSM-5* would lead to even more children being diagnosed as ill. "I bear partial responsibility for two other false 'epidemics'—of attention deficit and autistic disorders."[13] The normal age-appropriate bell curve whereby some children develop self-control earlier or later than others has been replaced with a label for those who are late bloomers. High school boys are no longer fidgety. Instead, 20 percent now have a diagnosis of attention-deficit hyperactivity disorder (ADHD) and are taking medications like Ritalin and Adderall.[14] There is no doubt that some children have a serious mental illness, but the humor newspaper the *Onion* was barely kidding when it announced "More U.S. Children Being Diagnosed with Youthful Tendency Disorder."[15]

The pharmaceutical industry is complicit. "The best way to sell psychiatric pills is to sell psychiatric ills."[16] Its ad campaigns convince consumers they have an illness and to "ask your doctor." But that is only after the pharmaceutical companies blanket the doctors—both psychiatrists and primary care doctors—with their free samples and sales pitches. While it is rare to find a doctor who will make a house call to a patient, the pharmaceutical company sales reps make daily house calls to doctors to convince them to prescribe whatever medication they are selling. The free samples handed out by pharmaceutical company reps do allow doctors to help some poor individuals who can't afford the medications, but they also encourage overprescribing. Primary care physicians prescribe well over 50 percent of all antidepressants.[17] Some of these medications are important effective medications for serious illnesses, but others are not.

For many mental health advocates and nonprofits, even the three hundred–plus disorders in the all-encompassing *DSM* are not enough. Advocates invent new diagnoses as needed. (Read: "as needed for fundraising.") Everyone loses a job or loved one or experiences something unpleasant at some point. Advocates had SAMHSA and the Center for Mental Health Services (CMHS) redefine that as an illness: "trauma." Trauma is not a mental illness. Post-traumatic stress disorder (PTSD) is, and even that can range from mild to severe.[18] Other recently invented illnesses are bullying and cyberbullying. Neither are mental illnesses, but it's a rare mental health industry nonprofit that won't take public money to "treat" them.

Decades ago, the government recognized that not everything in *DSM* is serious. "For most of the [adults in the United States who suffer from mental illness], the disorders are relatively mild and brief."[19] Today it is politically incorrect to suggest that all illnesses are not serious. John Grohol, who bills his PsychCentral website as the "internet's largest and oldest independent mental health social network," claims the division between "serious" mental illness and others is a "myth."[20]

Poor mental health and mild mental illness are not the most pressing problems we have, yet they receive the bulk of our attention. Serious mental illness, discussed in the following chapter, is largely ignored.

Chapter 5

WHAT SERIOUS MENTAL ILLNESS IS AND HOW THAT SHOULD DRIVE POLICY

"While the line between serious mental illness and the other mental illnesses is debatable, the extremities are clear."

—Unknown

"Serious" mental illnesses are a small subset of the three hundred mental illnesses in the *DSM* and are experienced by ten million adults (4 percent of the US population over eighteen).[1] Put another way, less than one-quarter of those with *any* mental illness have a *serious* mental illness.

Navy veteran Scott Panetti has schizophrenia. In 1986, it caused him to believe the devil was in his furniture. "Naturally" he took some of it out of the house, buried it in the backyard, conducted an exorcism over the furniture left in the house, and then nailed the curtains shut so the buried furniture couldn't get back in. His schizophrenia was left untreated, and in 1992 his delusional thinking caused him to kill his wife's parents. After twenty-five years of incarceration, Mr. Panetti is still on death row.[2]

Serious mental illness is obvious to families who experience it in loved ones. No special training is needed to identify it, as these families told me:

- "My brother once talked to clothes hanging on a rack behind the door. He believed the clothes to be God, and he seemed to be taking orders from Him. We always listened carefully to his conversations with inanimate objects in case 'God' told him something completely unacceptable to do, we wanted to be [the] first to know."—Mary Neal

- "Once my son thought half of his body was evil, and he tried to kill that half by running out into the middle of the interstate. Fortunately he was not hit, but picked up by police and taken to the hospital."—Danielle
- "My mother would mix cigarette butts and tobacco in the ice cream and put it back in the freezer. She would also go to the neighbors and eat their flowers."—Dominique

People with poor mental health or mild mental illness don't do those sorts of things.

DEFINITION OF SERIOUS MENTAL ILLNESS

The government made multiple attempts to define serious mental illness. See appendix A. Interestingly, different government entities came to similar conclusions as to what it is and—give or take a percentage or two—how many Americans have it. Paraphrasing Associate Supreme Court Justice Potter Stewart's definition of pornography, "I know it when I see it." Serious mental illnesses can be described as mental illnesses listed in *DSM* that "resulted in functional impairment which *substantially* interferes with or limits one or more *major* life activities."[3]

That definition was created by the Center for Mental Health Services (CMHS) within the Substance Abuse and Mental Health Services Administration (SAMHSA) to guide their distribution of federal mental health funds to states, and it generates the 4 percent prevalence rate quoted above. By all accounts, serious mental illnesses include "schizophrenia-spectrum disorders," "*severe* bipolar disorder," and "*severe major* depression" as specifically and narrowly defined in *DSM*.[4] People with those disorders comprise the bulk of those with serious mental illness. However, when other mental illnesses cause *significant* functional impairment they also count as a serious mental illness. For example, some people with obsessive-compulsive disorder (OCD) can hold down a job and have a good social life, while others may be afraid to leave home because they are obsessed with the idea they might not turn out the light. Clearly, one is seriously ill while the other is not. PTSD and eating disorders have both mild and severe forms.

**Rough Estimate of One Year Prevalence of
Serious Mental Illnesses in Adults by Diagnosis**

Disorder	Prevalence in Adults	Calculation of Number of adults affected (Column 2 times US census of adults over 18) (E)
Schizophrenias (NIMH defines all schizophrenias as "severe")	1.1% (A)	2,640,000
The subset of bipolar disorder classified as "severe"	2.2% (B)	5,280,000
The subset of major depression called "severe, major depression"	2.0% (C)	4,800,000
Calculated Totals	**5.3%** (D)	**12,720,000** (D)

Fig. 5.1.

(A) National Institute of Mental Health (NIMH), "Schizophrenia (Statistics)," 2005, http://www.nimh.nih.gov/health/statistics/prevalence/schizophrenia.shtml (accessed July 10, 2016). (B) NIMH, "Bipolar Disorder among Adults (Statistics)," http://www.nimh.nih.gov/health/statistics/prevalence/bipolar-disorder-among-adults.shtml (accessed July 10, 2016). (C) NIMH, "Major Depressive Disorder among Adults (Statistics)," http://www.nimh.nih.gov/health/statistics/prevalence/major-depression-among-adults.shtml (accessed July 10, 2016). (D) The actual total is less than 5.3% because some individuals have more than one disorder. The total does exclude other disorders that may be serious, although the number of people with those is not large. (E) US Census Bureau, "Annual Estimates of the Resident Population for Selected Age Groups by Sex: April 1, 2010, to July 1, 2013," June 2014.

The number of people with serious mental illness who don't have schizophrenia, severe bipolar disorder, or severe major depression is relatively small.[5] Therefore many think a better definition of serious mental illness would be based solely on the diagnosis, not any functional impairment. But because there is massive data using the CMHS definition relying on impairment, it is the one used in this book. The table in Fig. 5.1 gives a *rough* breakdown of serious mental illness by diagnosis, understanding that some people have more than one disorder.

Focusing on this small group can help eliminate the consequences described in section 1. Following are important facts about serious mental illnesses that should be reflected in policy.

SERIOUS MENTAL ILLNESSES ARE BRAIN DISORDERS

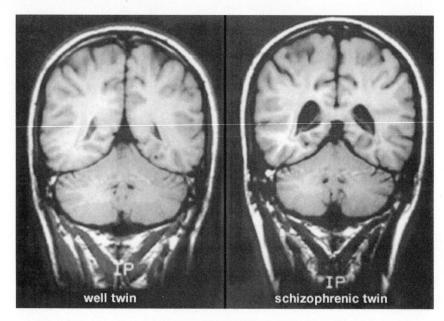

well twin   **schizophrenic twin**

Schizophrenia Scan

Fig. 5.2. MRI of individual with schizophrenia
shows larger fluid-filled cavities (ventricles) than a twin.
(MRI courtesy of Drs. E. Fuller Torrey and Daniel Weinberger.)

There is overwhelming scientific evidence that serious mental illnesses are
physical brain disorders.[6] Every organ of the body can malfunction, and
the brain is no exception. Thus, care and treatment of people with serious
mental illness is largely, but not exclusively, a medical issue requiring easy
access to doctors. Magnetic resonance images (MRIs) of the brains of
people who have depression, bipolar disorder, and schizophrenia look different from MRIs of controls.[7] Some of these differences are due to the
illness, not the treatment, as they appear in those never treated. Individuals
with schizophrenia who have never been treated have enlarged ventricles,
reduced volume of gray matter, more neurological and neuropsychological
abnormalities, and decreased function of the prefrontal area.[8] People with
bipolar illness who have never been treated have decreased white matter in

certain parts of the brain.[9] The areas in depression that play a role are the amygdala (often smaller), the thalamus, and the hippocampus.[10]

However, in addition to the illness itself, the medications used to treat mental illnesses, like those for Parkinson's and Alzheimer's, can also change some aspects of brain structure. Some of these medication-induced brain changes are likely beneficial and explain why the drugs are effective, while other medication-induced changes may be the cause of their side effects.[11] Numerous genetic differences between those with serious mental illness and those without are also being discovered.[12] These differences are not yet understood well enough to be useful in diagnosis, nor are they present in everyone with the disorders.

HALLUCINATIONS, DELUSIONS, AND HEARING VOICES

Leaving schizophrenia, severe bipolar disorder, and psychotic depression untreated can cause people to hallucinate, hear voices, become delusional, and lose touch with reality.[13] Sensory processing can be radically compromised. Listening can be impossible, as the sound they are trying to focus on simply blends with all the other sounds in the room and the universe, making it impossible to follow a conversation. Visual misperception can cause people and objects to take on a frightening satanic patina, or appear liquid or psychedelic. Sense of taste and smell can be so heightened that food tastes poisoned and air smells disgusting and gaseous. They may "feel" insects crawling in their bodies. This is generally not true for individuals who simply need their mental health improved or have minor mental illnesses.

- Joseph Bowers of Pueblo, Colorado, was diagnosed with schizophrenia and told me that when not in treatment, "I knew that the devil's soul had taken over my grandmother's body." Bowers wrote *Life Under a Cloud: The Story of a Schizophrenic*, about what the illness did to him.
- Joy Torres, an advocate for the seriously mentally ill in Santa Ana, California, with a diagnosis of paranoid schizophrenia, told me that during an untreated episode, "I knew I was the devil and I had to burn everything."
- Annie Allen's relative feels an evil witch named "Georgia" periodi-

cally getting angry and destroying her insides by punching, kicking, and eating them.

- Katherine Flannery Dering wrote in *Shot in the Head* how her brother Paul "knew" his teeth had somehow fallen out of his mouth and onto the ground and from them sprang up hundreds of babies, who cried out to him for help. He would get distraught listening to them and cover his ears and cry, "My children, they're crying for me!"
- Kathy Day is a caretaker to someone who often believes aliens are harvesting his organs.
- Anna's son in Odessa, Texas, has schizophrenia and knows he had a long-term relationship with Marilyn Monroe.

These hallucinations and delusions can compel people to take dangerous and sometimes deadly action. Mary Barksdale told me her son went without treatment and killed two police officers because he believed they were aliens from space.

People with serious mental illnesses, especially those with untreated severe bipolar disorder in the manic phase, may "know" that they are the Messiah, loved by a celebrity, or have the key to the universe. A mom in New Jersey told me, "My son knows he's smarter than Einstein and has invented some type of method of traveling in space with no time lapsed. He came home from CVS and told me Warren Beatty and Shirley MacLaine were behind him in line and told him not to worry, that they were going to take care of all his problems."

Others with untreated serious mental illness may have paranoid or persecutory delusions and "know" television sets are directing special messages to them, radio stations are broadcasting their thoughts aloud to others, and people are using magnetic waves to read their minds or control their behavior. Joel Sax, who has bipolar disorder, wrote me about his experience: "I believed that I knew what everyone was going to say before they said it and I believed I made them say it

People with untreated serious mental illness may believe others are trying to harm them, and act out violently to save themselves. One study put it succinctly. "Untreated schizophrenia was associated with the emergence of persecutory delusions which were associated with violence."[14] Policy makers need to understand that many people with psychotic delusions will not volunteer for psychiatric services.

"NEGATIVE" SYMPTOMS

People with serious mental illness, especially schizophrenia, often can't express emotion. This is known as a "negative" symptom. Those with it often have a blank, expressionless face, are unable to make eye contact, and speak in monotones and monosyllables. They lack interest in anything and are unable to feel pleasure (anhedonia) or unable to act spontaneously.[15] They often ignore basic personal hygiene and may be perceived as lazy or unwilling to help themselves. Some people with negative symptoms withdraw into mutism and freeze in one position, sitting for hours without moving or talking. These are not "lifestyle choices." They are symptoms of the illness. These individuals may be unable to "pick themselves up by their bootstraps." Policy makers must recognize that many seriously mentally ill need intensive case management to help them navigate the confusing mental health and insurance systems, and to apply for income support, housing, and other services they need in order to access food, clothing, treatment, and shelter.

DEFICITS IN COGNITIVE FUNCTION

Some people who have untreated serious mental illness may lose cognitive abilities they once had. I was shocked to learn that someone I knew as a healthy high school student later developed schizophrenia and lost the ability to recognize that in order to take off his pants, his shoes had to come off first or his pants wouldn't fit over them. Some people with untreated serious mental illness can't think straight, or organize, connect with or gain control of their thought process.[16] Thoughts may come so fast and furious and disconnected that they spew a flood of impossible-to-understand gibberish, what psychiatrists call "word salad," like my sister-in-law in the introduction did, or meaningless words (neologisms).[17] This cognitive dysfunction is likely associated with neurobiology.[18] Instead of controlling their thoughts, their thoughts control them. Loss of cognition affects over 70 percent of the homeless who have serious mental illness.[19]

Because of cognitive dysfunction, such individuals may laugh when talking about death or for no reason at all. This is the well-known maniacal laugh often portrayed in novels and movies. Many thought the smirking mug shot of Jared Loughner who shot Representative Gabrielle Giffords showed evidence of this.

People with serious mental illness may remain able to speak even when they've lost the ability to formulate thoughts. They open their mouths, but nothing rational comes out. They may say there are cats eating their brains, but they don't want treatment because they think the medication will poison the cats. The illness hijacks free will. It is a "thought disorder." Cognitive difficulties also cause noncompliance with treatment.[20] For the patient's own safety, policy makers must ensure there is a mechanism to overcome their objections to treatment if needed. Following the directions of those who lack cognitive function by refusing to treat them—even if it's done under the guise of protecting their civil rights—is cruel. As Clayton Cramer wrote in *My Brother, Ron*, "the greatest mercy is getting them into treatment."[21]

ANOSOGNOSIA

When people with mental illness walk down the street screaming, "I am the Messiah," it is not because they believe they are the Messiah. They *know* it. They are totally unaware they are ill. It is not surprising that some people with serious mental illness do not recognize they are ill. The organ needed for awareness, the brain, likely its right hemisphere, is not functioning properly. This same lack of awareness is sometimes seen in stroke victims. Anosognosia is the clinical term for lack of awareness of being ill, and it has major policy implications.

Anosognosia rarely affects those with poor mental health. But as shown in appendix C, anosognosia is present in up to 50 percent of those with untreated schizophrenia and 40 percent of those with untreated bipolar disorder. It has been photographed using various brain-scanning technologies, and anosognosia, not stigma, is a primary reason some people with serious mental illness refuse treatment.[22]

As a result of anosognosia, when a mother urges a son or daughter with serious mental illness to see a psychiatrist, the mother will often hear, "I'm not crazy. I don't need help! You do!" Dr. Xavier Amador, who evaluated Ted Kaczynski, the Unabomber, is best known for being the psychologist on the Bravo series *Bethany Ever After* and for his multiple appearances on

CNN. He heard "I'm not sick, I don't need help" so often from his brother who had schizophrenia that he wrote a book with that title focusing on how to get treatment to persons with mental illness who don't believe they are ill.[23] Anna-Lisa Johanson contributed to the effort. Her mother, Margaret Mary Ray, suffered from serious mental illness, but did not believe she was ill. She made headlines and became fodder for late-night talk shows when she became obsessed with and started stalking David Letterman. She was caught and, when released, later took her own life by lying down in front of an oncoming freight train.[24] Anna-Lisa has become an advocate for persons with serious mental illness.

Policy makers should not require everyone to be well enough to recognize they are ill before they can be treated. Failing to deliver treatment to those not well enough to recognize they are ill can often lead to danger.

SERIOUS MENTAL ILLNESSES START IN THE LATE TEENS AND EARLY TWENTIES, RARELY MUCH YOUNGER OR OLDER

In men, schizophrenia generally strikes in the late teens or early twenties, and in women, in their twenties or thirties.[25] The median age of onset for bipolar disorder is twenty-five, but like schizophrenia, it often starts in the late teens and early twenties.[26] The onset of major depressive disorder (as opposed to lesser depression) can develop at any time, but the median age is thirty-two.

To make the case for expanding "early intervention" programs aimed at children, mental health industry advocates tout research claiming "half of all lifetime cases of mental illness begin by age fourteen." That may be true for *any* mental illness, but it is not true for *serious* mental illnesses.[27] The illnesses experienced by those under eighteen or so are rarely the same as or become the serious mental illnesses experienced by adults. Early-onset and late-onset versions do exist, but they are the exceptions.

Many early intervention programs are worthy social services that masquerade as mental health programs to get mental health dollars. They may help improve grades, job outlook, social development, and other outcomes down the line, but policy makers should know that the bad grades and poor social development were likely *not* caused by serious mental illnesses, nor are they taken individually, "risk factors" for serious mental illnesses.

THE CAUSES OF SERIOUS MENTAL ILLNESSES ARE NOT KNOWN, SO THEY CANNOT BE PREDICTED OR PREVENTED

Policy makers are being misled by the mental health industry into wasting vast sums of money on prediction and prevention. It sounds so logical: intervene early and you can prevent serious mental illness. But it's generally not true. We don't know who will develop serious mental illness, so we don't know whom to target with the interventions. As former NIMH director Dr. Thomas Insel noted, "For mental disorders, we do not know the cause [and] we lack a biomarker that is 100% accurate for diagnosis."[28] Research is ongoing.[29] Until we find specific causes or a biomarker, like a blood or a spinal fluid test, serious mental illness is diagnosed by examining the symptoms *after* they've developed and by eliminating other illnesses that cause the same behavior—as is done with Parkinson's and Alzheimer's.[30]

"Early interventions" that are applied to people who haven't yet developed symptoms are mainly going to people who will never develop mental illness. That is wasteful and illogical. As far back as 1994, the Institute of Medicine (IOM) exposed the fact that "the nation is spending billions of dollars on [prevention] programs whose effectiveness is not known."[31] Nine years later, the President's New Freedom Commission acknowledged, "Preventing mental illnesses remains a promise of the future."[32] And in 2014, evidence that preventing serious mental illness is not yet possible was described in an IOM report on efforts to prevent mental illness in the military.[33] The *Wall Street Journal* headline summed up the findings: "Study Fails to Find Evidence That Programs for Soldiers and Families Prevent Psychological Disorders."[34]

The lack of biomarkers means that determining the correct diagnosis often takes time and that individuals may receive multiple diagnoses over their lifetime until the right one is found.[35] This "diagnosis du jour syndrome" frustrates families and patients as every new doctor declares a new diagnosis.

Serious mental illness is often first experienced during the same years people may start experimenting with illegal drugs, or perhaps lose a parent, so many conclude their illness was the direct result of the drugs or loss. That is likely not true. Millions try drugs and lose a parent and do not develop serious mental illness.

We can't prevent serious mental illness, but we are starting to learn how to prevent young people who *already* have prodromal symptoms or experienced First Episode Psychosis from going on to develop a full-blown illness.[36] Policy makers should be aware that that research is still in its early stages and has not been replicated. The PR for it is far ahead of the actual results. Further, preventing progression of an illness is much different than preventing the illness. Preventing progression requires policy makers to target people with the illness, not those without.

"Preventing mental illness" is a good sound bite, but unsound science.

SERIOUS MENTAL ILLNESSES TEND TO RUN IN FAMILIES

According to the Stanley Center for Psychiatric Research at the Broad Institute, "The largest known risk factor for bipolar disorder and schizophrenia is an inherited vulnerability."[37]

- Schizophrenia occurs in 27 percent of the population when both parents have it, 7 percent when one parent has it, and .86 percent when neither parent has it.[38] The risk is highest for an identical twin of a person with schizophrenia. That person has a 35–50 percent chance of developing the disorder. But most schizophrenia occurs in individuals who do not have family members with it.
- Bipolar disorder occurs in 25 percent of the population when both parents have it, 4.4 percent when one parent has it, and .48 percent when neither parent has it.[39] Children of parents with bipolar disorder are also more likely to have severe symptoms including suicidal ideation, depressive symptoms, and racing thoughts.[40]
- If someone has a parent or sibling with major depression, that person probably has a two or three times greater risk of developing depression compared with the average person.[41]

There is an increasing parade of "genetic breakthrough" headlines often emanating from the Broad Institute, a leading investigator of genetic vulnerability, but so far they have not proven useful in diagnosing or preventing mental illness. Most people with a family history of serious mental illness will not develop the illness, and most people with the illness do not have a family member with it, so mental illness is not entirely a genetic disorder. However, if policy makers are going to allocate funds based on risk factors, then they should prioritize people with mental illness in their families, not other fake high-risk groups.

SERIOUS MENTAL ILLNESSES MAY BE EPISODIC

Roughly one-third of schizophrenia may be chronic (always present), or episodic (occur once or a few times over a lifetime) or remit (disappear after a time).[42] People who have a mental illness that is episodic or remits sometimes attribute the cure to whatever they were doing at the time they felt better. They may attribute their cure to overcoming trauma, talking to someone who has had or has mental illness ("peer support"), using natural remedies, introspection, yoga, or dozens of other alleged "cures." Policy makers must be wary of diverting resources to interventions that lack scientific evidence of efficacy.

FAMILY INVOLVEMENT IMPROVES OUTCOMES AND CUTS COSTS

Many families want to provide free case management, medication management, housing, and transportation services for seriously mentally ill loved ones. That improves outcomes and saves the government money. But to do so, families need Congress to reform HIPAA (discussed in chapter 15) so families can get access to the information they need to help and are welcomed as part of the treatment team.

We know a lot, but not everything, about serious mental illnesses. They are often characterized by psychosis or delusions of grandeur. They differ from poor mental health and less serious illnesses like minor depression and anxiety, where sufferers understand they are not well, tend to seek treatment, and can often maintain a high level of functioning. The consequences of letting serious mental illness go untreated are significant, and sometimes tragic.

The following chapter discusses the treatments that policy makers should make available to the seriously mentally ill to prevent the consequences described in section 1.

Chapter 6

WHAT SCIENCE TELLS US ABOUT TREATMENT THAT SHOULD BE REFLECTED IN POLICY

"Joseph Olecki of Logan Township, PA, was 33 when he shot a husband and wife in their garden while he was off his medication. At his sentencing, he thanked the judge for his hospitalization and being given the right medication after he was incarcerated. 'The medication definitely works if you get the medication you need.'"
—*Altoona* (PA) *Mirror*, April 13, 2013

The treatments for serious mental illness are different than those for "poor mental health," and they are rarely proposed by the mental health industry. Our goal needs to be expanding approaches that help the seriously ill. Instead, we fund what's useless and stymie what's critical. The following is what we know about treatments.

MEDICATIONS ARE USUALLY THE MOST EFFECTIVE TREATMENT

Medications do not cure but can ameliorate some of the most severe symptoms of serious mental illness, such as delusions and hallucinations, and are the most effective treatments for schizophrenia and bipolar disorder.[1] They are the *sine qua non* for many. "Consequences of treatment nonadherence [to antipsychotics] include a fourfold increase in the risk of suicide, a near fourfold increase in relapse, and an increased risk of violent behavior. In addition, nonadherence is associated with increased rates of hospitalization, use of emergency psychiatric services, arrests, violence, victimizations, poorer mental functioning, poorer life satisfaction, greater substance use, and more alcohol-related problems."[2] As documented in appendix B, medications also reduce criminal justice involvement and violence.

Finding the best medications, giving them time to work, and trying different doses and combinations can take weeks to months.[3] Medicines stop working when someone stops taking them. Anyone who has schizophrenia for more than a year and deteriorates while off medication will likely deteriorate if that person goes off medications again.[4] That should not mean "once medicated, always medicated." A careful attempt to lower the dose of medications or wean off medications may be appropriate for some people after they have been stabilized for longer than a year and are doing well. First-generation schizophrenia medications are not as effective on its negative symptoms. Individuals who take them may no longer have hallucinations and delusions but may still have severe cognitive problems. All medications have side effects that need monitoring. They can be serious and lead to noncompliance. Side effects should not be minimized or hidden from patients, and patients wanting to change medications or dosage need doctors who will work with them.

It is critical for policy makers to understand that getting adults with serious mental illness on the right medications at the right dose—and keeping them there—is critical, takes time, and requires quick access to doctors when needed. Making a patient wait a month or even a day may be too late.

WE NEED PSYCHIATRIC HOSPITALS, NOT JUST COMMUNITY SERVICES

Even if there were perfect readily available community services, and access to doctors when needed, some of the sickest will still need to be hospitalized at some point. But there are not enough beds for them. According to the Treatment Advocacy Center, the minimum number of beds needed to serve the most seriously mentally ill is 147,000, roughly 50 beds per 100,000 citizens.[5] As of 2006 we were short 95,000 beds.[6] Beds continue to be closed, and more are being reserved for those in the criminal justice system.[7] As of 2016, the Treatment Advocacy Center found there were less than 6.2 non-forensic state hospital beds per 100,000 in the population. (See chart.)[8]

Key State Hospital Bed Trends

Year	Number	Type of Bed	Per 100,000 Population*	Percentage of Historical Peak*
2016	37,679	Total state hospital beds	11.7	3.50%
	20,078	Civil beds in state hospitals	6.2	**
	17,601	Forensic beds in state hospitals	5.5	**
2010	43,318	Total state hospital beds	14.1	4.20%
2005	50,509	Total state hospital beds	16.8	5.00%
1955	558,922	Total state hospital beds	337	

Fig. 6.1.

* Adjusted for the growth in US population.
** 1955 data are not available.

Data source: Doris A. Fuller, Elizabeth Sinclair, Jeffrey Geller, et al., *Going, Going, Gone: Trends and Consequences of Eliminating State Psychiatric Beds, 2016* (Arlington, VA: Treatment Advocacy Center, 2016), http://www.tacreports.org/storage/documents/going-going-gone.pdf (accessed July 12, 2016).

The shortage of long-term state beds has backed up county and city emergency rooms and forced them to adopt a Catch-22 policy—anyone well enough to walk into an ER and ask for care is deemed not sick enough to need it.[9] The consequences can be deadly.

- Virginia State senator Creigh Deeds became worried when his twenty-four-year-old son Gus stopped taking medications for his bipolar disorder and started deteriorating. Senator Deeds called police, who also recognized Gus needed help and took him to a psychiatric hospital for evaluation. The hospital claimed there were no psychiatric beds in their hospital or elsewhere and sent Gus back home. The next morning Gus stabbed his father multiple times in the face and head and committed suicide.[10]
- Andrew Goldstein had schizophrenia and a history of going off medications. When he went off his medications he tried to get into

a New York City hospital but was denied admission. Subsequently, he pushed Kendra Webdale onto subway tracks, leading to her death, his incarceration, and the passage of Kendra's Law.[11] Keeping him on his medications or giving him access to the hospital might have prevented the tragedy.

Patients who do get admitted are almost inevitably "dumped," or "streeted," i.e., discharged sicker and quicker with no community services in place. The average length of stay for those with psychosis who actually gain admission is only seven days, not enough time for doctors to collect records of previous hospitalizations, interview families, find the right medication at the right dose (titrate), decide if the medications are working, and develop a discharge plan.[12] Seventy-nine percent of emergency room medical directors said psychiatric patients are regularly kept (boarded) right in their emergency rooms because inpatient beds can't be found.[13] Thirty-three percent of the patients are boarded in ERs for over eight hours, and 6 percent for over twenty-four hours. Eighty-nine percent of the doctors transfer patients weekly due to the lack of available psychiatric beds at their own hospital. In late 2016, the American College of Emergency Physicians (ACEP) released a report that says it all: "Waits for Care and Hospital Beds Growing Dramatically for Psychiatric Emergency Patients."[14] In Nevada, the psychiatric bed shortage is so severe that hundreds were inhumanely kicked out with nothing more than a bus ticket to another state.[15] The effect of closing hospitals has caused an increase in homelessness, crime, violence, and arrest.[16] Bernard Harcourt found a direct connection between reduced hospitalization and increased incarceration.[17]

Fig. 6.2 shows that as the number of seriously mentally ill hospitalized decreased from roughly 535,540 in 1960 to 62,532 in 2014, the number incarcerated increased from roughly 55,362 to 392,037.

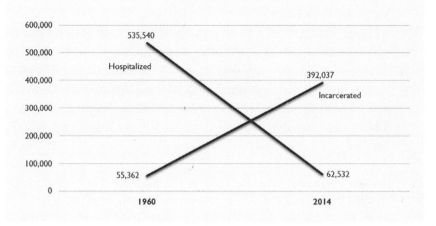

Fig. 6.2. As the number of mentally ill in hospital beds went down, the number incarcerated went up.

Hospitalization in 1960, 535,540. Data source: Gerald Grob, *From Asylum to Community* (Princeton University Press, 1991), p. 260. Hospitalization in 2014, 62,532. California Hospital Association quoting American Hospital Association. Consists of 1,176 general acute care hospitals with 36,909 beds and 223 acute psychiatric hospitals and psychiatric health facilities with 25,623 beds. Data source: California Hospital Assoc., "California's Acute Psychiatric Bed Loss," 2014, p. 3, http://www.calhospital.org/sites/main/files/file-attachments/psychbeddata.pdf) (accessed December 18, 2016).

Incarceration in 1960, 55,362. Calculated by combining the 226,344 in state and federal prisons (Department of Justice, "Historical Corrections Statistics in the United States, 1850–1984," December 1986, p. 29, https://www.bjs.gov/content/pub/pdf/hcsus5084.pdf) with the 119,671 who were in jails (Ibid., p. 76), and, for lack of a better number, applying today's 16 percent serious mental illness rate among incarcerated (chapter 2) to it. Incarceration in 2014, 592,037, per chapter 2, "overcrowded jails and prisons." Data not adjusted for population growth.

Police and sheriffs also find that the fewer hospitals, the more incarceration:

- Ohio: Summit County sheriff Drew Alexander announced his overcrowded jail would no longer admit people who needed hospitalization. Sheriff Alexander wrote, "The most common question to me is this . . . where else are we going to place them? My answer is this . . . I do not know! The mental institutions closed down in the mid 1980s because we did not want to institutionalize them. So now we arrest them and make them criminals. I do know that the Summit County Jail is not the answer."[18]

- Maine: "Sheriff Glenn Ross says his title may be 'Sheriff,' but he often feels like the CEO of the largest mental health facility. 'I'm just dealing with this over and over again.' The problem, Ross explains, is that none of the approximately 145 state psychiatric beds are available." His work-around is to send jail staff to the hospital.[19]

- Tennessee: Hamilton County Sessions Court judge Gary Starnes testified in favor of building a new psychiatric hospital since he has nowhere to send the seriously ill. "This week I have seen twelve individuals who needed care at Moccasin Bend [the state mental health facility] but they can't get in. . . . So we try to keep them in a jail cell."[20]

Closing hospital beds is not a relic of the past; it continues today. The Treatment Advocacy Center found the number of state psychiatric beds decreased by 14 percent from 2005 (50,509 beds) to 2010 (43,318).[21] In 2009, there were 29.9 emergency psychiatric beds per 100,000 in the population. In 2014, the number was down to 26.1.[22]

Policy makers should understand the primary reason that states shut down psychiatric hospitals is because Medicaid's Institute for Mental Disease (IMD) Exclusion generally precludes states from getting reimbursed for long-term treatment of adults in state psychiatric hospitals. When state governments can't get reimbursed for patients in psychiatric hospitals, they simply close them. As discussed in chapter 14, the single most important change Washington can make is to eliminate the IMD Exclusion, which is federally sanctioned discrimination against the seriously mentally ill. Discriminatory provisions in Medicare that limit hospitalization to 190 days should also be eliminated. State legislators and governors need to stop closing hospitals and start increasing the number of beds available.

CASE MANAGEMENT, SUPPORTED HOUSING, AND INCOME SUPPORT ARE CRITICAL

Access to hospitals is necessary for many at some point, but is rarely needed long-term except by a few. Even the most seriously mentally ill, if provided proper community support, can live in the community, and at less cost than in a hospital. Case management services from highly trained social workers are a necessary adjunct to help adults with serious mental illness navigate the treatment system, maintain access to benefits, secure and maintain a place to live, and avail themselves of other supports. Two case management models are most effective for the most seriously ill. Intensive Case Managers (ICMs) have better training and are given lower caseloads than ordinary case managers, which allows them to provide the intensive time-consuming support people with serious mental illness often need. Assertive Community Treatment (ACT) teams are even better. An ACT team consists of doctors, nurses, social workers, and substance abuse professionals working together. Someone on the team is available 24/7 so they can deescalate off-hour emergencies immediately. The team goes out to the client, rather than requiring the client to come to it. Unfortunately, many states call their case managers ACT or ICM without maintaining fidelity to the models.

Rehabilitation services can help people with serious mental illness regain important social skills. Access to scheduled activity can also be very important. Job-training programs may provide hope and activity but only rarely help someone with schizophrenia obtain competitive, nonsubsidized employment outside the mental health field. Because many can't work, the seriously ill need income supports like Supplemental Security Income (SSI) and case managers to help them access those benefits.

Supported housing is important for those who are too symptomatic to live with family members, do not have family, or have a dysfunctional one. Good supported housing can be provided by small group homes, adult homes, and clubhouses like Fountain House in New York that provides integrated housing, case management, and rehabilitation services. Some people with mental illness can live independently if provided with ACT or ICM services.

When these housing, case management, and psychotherapy services are working for someone, mental health officials should not withdraw them. Officials often tell patients that they have "graduated," an industry euphemism for having their intensive services taken away and replaced by less expensive ones. Someone I am close to lived successfully in a group home with onsite 24/7 support. But he was prematurely "graduated" to cheaper independent living without onsite support. He did not have the concentration to read or follow up on multiple letters requiring him to be reevaluated for continued Medicaid eligibility. When he went to refill his prescription for his antipsychotic, the pharmacist told him Medicaid discontinued his coverage because he never responded to its letters. He deteriorated, and neighbors called the police two weeks later after smelling the stench of uncollected garbage from his apartment and hearing him loudly arguing with himself. He was involuntarily admitted to the hospital, and while he was committed we feared his landlord would try to have him evicted. The involuntary admission to the hospital could have been avoided if he had been allowed to continue to live at the group home. As Alabama doctor and advocate Pippa Abston told me, "The system works under the crazy idea that because services are effective we should take them away." Policy makers must resist that.

PSYCHO-EDUCATION AND PSYCHOTHERAPIES

Psycho-education teaches important coping strategies like how to monitor symptoms and self-manage care. Psychotherapy, also known as "talk therapy," is useful for some, but not all. Some versions may help people with moderate depression or ADHD, or work in combination with medications to improve results in people with serious mental illness. Having someone to bounce ideas off of and listen to you can be helpful. NIMH lists many forms of talk therapy, including Cognitive Behavioral Therapy (CBT), Dialectal Behavioral Therapy (DBT), Interpersonal Therapy, and Family Therapy.[23] CBT is starting to gain press in the US as a treatment for psychosis mainly due to clinical recommendations promulgated by the UK's National Institute for Health and Care Excellence (NICE).[24] But CBT is not a stand-alone treatment for the seriously ill as it provides minimal, if any, benefits for people with schizophrenia or other psychosis.[25] Dialectal Behavioral Therapy seems to show some results in persons with Borderline Personality Disorder (BPD).

ELECTROCONVULSIVE THERAPY (ECT)

The Food and Drug Administration (FDA) investigated and found that electroconvulsive therapy (ECT) is a particularly important treatment for some people with severe major depression and depressive symptoms of bipolar disorder because it can help those who have not been helped by medications.[26] The FDA also found that because it is faster-acting than medications, it can be useful for treating patients who, due to the severity of their illness, require a more rapid response. Other research shows that ECT can also help some people with schizophrenia.[27] It may also be appropriate for some elderly people who have problems with the side effects of medications and for pregnant or nursing mothers who don't want to put medicines in their system.[28] While ongoing ("maintenance") ECT is often needed, unlike with medications, ECT can sometimes lead to permanent remission.

Like all treatments, ECT has side effects, and doctors often don't describe them adequately. Officials should make ECT easily available to those who can benefit from it as they are among the most seriously ill.

PEER SUPPORT IS NOT PROVEN TO HELP
PEOPLE WITH SERIOUS MENTAL ILLNESS

Peer support places someone with mental illness under the guidance of someone else whose qualification is that that person, too, has had a mental illness. It is a popular, well-funded, community-based service, but policy makers should keep in mind that unlike case management, supportive housing, hospitalization, involuntary interventions, and medications, there is no evidence it reduces homelessness, suicide, arrest, or incarceration of the seriously mentally ill.

Proponents often claim that peer support is an evidence-based practice, but few studies of peer support indicate the diagnosis of those being served, so while it may help substance abusers or those with mild mental illness, no conclusions about its utility for people with serious mental illness can be drawn. Most studies measure soft outcomes like increased "hopefulness," "self-esteem," "empowerment," "social network," "regard," "inclusion," and "acceptance." Peer support may improve those. But California mental health advocate Jeffery Hayden said those are not the important metrics. "For the seriously mentally ill, the metaphorical 'patient's temperature' is homelessness, arrest, incarceration, death, and suicide."[29] What is the impact of peer support on those? While studies of peer support do not limit themselves to the seriously mentally ill, even when looking at those with any mental health issues, the alleged benefits of peer support remain unsupported by scientific studies.

- The well-respected Cochrane Collaborative reviewed all the high-quality and low-quality data on peer support and concluded, "Involving consumer-providers in mental health teams results in psychosocial, mental health symptom and service use outcomes for clients that were no better or worse than those achieved by professionals employed in similar roles, particularly for case management services."[30] Simply put, peers are no more effective than professionals.
- The American Psychiatric Association found that "a majority of randomized trials that compare peer-delivered with non-peer-delivered services do not show differences on most outcome measures" and quoted four studies in support of its conclusion.[31]
- A recent study of eighteen trials of 5,597 participants found "there is little evidence from current trials about the effects of peer support for people with severe mental illness. ... [C]urrent evidence does not support recommendations or mandatory requirements from policy makers for mental health services to provide peer support programmes."[32]
- The Centers for Medicaid and Medicare Services (CMS) found peer support is expensive but doesn't improve outcomes.[33]

SAMHSA and the Western Massachusetts Recovery Learning Center set up a group specifically to promote peer support. It too was forced to recognize the paucity of *evidence* for peer support.[34]

The mental health industry has convinced officials to make a large investment in peer support networks. As will be seen in sections four and five, those networks rarely represent people with the most serious mental illnesses and often engage in extramural activities that are harmful to those with serious mental illness. Policy makers should direct the funds elsewhere.

STIGMA IS NOT A MAJOR REASON PEOPLE WITH SERIOUS MENTAL ILLNESS AVOID TREATMENT

Policy makers and the media have been taught by the mental health industry and advocates that stigma is an important reason seriously mentally ill people do not receive care. Research shows stigma is not a major reason they avoid treatment:

- As the chart in Fig. 6.3 shows, a 2011 survey by the SAMHSA Center for Behavioral Health Statistics and Quality found stigma (mentioned by 7 percent of respondents) was low on the list of why people with mental illness do not receive care, far behind cost (50 percent).[35] Stigma also came behind "could handle problem without treatment," "did not know where to go for services," "did not have time," belief that "treatment would not help," "did not feel need for treatment," and lack of adequate insurance.
- A 2014 Rand study, "Mental Health Stigma in the Military," reported, "[W]e are unable to link military mental health stigma to changes in treatment seeking behaviors" and "decreasing (or completely eliminating) stigma would not increase the number of service members seeking mental health treatment."[36]
- In a survey of Californians who had difficulty getting care for mental illness, three times as many (63 percent) said cost was a reason as those who said they were afraid or embarrassed to ask for help (21 percent).[37]
- A recent study, "What is the Impact of Mental Health-Related Stigma on Help-Seeking," found stigma was only the fourth-highest reason people didn't seek care.[38]
- A 2011 study, "Barriers to Mental Health Treatment," found "low perceived need for treatment" was the primary barrier to treatment, with everything else—including stigma—far behind.[39]

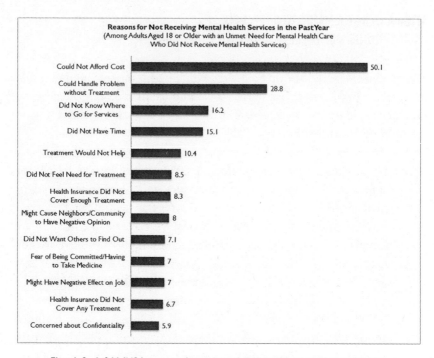

Fig. 6.3. A SAMHSA survey found cost, failure to perceive need for treatment, and other factors were more significant impediments to treatment than stigma ("did not want others to find out").

Another indication that stigma does not play a significant role in lack of care is that the number of people who go to a doctor and get a diagnosis of mental illness has exploded. If stigma were a strong factor in keeping people from seeking treatment, wouldn't this number be stable or decreasing? Likewise, the use of antidepressants increased 400 percent from 1988 to 2008; so stigma is likely not inhibiting people from seeking care.[40]

On Facebook, Dr. Tracey Goodman Skale sagely coined "Skale's Rule: The role of stigma in preventing care is inversely related to severity of illness." High-powered executives may worry what other executives will think if they get care, but the psychotic do not have such worries. Politicians should not be tricked into funding stigma campaigns when the funds can be used for treatment.

ALTERNATIVE THERAPIES DON'T WORK

When an alternative therapy is proven to work, it is no longer alternative; it is an evidence-based primary treatment. The National Center for Complementary and Integrative Health (NCCIH) at the National Institutes of Health (NIH) investigates complementary treatments to see if they confer any benefits when used in combination with conventional treatments and investigates alternative treatments to see if they can be used in lieu of conventional treatments. Open Dialogue, Soteria, mindfulness, peer support, Mental Health First Aid, vitamin B supplements, and various orthomolecular approaches have been falsely touted as either complementary or alternative, although none have evidence they reduce homelessness, arrest, incarceration, and other important outcomes in people with serious mental illness.

The government should support research into complementary and alternative treatments, but stop SAMHSA and the Center for Mental Health Services (CMHS) from funding mass implementation of unproven approaches.

WHEN ALL ELSE FAILS, INVOLUNTARY INTERVENTIONS CAN HELP SOME OF THE MOST SERIOUSLY ILL, INCLUDING THOSE WITH ANOSOGNOSIA

For a very small group of the seriously mentally ill who are too sick to recognize their need for treatment, temporary involuntary commitment can keep them safe and reduce homelessness, arrest, violence, suicide, and incarceration. In most states, people who are deemed a "danger to self or others" and are involuntarily committed still maintain the right to refuse treatment and cannot be medicated over objection until after another hearing is held to determine if they have the mental "capacity" or "competency" to refuse medications. During the delay between the commitment hearing based on dangerousness and a later hearing to determine capacity, some patients act out, so hospital security calls the police and patients who should be hospitalized and treated are instead taken off to jail.

Involuntary inpatient commitment is the most restrictive and expensive form of commitment. Each state has its own laws for short-term ("emergency detention" or "involuntary examination") and long-term commitments. Typically, short-term commitment is for no longer than seventy-two hours, and is the result of police being called to respond to an emergency crisis situation and taking the ill individual to a hospital, or because a mental health professional arranges hospitalization, sometimes after being called by family members during the emergency. These emergency detention procedures are designed to protect individuals from harming themselves or others and to get a psychiatric evaluation to determine if longer term commitment is needed. Continuing that emergency detention for a longer period appropriately requires a court or judicially sanctioned process to decide if the person meets the state's commitment standard.

State commitment standards vary. Some states had to enact narrow commitment standards to free themselves from lawsuits and pressure emanating from chapters of the American Civil Liberties Union and federally funded Protection and Advocacy lawyers. The result is that many individuals go without necessary treatment until it's too late.[41] Treatment before tragedy is discouraged, while treatment after tragedy is grudgingly allowed. All states allow the involuntary commitment of someone who is a "danger to self or others" as defined by state law. Some states and courts interpret "danger" broadly, but others interpret it narrowly, requiring someone to be "imminently" dangerous. Some states supplement or expand the definition of dangerousness with the "grave disability," "in need of treatment," and "lack of capacity" standards discussed in chapter 15.

In general, to facilitate involuntary inpatient commitment, a police officer or mental health official in some states has to be willing to come out and make a determination that the person meets the state's emergency detention or commitment standard. Unfortunately, many will only do that if the person meets the dangerousness standard, and will ignore other useful standards the state may have in place. If initiated by a police officer, that officer must also have a chief who will tolerate the officer deciding to take the person to the hospital, often hours away, leaving the chief with at least one less officer on patrol. The officer must find a doctor at the hospital willing to help the patient, agree to admit, and also have a supervisor who won't be critical if the doctor elects to admit the person. Then the hospital has to be willing to petition the court for continuing commitment beyond the seventy-two-hour emergency detention, argue the case against publicly funded lawyers who will represent the patient, and possibly be willing to go back to the court for a second hearing to allow medication over objection if the person refuses the medication, again, arguing with lawyers who will oppose it.

And then there is the lack of hospital beds to contend with. As a result of the cumbersome procedures and the shortage of psychiatric beds, a common scenario is that hospitals simply discharge patients at the end of the short-term commitment. They don't want to or cannot afford to pay for holding the hearings, or know that even if they prevail in the hearings, they will be unable to find a long-term psychiatric bed to place the patient in. Likewise, law enforcement officers know the drill and don't want to waste their time bringing someone to a hospital who desperately needs care, if they know the person is not likely to receive it and will simply become a revolving door patient. It's easier and less time consuming to arrest the patient.

ASSISTED OUTPATIENT TREATMENT

Assisted Outpatient Treatment (AOT) is a useful alternative to inpatient commitment, especially for those with anosognosia. State laws vary, but generally AOT allows judges, after full due process, to order untreated seriously mentally ill people who meet narrow and specific criteria to stay in, say, six months of mandated and monitored treatment while they continue living freely in the community. In some states the outpatient standard is identical to the inpatient commitment standard, and in other states they are different. AOT is an exceedingly effective option that exists in every state except Connecticut, Maryland, Massachusetts, and Tennessee but is rarely used due to opposition from the mental health industry described in chapter ten.

To demonstrate how AOT works in practice, look at New York where AOT is called "Kendra's Law."[42] In New York, certain persons, including family and mental health workers, can petition the court to place someone with serious mental illness in AOT. There is a medical examination, a hearing, and the patient is given free counsel. If the judge finds the person meets the criteria of having a serious mental illness plus multiple prior arrests, incarcerations, or hospitalizations within a specific time frame that were caused by going off treatment—and the judge believes the patient will not comply with the treatment needed to keep him safe—the judge can order AOT for up to six months.[43] The judge then orders the mental health system to provide the treatment. Patients help develop their own treatment plan, but it must include case management services so their compliance can be monitored. It may also include other services, such as supported housing, psychotherapy, and substance abuse counseling. The judge may require the patient to take medications, but the court order does not allow the forcible administration of medications. The only consequence of failing to take medications or meet other court-ordered conditions is that the individual can be examined to see if he meets the preexisting inpatient commitment criteria. But that provision is very significant, because it allows an individual to be evaluated *before* becoming a danger to self or others rather than forcing the treatment system to stand back until *after* the person becomes dangerous. In spite of the fact that the order does not allow forced medication, both opponents and proponents have recognized that the "black robe" effect of going in front of a judge coerces most patients to not violate the order.[44] The order can be renewed six months at a time if necessary.

As summarized in appendix D, the research on AOT is extensive and overwhelmingly positive. It reduced homelessness by 74 percent, hospitalization 77 percent, arrest 83 percent, incarceration 87 percent, physical harm to others 47 percent, property destruction 46 percent, suicidal behavior 55 percent, substance abuse 48 percent, in the most difficult to treat patients who *already accumulated multiple* hospitalizations or acts of violence associated with going off treatment. By replacing expensive hospitalization and incarceration with less expensive community services, AOT cuts costs to taxpayers in half. Results from California, Ohio, Arizona, and many other states are similar.

Assisted Outpatient Treatment is supported by those who have experienced it. Seventy-five percent of patients in AOT in New York reported that AOT helped them gain control over their lives, 81 percent said AOT helped them get and stay well, and 90 percent said AOT made them more likely to keep appointments and take medication.

AOT has been endorsed by the National Sheriffs' Association, the International Association of Chiefs of Police (IACP), the US Department of Justice, and others in criminal justice.[45]

In 1995, National Alliance on Mental Illness (NAMI) membership overwhelmingly endorsed AOT in a direct vote of members.[46] AOT has been declared an evidence-based practice by SAMHSA and the Agency for Healthcare Research and Quality.[47] Because AOT is more humane and less restrictive and expensive than the alternatives—involuntary inpatient commitment or incarceration—it's been endorsed by the United States Conference of Catholic Bishops.[48]

Courts have ruled that it is an appropriate use of the state's police powers and *parens patriae* powers.[49] For many, it's the last off ramp before jail. Linda Dunn became an advocate in California as a result of having a son with a psychotic disorder. She said, "AOT is like putting a fence by the edge of the cliff rather than an ambulance at the bottom."[50] AOT is not an alternative to voluntary treatment; it is a way to see that voluntary services get used by those who lack the ability or refuse to accept voluntary treatment. In a letter to the editor of the *Wall Street Journal*, Pat and Bruce Goodall explained how AOT worked for their son:

> [O]ur schizophrenic son went off his meds. He was hospitalized four times and picked up by the police for a variety of infractions. He wandered the streets inadequately clothed, hallucinating and begging cigarettes and money from strangers. For a year and a half this continued until one day he threatened his mother with a jagged shard of broken glass. This was the "threat to others" that finally brought him to court where an order for assisted outpatient treatment (AOT) was given. What a lifesaving action! ... The AOT order continues and he is able to live in his own apartment and take care of himself. He is an artist and has started painting again.[51]

Because AOT requires a court, it is cumbersome and expensive for families to access. The "easiest" way in is to convince the hospital or community program that is serving the patient to file the petition, attend the hearings, and assist in developing the treatment plans. But the hospitals and programs often resist, preferring to sever their connection to difficult patients, rather than going to court to ensure they receive continuing treatment.

Before AOT, families, clinicians, and criminal justice had to make a binary choice between total removal of rights via involuntary commitment or incarceration on the one hand, and unfettered living in the community on the other. AOT is a useful middle ground. After someone with mental illness climbed over the White House fence and made it inside the East

Room, the director of the Secret Service told Congress, "We don't take it lightly [but] there is not a lot we can do with mentally ill individuals who do not commit a crime. We are limited by the laws."[52] AOT can help fix that. By supplementing community living with an obligation to stay in treatment, AOT allows patients more freedom, saves taxpayers money, and protects everyone. A primary responsibility of every policy maker should be to fund AOT and foster greater use of it.

The next section shows how SAMHSA, CMHS, and the mental health industry ignore the facts described in the preceding chapters and convince the government to do the same.

Section 3

THE MENTAL HEALTH INDUSTRY

SUBSTANCE ABUSE AND MENTAL HEALTH SERVICES ADMINISTRATION (SAMHSA)

"SAMHSA has not made the treatment of the seriously mentally ill a priority. In fact, I'm afraid serious mental illness such as schizophrenia and bipolar disorder may not be a concern at all to SAMHSA."

—Representative Tim Murphy (R-PA)

The Substance Abuse and Mental Health Services Administration (SAMHSA) has a disproportionate influence on mental health policy because it is the major federal agency responsible for developing and coordinating it. It also provides funds directly. Congress established SAMHSA in 1992 and directed it "to target . . . mental health services to the people most in need."[1] Priority populations were defined as adults with a serious mental illness and children with a serious emotional disturbance.[2]

SAMHSA refuses to focus on the most seriously ill.[3] SAMHSA's 2011–2014 strategic plan directed its mental health resources toward a terribly vague and impossibly broad mission that reads a lot like a cheap self-help book: "creating a high-quality, self-directed, satisfying life integrated in the community for *all Americans*."[4] (Emphasis added.) A top SAMHSA official told *Time* magazine, "The behavioral health of the *entire population* is a priority for SAMHSA."[5] (Emphasis added.) Of SAMHSA's six 2015–2018 "strategic initiatives" only one mentions serious mental illness, and that is limited to preventing it, something that cannot be done.[6] The result? SAMHSA fails to serve the most seriously ill and encourages states to ignore them too.

SAMHSA focuses on irrelevant and tangential issues and ignores con-

A Brief History of SAMHSA

The Alcohol, Drug Abuse and Mental Health Administration (ADAMHA) was the predecessor agency to SAMHSA, responsible for both mental health research and providing mental health services.* In the 1980s, many realized mental illness research should be housed within the National Institute of Mental Health (NIMH), part of the National Institute of Health (NIH), which had extensive research capabilities. In 1992, the ADAMHA Reorganization Act (Public Law 102-321) moved research to NIMH, technically dissolved ADAMHA, and transferred its service responsibilities to SAMHSA, which is located within the Department of Health and Human Services (HHS). Congress established the Center for Mental Health Services (CMHS) within SAMHSA to conduct most of SAMHSA's mental illness–related responsibilities. The 2016 21st Century Cures Act made the SAMHSA Administrator an assistant secretary within HHS. Roughly two-thirds of SAMHSA's budget is focused on substance abuse and one-third on mental illness. *Insane Consequences* focuses exclusively on the mental illness component of SAMHSA.

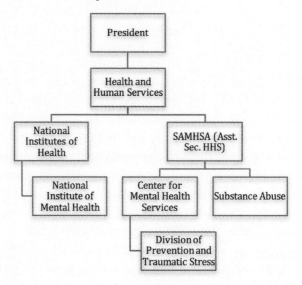

The Center for Mental Health Services administers the mental health programs within SAMHSA. It has a division to address "prevention" and "traumatic stress" but not one specifically tasked to address serious mental illness, a subject it has shown little interest in.

*ADAMHA was established on May 21, 1972 (88 Stat. 134), effective as of September 25, 1973. It was reorganized and moved around numerous times.

sequential ones like reducing violence, incarceration, hospitalization, and homelessness. After reviewing SAMHSA's 2015–2018 strategic plan, Dr. Paul Summergrad, then president of the American Psychiatric Association (APA), concluded, "The proposed plan is striking for what it leaves out: a focus on the appropriate medical care of patients with serious mental illness." The "APA is strongly concerned about the lack of explicit recognition of the psychiatric treatment needs for Americans suffering from mental illness and substance use disorders, and in particular for the 13 million Americans who suffer from debilitating serious mental illnesses (SMI)."[7] Representative Tim Murphy (R-PA), a child psychologist, read an earlier plan and noted,

> The 2011–2014 SAMHSA strategic plan … think[s] in broad terms of "behavioral" and "emotional" health, promoting such concepts as "wellness" and "recovery." Not once in this entire 117-page document will you find the words schizophrenia or bipolar disorder. Nowhere in the testimony that was provided to this committee yesterday by the SAMHSA administrator do those words appear. And nowhere on SAMHSA's web site or in their publications can you learn about the increased risk of violent behavior by persons with untreated serious mental illness. It's as if SAMHSA doesn't believe serious mental illness exists.[8]

The editorial board of the *Wall Street Journal* went further: "SAMHSA uses its $3.6 billion annual budget to undermine treatment for severe mental disorders."[9] They are right. Developing a plan to eliminate SAMHSA, to reassign its mental health responsibilities to other agencies, or focus it on serious mental illness should be an issue that unites Democrats and Republicans. It would save money, improve care, and keep patients, the public, and the police safer. There is virtually no support for SAMHSA other than from those who receive funds from it.

For years, SAMHSA had no doctors on staff or in leadership positions. Even CMHS, the mental illness unit, is headed by a consumer, not a doctor.[10] After coming under outside pressure to hire at least a single doctor, SAMHSA did hire Dr. Elinore McCance-Katz to be its first chief medical officer. She left after only two years and told why in a scathing piece in *Psychiatric Times*:

Unfortunately, SAMHSA does not address the treatment needs of the most vulnerable in our society. Rather, the unit within SAMHSA charged with addressing these disorders, the Center for Mental Health Services, chooses to focus on its own definition of "recovery," which generally ignores the treatment of mental disorders. . . . There is a perceptible hostility toward psychiatric medicine: a resistance to addressing the treatment needs of those with serious mental illness and a questioning by some at SAMHSA as to whether mental disorders even exist—for example, is psychosis just a "different way of thinking for some experiencing stress?"[11]

In a 2015 survey of federal employees, SAMHSA employees ranked SAMHSA the 317th worst place to work out of 320 government agencies.[12] That's down from 298th in the 2014 survey. Employees cited ineffective leadership, something confirmed by a 2015 General Accountability Office (GAO) audit that found SAMHSA fails to coordinate the nation's mental health policies and that most programs go unevaluated.[13]

Following is how SAMHSA undermines treatment of the seriously mentally ill.

SAMHSA REPLACED THE SCIENTIFIC "MEDICAL MODEL" WITH A SAMHSA-INVENTED "RECOVERY MODEL"

To compensate for the lack of psychiatrists among its 589 employees, SAMHSA relies on popularity contests to develop policies. It convenes meetings of "stakeholders" and lets them vote in online polls. While SAMHSA claims to collect the input of people with mental illness, it does not hold hearings where people with serious mental illness are: in jails, shelters, prisons, and forensic hospitals. There is no outreach to get police, sheriffs, psychiatrists, and others concerned about serious mental illness and issues like hospitalization, arrest, violence, homelessness, and incarceration to vote in the polls. Instead, SAMHSA stacks online meetings with high-functioning consumers and mental "health" organizations, many of which they fund. That's what SAMHSA did when it wanted to replace the proven medical model with its own internally invented politically correct "Recovery Model."[14] The make-work process went on for sixteen months and resulted in an 1,100-word definition of "recovery" and a model that puts every patient in charge of crafting his own recovery plan. It stresses "empowerment" over treatment no matter how psychotic the individual is.

SAMHSA summarized recovery as,

> A process of change through which individuals improve their health and wellness, live a self-directed life, and strive to reach their full potential.[15]

Before SAMHSA, recovery meant "a return to health." But research suggests only 14 percent of those with schizophrenia recover.[16] By inventing a new definition, SAMHSA was able to declare that everyone recovers. Voila! Recovery is simply a "process of change." Improving "health and wellness" is in; treating serious mental illness is out. SAMHSA's Recovery Model is used to justify spending mental health funds on anything people believe will help them "reach their full potential." The fact that some people with schizophrenia and bipolar disorder do not recover is simply ignored.

SAMHSA's Recovery Model includes "10 Guiding Principles of Recovery." The most important is that "self-determination and self-direction are the foundations for recovery." The Recovery Model is dangerous to some as it makes no allowance for the fact that there are individuals with severe mental illness who cannot self-direct their care. Dr. Torrey and I wrote that "Under the 'Recovery Model,' John Hinckley was defining his own life goal—the attention of Jodie Foster—when he shot President Reagan."[17] Dr. Sally Satel of the American Enterprise Institute and Mary Zdanowicz, former executive director of the Treatment Advocacy Center, wrote an op-ed astutely observing,

> [The Recovery Model] is a dangerously partial vision. It sets up unrealistic expectations for those who will never fully "recover," no matter how hard they try, because their illness is so severe. What's more, exclusive emphasis on recovery as a goal steers policymakers away from making changes vital to the needs of the most severely disabled.[18]

Dr. Satel was a former member of the Center for Mental Health Services (CMHS) National Advisory Council. She believes if a psychiatrist followed the principles of recovery, "he would be at risk of committing malpractice."[19]

SAMHSA encourages states to replace the medical model with the Recovery Model and to use federal Mental Health Block Grants (MHBG) for it.[20] SAMHSA led large segments of the mental health industry into abandoning the medical model for the Recovery Model.[21] "People Recover" became part of SAMHSA's formal motto and a key strategic initiative.[22]

This is not some minor league bureaucrat run amok. The process was driven by former SAMHSA administrator Pamela Hyde and current CMHS director Paolo del Vecchio. Mr. del Vecchio wrote that the definition is consistent with SAMHSA's mission "to promote a high-quality, self-directed, satisfying life integrated in a community for all Americans."[23] That is a gross misrepresentation of SAMHSA's mental health mission, which is to help the seriously mentally ill, not "all Americans." The new SAMHSA acting administrator, Kana Enomoto, has not taken steps to right the ship.

Charlotte Walker, a person with mental illness who writes the mental health blog *purplepersuasion*, described the problem with the "sanitized" Recovery Model in "Jagged Little Pill: Has the Recovery Narrative Gone Too Far?"

> I am not going to completely recover. It's just not going to happen. . . . I will relapse at some point. . . . It's no good portraying me as "just like anybody else." . . . I have rocked back and forth on the bus because I was manic and trying to hold in the urge to run around the bus screaming. . . . I have cried in public. . . . When I am hypomanic I am not very good at keeping my temper. It's rare, but I sometimes exhibit what services call "challenging behaviour." . . .
>
> It is hopeless to say that I am now "recovered." If the dominant discourse is allowed to become about the more palatable, sugar-coated "complete recovery," it is shutting out those with long-term mental illness.[24]

SAMHSA REFUSES TO CERTIFY PROGRAMS THAT HELP THE SERIOUSLY MENTALLY ILL AND CERTIFIES PROGRAMS THAT DON'T

In the United States, there is no licensing or regulation of education modules or talk therapies. Anyone can claim she has one that works, and SAMHSA helps that person. SAMHSA maintains what they call a National Registry of Evidence-Based Programs and Practices (NREPP).[25]

It is little more than a collection of privately developed workshops and training sessions, that SAMHSA essentially certifies as being evidence-based.[26] SAMHSA encourages states to use their federal and state funds to buy the listed "programs and practices" from the vendors.

Little of what's in NREPP are actual treatments, and the "evidence" often comes straight from those who invent, sell, and profit from them. Mental Health First Aid (MHFA) is an all-day training program complete with course materials that ostensibly teaches people to identify the symptoms of mental illness in others and connect them to help. The three studies SAMHSA relied on to certify it were all done by the owners/vendors of the program, Betty Kitchener or Anthony F. Jorm.[27] Those studies show only that the trainers and trained like MHFA; they do not show that it improves outcomes for people with mental illness. There is a study that found no benefit for people with mental illness, but it was not submitted by Ms. Kitchener or Mr. Jorm to SAMHSA, and therefore it was not considered by SAMHSA.[28] First Lady Michelle Obama took part of the course, after the Newtown shootings President Obama promised $15 million to expand it, and in September 2016, the House Energy and Commerce Health Subcommittee authorized $60 million for it.[29] New York City's mayor Bill de Blasio allocated $8 million to provide MHFA training to 250,000 city residents.[30] Why such top-level attention for a program that doesn't help the mentally ill? Mental Health First Aid is sold in the United States by the powerful National Council for Community Behavioral Healthcare, which also licenses others to be trainers for a fee. Here are other programs that SAMHSA lists as evidence-based by relying on information that came from the people who sell them:

- Four of the five "studies" SAMHSA used to certify Triple-P Positive Parenting, a program that teaches parents of misbehaving children how to be better parents, were conducted by the vendor of the program.[31] Numerous independent studies show it doesn't work.[32]
- The two studies used to certify the Wellness Recovery Action Plan (WRAP), which teaches people to develop a wellness plan, were conducted at least partially by Mary Ellen Copeland, the vendor of the program.[33] Like MHFA, WRAP is not proven to benefit the seriously mentally ill.[34]

- TeenScreen a program purporting to teach ways to reduce suicide in schools, is used in forty-seven states, partially as a result of the owner promoting its NREPP certification. The NREPP certification was granted based on "manuscripts in preparation," not peer-reviewed research. TeenScreen doesn't reduce suicide.[35] SAMHSA removed certification only after Mental Illness Policy Org. informed it that the program is no longer sold. However, states are still using public funds for it.
- SAMHSA certified Kognito-At-Risk for College Students, a half-hour video that ostensibly trains college students how to identify classmates with "psychological distress" and get them into care. SAMHSA cites a single marketing brochure written by the manufacturer of the program, consisting of unsubstantiated, non-peer-reviewed claims by the program vendor, stating that it works.[36]

One trick used by SAMHSA is to certify programs as being "effective" even when they don't improve meaningful outcomes, such as reducing violence, arrest, incarceration, suicide, homelessness, and hospitalization. Many programs SAMHSA certifies as effective only improve soft outcomes, like "satisfaction," "feeling of wellness," "empowerment," "hopefulness," and "resiliency." Taking people bowling could probably gain NREPP certification because it makes people happier. Dr. Satel told a congressional committee, "Of the 288 programs listed [in NREPP], four by my count specifically designated people with severe illness as their recipients."[37]

While certifying ineffective workshops as evidence-based practices, SAMHSA does not evaluate programs that actually do improve meaningful outcomes in the seriously mentally ill. Assertive Community Treatment (ACT), Intensive Case Managers (ICM), Crisis Intervention Teams (CIT) to train police on how to deescalate a crisis, and Mental Health Courts are programs that help the seriously mentally ill that SAMHSA has refused to certify.[38]

SAMHSA PREVENTS STATES FROM USING MENTAL HEALTH BLOCK GRANT MONEY TO HELP PEOPLE WITH SERIOUS MENTAL ILLNESS

SAMHSA regulates how states spend $532 million (2016) in federally funded Mental Health Block Grants (MHBG).[39] The legislation requires the funds to be used for "adults with serious mental illness" and "children with serious emotional disturbance" and, as described in appendix A, narrowly defines those terms. But the SAMHSA MHBG instructions and application process encourages states to use the funds for people without mental illness.[40]

> SAMHSA strongly recommends that Block Grant funds be directed . . . to fund primary prevention: universal, selective, and indicated prevention activities and services for persons not identified as needing treatment.
>
> The focus is about everyone, not just those with an illness or disease, but the whole population.[41]

SAMHSA's block grant instructions tell states to fund trauma (not a mental illness); peer support (not proven to improve a meaningful outcome in people with serious mental illness); prevention (no one knows how to prevent serious mental illness); early intervention (no one knows who will develop serious mental illness until symptoms become manifest); employment training (most people with the most serious mental illnesses will not be able to work); people with different levels of risk (rather than those at highest risk); self-directed interventions (thereby excluding those too ill to self-direct); "everyone" (not just those with an illness); and of course, the Recovery Model.

Arthur T. Dean, chairman and CEO of Community Anti-Drug Coalitions of America (CADCA), tried to warn SAMHSA about its requirement to spend block grants on mental health promotion:

> The new Uniform Block Grant Application makes the case for and explicitly includes mental health promotion as a "priority area" for planning and resource allocation purposes, despite the fact that current law for neither the [substance abuse block grant] nor the [mental health block grant] includes any language to authorize expenditures for this purpose.[42]

SAMHSA ignored his warning. States are also required to exercise their own oversight of how block grants are spent to ensure they go to the seriously ill, but their efforts are no better than that of SAMHSA.[43]

The diversion of funds is ongoing. In 2014, Congress directed SAMHSA to set aside 5 percent of the mental health block grant over the following years to support "evidence-based programs that address the needs of individuals with early serious mental illness, including psychotic disorders."[44] CMHS issued guidance to states suggesting they use the set-aside for "peer support," which has not been shown to help people in early psychosis.[45]

SAMHSA INVENTED A NEW MENTAL ILLNESS: TRAUMA

Beyond its corrosive endorsement of treatments that fail to help the seriously mentally ill and its support for junk science, SAMHSA invented a new mental illness it calls "trauma." No reputable psychiatrist considers it an illness. Post-traumatic stress disorder (PTSD) is an illness, but even that can run from mild to severe. SAMHSA is not limiting its efforts to helping people with severe PTSD or even mild PTSD. In 2009, SAMHSA gave trauma the full monty by again conducting an online poll and letting "stakeholders" vote. They voted to make trauma an illness.[46] "Trauma and Justice" is now one of SAMHSA's most important strategic initiatives, and CMHS established a "traumatic stress" department. SAMHSA never exactly defined trauma, but declared,

> Individual trauma results from an event, series of events, or set of circumstances that is experienced by an individual as physically or emotionally harmful or threatening and that has lasting adverse effects on the individual's functioning and physical, social, emotional, or spiritual well-being.[47]

SAMHSA's "trauma" can therefore include anyone who got divorced, found a spouse was cheating, knows someone who died, was in a storm, or had any event she "experienced as . . . emotionally harmful" if it affected her "spiritual well-being." In an exposé of the trauma-informed care sham that caused his hospital to divert funds to opening "empathy rooms," Dr. Boris Vatel wrote,

Trauma-informed care training teaches that traumatic stress already constitutes an injury, and since the definition of traumatic stress is whatever one may find stressful, we are all potential trauma victims. . . . Traumainformed care actually trivializes severe trauma by placing it on par with experiences that objectively would be classified as merely unpleasant.[48]

SAMHSA is pouring millions into preventing trauma.[49] It is largely responsible for the growth of the trauma industry, grief industry, and bereavement industry that was documented in *One Nation Under Therapy*.[50] It has worked to "promote the idea that seemingly content and well-adjusted Americans—adults as well as children—are emotionally damaged." SAMHSA made trauma-informed care a core component of the Recovery Model, created a National Center for Trauma Informed Care, and awarded major trauma grants to organizations like the National Association of State Mental Health Program Directors (NASMHPD).[51] That is money diverted from treating serious mental illness.

SAMHSA FUNDS ANTIPSYCHIATRY AND ANTIPSYCHIATRISTS

SAMHSA is responsible for distributing funds that Congress appropriated for programs of "Regional and National Significance." As Mental Illness Policy Org. documented, some of those funds go directly from SAMHSA to antipsychiatry organizations that don't believe mental illness exists and often oppose treatment.[52] Other than Scientology, it is hard to find an antipsychiatry organization that does not receive financial or public relations support from SAMHSA. SAMHSA's own *Mental Illness Awareness Week Guide* suggests that schools invite MindFreedom, the Icarus Project, and the National Coalition for Mental Health Recovery (NCMHR) into classrooms to teach children about mental illness.[53] MindFreedom believes "mental illnesses are not brain diseases."[54] The Icarus Project believes "these experiences—commonly diagnosed and labeled as psychiatric conditions— are mad gifts needing cultivation and care, rather than diseases or disorders."[55] The National Coalition for Mental Health Recovery (NCMHR) believes "psychiatric labeling is a pseudoscientific practice of limited value in helping people recover."[56] Are these whom we want teaching our children?

- SAMHSA provided $329,000 to the Mental Health Association of Oregon, whose former board president lent her support to a group in New York that wanted to have involuntary mental health treatment classified as "torture."[57]
- SAMHSA gave $70,000 to the Pennsylvania Mental Health Consumers Association. The head of the association wanted to close all state psychiatric hospitals, thereby preventing the most seriously ill from receiving treatment when needed.[58]
- SAMHSA gave Advocates for Human Potential over $8 million.[59] A senior research associate at Advocates for Human Potential told her Facebook followers that everything in the *DSM* is made up.
- SAMHSA invited Pat Risser to serve on its advisory board to review SAMHSA grants to ensure they were, in his mind, appropriate.[60] Mr. Risser was past president of the radical National Association for Rights Protection and Advocacy (NARPA). His homepage features such articles as "How to Escape a Mental Hospital" and "Stopping Psychiatric Drugs." He also claimed credit for having "deprogrammed them [consumers] from the brainwashing cult of psychiatry."[61]

SAMHSA's and CMHS's unrelenting support of individuals and organizations opposed to the medical model has made incarceration of seriously mentally ill people more likely. SAMHSA once let people who were not antiscience join the CMHS advisory board. Those individuals advised SAMHSA and CMHS against funding antipsychiatry and unproven interventions, but both organizations ignored them, leading the advisors to resign.[62]

SAMHSA WASTES MONEY INTENDED TO HELP PEOPLE WITH SERIOUS MENTAL ILLNESS

SAMHSA wastes money. It uses its budget to publish and distribute children's books, such as *Play Day in the Park* for three-year-olds and four-year-olds; *Look What I Can Do!* for five-year-olds and six-year-olds; coloring books, such as *Wally Bear and Friends*; and, my favorite, *The Lion and the Mouse* sing-along.[63] We are unaware of any evidence that these reduce either substance abuse or mental illness, and the administrator of SAMHSA couldn't produce any when asked by Representative Markwayne Mullin (R-OK) at a congressional hearing.[64]

SAMHSA has scores of free publications covering non–mental illness. These include "What a Difference a Friend Makes" and publications on oil spill response, hurricane recovery, American Indian and Alaska native culture, peer pressure, social marketing, employment services, and health promotion. But SAMHSA has only a single publication on schizophrenia, and it is out of stock.

Dr. Torrey reported that the SAMHSA-led "National Wellness Week" encouraged "visiting a farmers' market, taking a class on nutritional cooking, 'drinking a veggie or fruit smoothie,' reading poetry, making a collage, taking a walk, joining a song circle, taking a class on how to make sacred drums . . . and join[ing] the Line Dance for wellness . . . because 'dancing is a great stress reliever and also provides social interaction.'"[65]

SAMHSA commissioned a $22,500 painting of Native Americans to help raise awareness about the roles of families and the community in mental health and in substance abuse disorder prevention.[66] It sits in SAMHSA's headquarters. SAMHSA spent $200,000 to put on a party at Paramount Studies in Hollywood, winning it a place in former senator Tom Coburn's (R-OK) *Wastebook*.[67]

Things are so bad at SAMHSA that in December 2016, Republicans and Democrats came together and incorporated Representative Tim Murphy's ideas to fix SAMHSA in the 21st Century Cures Act.[68] It attempts to get SAMHSA and CMHS more focused on the seriously mentally ill and to rely on science rather than popularity contests to construct policy. It creates a chief medical officer within SAMHSA and ties it more closely to other federal departments, like DOJ and NIMH. The position of SAMHSA administrator is eliminated and replaced with an assistant secretary within HHS. The success of the plan will depend on whom President Trump nominates to be the assistant secretary. NIMH had similar problems of mission creep that started to get solved when its previous director was replaced by Dr. Thomas Insel. New leadership at SAMHSA and CMHS could be just what the doctor ordered.

The following chapter describes the mental health organizations, many SAMHSA-funded, that fail the most seriously ill and the few organizations trying to help.

Chapter 8

THE MENTAL HEALTH NONPROFIT COMPLEX AND ITS CRITICS

"The military industrial complex has nothing on the mental health non-profit complex."

—Unknown

The behavioral health landscape has largely split into two with some overlap. On one side are the mental health industry and mental health advocates who focus on improving the mental health of the 100 percent with poor mental health or empowering the 18 percent with some form of mental illness. On the other side are a few organizations trying to help the 4 percent who have serious mental illness. The government has sided with the mental health industry. It gives the industry what it wants: entrée to policy meetings and mental health funds without an obligation to serve the seriously ill.

Following is an introduction to some of the major mental health organizations that prevent prioritization of the most seriously ill and those that are working to improve their treatment. The chapters after this document their anti-treatment activities.

Organizations in the left column either don't admit mental illness exists, work to prevent prioritizing seriously ill adults, favor funding non-evidence-based practices, believe the causes of serious mental illness are known and that it can be predicted and prevented, favor spending mental health funds on people without mental health problems, oppose more hospital beds, or oppose AOT. The organizations in the right column support helping the most seriously ill by creating more hospital beds, improving civil commitment and HIPAA laws, or expanding AOT. Organizations in the middle tend to engage both activities.

Mental Health Industry vs. Advocates for Seriously Mentally Ill

Mental Health Advocates (Generally not focused on serious mental illness)	Mental Health and Serious Mental Illness	Advocates for the Seriously Mentally Ill
SAMHSA-FUNDED TECHNICAL ASSISTANCE CENTERS National Coalition for Mental Health Recovery (NCMHR) National Empowerment Center (NEC) National Mental Health Consumers Self-Help Clearinghouse Copeland Center for Wellness and Recovery National Alliance on Mental Illness— national office (NAMI)	**TRADE ASSOCIATIONS** Pharmaceutical Research and Manufacturers of America (PHrMA) National Association of Psychiatric Health Systems (NAPHS) National Association for Children's Behavioral Health	**MENTAL ILLNESS ORGANIZATIONS** Treatment Advocacy Center Mental Illness Policy Org.
MENTAL HEALTH LAWYERS American Civil Liberties Union (ACLU) Bazelon Center Protection and Advocacy (P&A/PAIMI) National Disability Right Network National Alliance for Rights Protection and Advocacy (NARPA)	**GUILDS** American Psychiatric Association (APA) 1199 Service Employees International Union	**CRIMINAL JUSTICE** International Association of Chiefs of Police (IACP) National Sheriffs Association (NSA) **TRADE ASSOCATIONS** American Hospital Association (AHA) Clubhouse International
MENTAL HEALTH DIRECTORS National Association of State Mental Health Program Directors National Association of County Behavioral Health & Developmental Disability Directors	**CELEBRITY-CENTRIC ORGANIZATIONS** One Mind for Research Kennedy Forum on Mental Health	**GUILDS** American College of Emergency Physicians American Psychiatric Nurses Association American Association of Psychiatric Technicians
TRADE ASSOCIATIONS Mental Health America (MHA) National Council for Behavioral Health New York Association of Psychiatric Rehabilitation Services (NYAPRS)	**OTHER** National Alliance on Mental Illness state orgs.	**CELEBRITY-CENTRIC ORGANIZATIONS** Bring Change 2 Mind
GUILDS American Academy of Child and Adolescent Psychiatry American Psychological Association		**OTHER** National Alliance on Mental Illness—local chapters
CELEBRITY-CENTRIC ORGANIZATIONS Carter Center		
OTHER The Icarus Project Foundation for Excellence in Mental Health Care Scientology and Citizens Commission on Human Rights		

Fig. 8.1.

SAMHSA-FUNDED TECHNICAL ASSISTANCE CENTERS

SAMHSA's Technical Assistance Centers ("Programs of Regional and National Significance") are funded through the Center for Mental Health Services (CMHS). Most Technical Assistance Centers fund groups of people SAMHSA calls "peers." SAMHSA uses that term, or "consumers," or "persons with lived experience" instead of "patients" or "persons with mental illness" so the organizations that receive the funds don't have to admit mental illness exists. In addition to their direct funding, SAMHSA and CMHS pay stipends and honoraria to peer Technical Assistance Centers, fund "scholarships" to their workshops, hire their leaders to give presentations and webinars, and funnel money to them, through the National Center for Trauma Informed Care and other programs. SAMHSA funding and publicity give the Technical Assistance Centers a lopsided influence on state and federal policies and seems to buy their silence on SAMHSA's failures.

Most SAMHSA-funded Technical Assistance Centers—peer and non-peer—support the broadest definition of "mental health," oppose prioritizing the most seriously ill, support the Recovery Model over the medical model, oppose Assisted Outpatient Treatment or making hospital beds available for the seriously ill, claim persons with untreated serious mental illness are not more violent than others, everyone recovers, prevention works, there is a stigma to being mentally ill, and the most important thing for the government to do is to give them money and jobs. The following are direct and indirect recipients of SAMHSA Technical Assistance Center grants. They are practically the only groups that support SAMHSA as-is.

The National Coalition for Mental Health Recovery and member organizations

The National Coalition for Mental Health Recovery (NCMHR) acts as the umbrella trade association for peer groups, including the SAMHSA-funded peer Technical Assistance Centers.[1] SAMHSA funds go indirectly to NCMHR in the form of dues paid by members. Their battle cry, "Nothing About Us Without Us," reflects their belief that medical mental health policy should be dictated by those who at one point in their lives may have been told or believed they had a mental health issue rather than by doctors with medical degrees. It has been headed by Dan Fisher of the National Empowerment Center (NEC) and others who hold anti-psychiatry positions. In 2012, NCMHR associate director Lauren Spiro wrote, "Mental health services should move away from a bio-psychiatric approach, such as the one enshrined in the DSM. . . . We need to better understand the oppressive dynamics embedded in our culture that bring about great emotional distress. . . ."[2] NCMHR eschews the terms "mentally ill" and "mental illness," substituting "people with lived experience" to describe the population it serves.[3] I am not aware of any person anywhere without "lived experience." NCMHR also uses the tortured phrase, "non-consensus reality," rather than "psychotic" to avoid admitting delusions and hallucinations are symptoms of an illness that needs treatment. Deputy Policy Director Raymond Bridges previously served as policy director for the Virginia Organization of Consumers Asserting Leadership (VOCAL), which believes mental illness is merely "an extreme state of consciousness."[4] It claims not to be biased against medications, but NCMHR distributes information about side effects, not efficacy.

I am unaware of any NCMHR leader acknowledging that schizo-phrenia or other brain disorders exist. Instead, NCMHR leaders, and many of its members, refer to people as being "diagnosed" with mental illness. That phrase allows NCMHR to acknowledge that a doctor may have said someone has a mental illness, without accepting that the patient is indeed ill. It's a neat trick: get government funds by claiming to represent those who are mentally ill without acknowledging that mental illness exists. NCMHR asserts that patients shouldn't be diagnosed with mental illness because "psychiatric labels obscure the socioeconomic and political roots of much of human suffering, and discount the lived experience of people struggling to cope with the effects of trauma in their lives."[5]

Members of NCMHR are a major force in driving funding away from people with serious mental illness and often in driving people with serious mental illness away from treatment. Its members are SAMHSA's biggest cheerleaders and lobbyists.

National Empowerment Center

The National Empowerment Center (NEC) is a nonprofit based in Law-rence, Massachusetts, that collects at least $330,000 in SAMHSA funding annually and double that in the years it puts on conferences about alterna-tives to the medical model of treatment for mental illness.[6] NEC CEO Dan Fisher claims severe mental illness is just "severe emotional distress" and "a spiritual experience" and that "the covert mission of the mental health system . . . is social control."[7] Fisher originated the description of the seri-ously mentally ill as "people with 'lived experience.'"[8] NEC chief operating officer Oryx Cohen previously cofounded the Freedom Center, dedicated to entirely eliminating the ability of children with mental illness to receive medications ("to end all psych drugging of children") and to end the use of medications in treating schizophrenia ("to change drugging as the medical standard of care for psychosis").[9] As an alternative to medical treatment, NEC promotes "Emotional CPR" (eCPR), a pop psychology educational program it describes as a "Tool of Peacekeeping and Bringing Healing to Communities" based on the idea that "inner peace creates global peace."[10] They claim it "saves lives."

National Mental Health Consumers' Self-Help Clearinghouse

Based in Philadelphia, the National Mental Health Consumers' Self-Help Clearinghouse ("The Clearinghouse") was until recently a SAMHSA-funded Technical Assistance Center that received over $400,000 a year from SAMHSA and more when it put on the Alternatives Conference, where among other issues people with "lived experience" are taught how to go off medications.[11] Executive Director Joe Rogers is on the NCMHR board, is chief advocacy officer of the SAMHSA-funded Mental Health Association of Southeast Pennsylvania, and leads the SAMHSA-funded Pennsylvania Mental Health Consumers Association, which is working to eliminate state psychiatric hospitals.[12] The Clearinghouse rejects the concept that there are "those who cannot help themselves."[13]

National Alliance on Mental Illness

The National Alliance on Mental Illness (NAMI) in Arlington, Virginia, was founded in 1979 by families, primarily moms of the most seriously mentally ill, to provide support to each other and to advocate for better care for the most seriously ill. The NAMI Family-to-Family program is a useful program that teaches families the basics of serious mental illness. But at the national level, NAMI now claims to represent sixty million people who experience any mental health "condition," shuns issues that help the most seriously ill, and has largely embraced the professional patients' (peer) agenda.[14] SAMHSA grants NAMI at least $330,000 a year and provides more via stipends, honoraria, scholarships, and other payments.

Some state NAMI organizations still focus on serious mental illness, but many limit themselves to teaching people that there is stigma to having a mental illness. Many receive funds from state mental health departments, and fear of losing that money caused them to sit on the sidelines as the state mental health commissioners shut psychiatric hospitals. The admirable desire to incorporate patients on their boards has led to the election of people who fail to advocate for those who are more symptomatic. Many of the local NAMI chapters still focus on serious mental illness and do a good job of running support groups and Family-to-Family classes, but with notable exceptions, they are often underfunded mom-and-pop operations that lack capacity to advocate for policy change. There is a tremendous need for a grassroots membership organization to do what NAMI used to do: advocate for improved services for the most seriously mentally ill.

Copeland Center for Wellness and Recovery

In 2016, the Copeland Center, run by Mary Ellen Copeland, received the Technical Assistant Grant that formerly went to the Consumer Clearinghouse. Ms. Copeland is the inventor and distributor of the Wellness Recovery Action Plan (WRAP). There is a lot of research on it, but not that it improves meaningful outcomes in the seriously mentally ill.[15]

MENTAL HEALTH LAWYERS

The role of the mental health bar in impeding treatment of the most seriously mentally ill was documented in *Madness in the Streets: How Psychiatry
and the Law Abandoned the Mentally Ill* and in *Nowhere to Go: The Tragic
Odyssey of the Homeless Mentally Ill*.[16] Amanda Peters meticulously captured
the issue in "Lawyers Who Break the Law: What Congress Can Do to
Prevent Mental Health Patient Advocates from Violating Federal Legislation," in the *Oregon Law Review*.[17] The mental health bar grew out of the
work of Dr. Morton Birnbaum, an attorney who wrote a law journal article
in 1960 positing that the mentally ill had a right to be treated while hospitalized; otherwise hospitalization was no different than incarceration.[18] He
helped establish a short-lived legally recognized "Right to Treatment."[19]
But, during the 1960s, the mental health bar broke into two streams. One
worked to improve care for the seriously ill, and the other to free them
from care, believing that being psychotic was a civil right to be protected.
The federal government funded the free-them-from-care branch, and as
discussed in chapter 15, the lawyers succeeded in having the courts place
so many roadblocks between patients and treatment that families wanting
treatment for a seriously mentally ill loved one are forced to find a lawyer
rather than a doctor.

Anti-treatment lawyers prevent care by raising specious claims of civil
rights violations backed with threats to sue doctors, programs, and state
governments that provide care.[20] Anti-treatment lawyers have replaced the
right to receive treatment with what Darold Treffert called the "right to die
with rights on."[21]

American Civil Liberties Union (ACLU) and the
Bazelon Center for Mental Health Law

The ACLU is the umbrella organization for state and local civil liberties
union chapters that hold that people with mental illness should never be
treated over their objection until *after* they become a danger to themselves
or others, that "danger" should be defined as narrowly as possible, and that
there should be cumbersome procedural hurdles to declaring someone
dangerous or incapacitated.

The Bazelon Center for Mental Health Law (Bazelon) in Washington, DC, also takes a civil liberties perspective to mental illness, i.e., it works to defend the right of the psychotic to stay psychotic, something it describes as a "progressive mental health policy agenda."[22] The two organizations use the implied threat of legal action to force states to implement non-evidence-based practices like peer support.[23] Bazelon and the ACLU are in the lead of a cruel phenomenon within the industry: they work to prevent the mentally ill from receiving treatment that could prevent incarceration and then want kudos for working to improve the treatment once incarcerated.

Protection and Advocacy Programs and the National Disability Rights Network

In 1986, Congress created the Protection and Advocacy for Individuals with Mental Illness (PAIMI or P&A) program, which has an annual SAMHSA-administered budget of $36 million that is supplemented by state and private funds.[24] PAIMI was originally conceived for the noble purpose of protecting institutionalized patients from abuse and neglect. Then its mission was expanded to cover people with mental illness living outside institutions. PAIMI created fifty state-centric, public interest law firms—many of which go by the name of "Disability Rights [Name of State]" that have essentially become the legal arm of those who want to free people with serious mental illness from treatment. Its Washington, DC–based trade association, the National Disability Rights Network (NDRN), lobbies in Washington and arranges for the sharing of papers among state PAIMIs so that a suit or threat of a suit in one state can be replicated in others.

PAIMI has done some good work on individual cases, but its systemic impact has been to make treating people with serious mental illness more difficult. They regularly define treatment as abuse. In Maine, PAIMI lawyers worked to "free" William Bruce from a psychiatric hospital treatment over the objections of his parents. William left the hospital and subsequently killed his mother, leading to Willie's father, Joe Bruce, becoming a leading advocate for PAIMI reform.[25] Between 1989 and 1995, New York PAIMI lawyers were involved in twenty-nine cases to free people from treatment. Some of the cases were likely meritorious, but none we know of helped people who needed hospitalization access it.[26] PAIMI lawyers bring Olmstead suits (discussed in chapter 15) to pressure states to empty hospitals and adult homes of the seriously mentally ill. These places are less than ideal for some but do provide housing. PAIMI lawyers advocate for prohibitions against treating the seriously ill before they become a danger to themselves or others, thereby causing many to become dangerous.

STATE, COUNTY, AND LOCAL MENTAL HEALTH DIRECTORS

The National Association of State Mental Health Program Directors (NASMHPD) website notes that it represents state mental health commissioners responsible for $41 billion in public federal and state mental health spending. The National Association of County Behavioral Health & Developmental Disability Directors (NACBHDD) represents officials responsible for county and local mental health services. They frequently point fingers at each other and the federal government.

The primary job of mental health directors—now often called "Behavioral Health" directors—is not to improve care for the seriously mentally ill. Their primary task is financial: to shift costs away from their own departments without generating an uproar that would reflect negatively on their governors or mayors. To cut costs, state commissioners cut state funding of psychiatric hospitals even as they lobby the federal government to fund them.[27] Commissioners tell their governors how much money they saved by closing psychiatric hospitals, without disclosing that doing so shifts bodies and costs to jails and prisons. If commissioners award even small $10,000 contracts to the state NAMI, MHA, or consumer groups for, say, "stigma education" or "peer support," commissioners can then say the money "saved" by closing institutions is going into the community (reinvestment) and prevent complaints from the groups that receive the funds.

TRADE ASSOCIATIONS REPRESENTING PROVIDERS OF SERVICES

Trade associations representing organizations that provide behavioral health services have well-funded lobbying machines that exert a tremendous influence on government policies. Most focus on increasing the income of member organizations and decreasing government regulation. A few do focus on serious mental illness, but most prefer higher-functioning patients because they cost less. The ad hoc Mental Health Liaison Group, a trade association of trade associations, chimes in whenever there is more money to be had.[28] Following are some of the major trade associations.

Mental Health America (MHA)

Mental Health America (MHA), formerly called the Mental Health Association, is a trade association for providers of mental health services many of which don't serve the seriously ill. It is "dedicated to helping all Americans achieve wellness by living mentally healthier lives" and embracing "prevention for all."[29] It accomplishes its mission by "educating the public about ways to preserve and strengthen its mental health."

MHA of New York State argued that hospitals that serve the seriously mentally ill should be closed and the savings given to its member organizations.[30] But many of its members are notoriously unwilling to serve the most seriously ill. The executive director of MHA of San Francisco refuses to use the term "mental illness" and regularly writes misleading op-eds and spreads information inconsistent with science. He told a panel that rather than medications, "people respond to dignity and fair treatment" and that "the psychophysiology of [anosognosia] is very conjectural."[31]

It is rare to find an MHA state or local chapter working to help the seriously mentally ill. MHA of Essex County, New Jersey, led by Robert Davison, is a rare exception.[32] MHA members solicit funds to teach people that there is stigma to mental illness and then use the existence of stigma to make the case that the government should give it more funds.

National Council for Behavioral Health

The National Council for Behavioral Health (National Council) is the trade association for the big behavioral healthcare conglomerates and local programs. Located on K Street in Washington, DC, alongside some of the nation's most powerful lobbying organizations, it does not have the name recognition as MHA but claims to have 2,800 member organizations employing 750,000 staff, serving ten million people, enabling it to generate significant support or opposition to whatever it chooses.[33] SAMHSA gave the National Council a five-year grant of $1.75 million annually as well as other grants.[34] According to Dr. E. Fuller Torrey, the council holds conferences on using "relaxation response" and other "holistic," "recovery-oriented" approaches for people who do not have the most serious mental illnesses.

Its primary legislative objective is to send more government money to member organizations.[35] It owns the rights to and sells Mental Health First Aid (MHFA) training and lobbied for the Mental Health First Aid Act of 2016 (H.R 1877) to allocate tens of millions to it.[36] It claims to have trained 600,000 people in this feel-good, but largely useless program.

American Hospital Association

The American Hospital Association (AHA) is a powerful voice in Washington, representing five thousand hospitals, health systems, and other healthcare organizations. "Behavioral health" is a small part of its portfolio, but because the most seriously ill are hospitalized, to the extent that AHA does focus on mental illness, it is often focused on the seriously ill. AHA tries to bring attention to the dangerous reductions in hospital bed capacity and state mental health budgets, and asked Congress to eliminate the Medicaid's Institute for Mental Disease (IMD) Exclusion, increase reimbursement rates, and fix provisions in the Affordable Care Act that reduce certain payments to Disproportionate Share Hospitals (DSH) that serve uninsured persons with mental illness.[37]

National Association of Psychiatric Health Systems

The National Association of Psychiatric Health Systems (NAPHS) represents any organization connected to "behavioral health." These include "integrated health systems, hospitals, units and behavioral health divisions of general hospitals, partial hospitalization programs, community mental health centers, residential treatment centers, youth services organizations, and behavioral group practices."[38] It advocates for more money for all of the above, regardless of the severity of the conditions in the populations being served. To its credit NAPHS did support the Helping Families in Mental Health Crisis Act, which included numerous provisions prioritizing the most seriously ill.

National Association for Children's Behavioral Health

The National Association for Children's Behavioral Health (NACBH) represents providers of services to children. Some work with children who have serious illnesses, and others work to diagnose quite normal children as having illnesses. As a result of pressure from NACBH, massive funding pours into labeling children, many of whom may have a learning disability or need social services, or are not at the exact right place on the bell curve, but do not have a mental health problem that will become a serious mental illness. By funding "early intervention," "detection," and "prevention" services for children, officials can say they are doing something important, while ignoring adults with serious mental illness. NACBH also exerts influence over organizations of parents trying to get attention for their children.

Pharmaceutical Research and Manufacturers of America

Pharmaceutical Research and Manufacturers of America (PhRMA) is a Washington, DC–based trade association representing companies that research, manufacture, sell, and distribute medications, including those that treat psychiatric disorders. In 2011, these companies earned "over $18 billion for antipsychotics (six percent of all drug sales); $11 billion on antidepressants, and nearly $8 billion for ADHD drugs."[39] Their products include the most important treatments for serious mental illness, but they will engage in sometimes unethical, if not illegal practices to keep prices high. Through their purchase of advertising in American Psychiatric Association publications and their hiring of psychiatrists to conduct research, they exert massive influence on the APA and its members. Their aggressive marketing to doctors has included bringing them free lunches (often delivered by pretty and handsome sales reps), providing high-prescribers trips to vacation destinations under the guise of hiring them to speak at a "conference," and slyly suggesting their medications be prescribed for un-researched "off-label" uses. Their direct-to-consumer (DTC) advertising convinces people with no illness to believe that they have one ("disease mongering"). They support research that too often makes ineffective medicines appear effective and fails to highlight side effects.[40] The FDA has tried to crack down on these practices in the past, but Senators Bernie Sanders (D-VT) and Elizabeth Warren (D-MA) believe the 21st Century Cures Act passed in December 2016 will make these practices even more common.[41] PhRMA continues to work to prevent the government from regulating efficacy claims, or negotiating prices, and successfully prevents Americans from importing medicines from Canada where they are less expensive. John Oliver summed it up: "Pharmaceutical companies are like high school boyfriends. They are much more interested in getting inside you, than being effective once in."[42]

New York Association of Psychiatric Rehabilitation Services

The New York Association of Psychiatric Rehabilitation Services (NYAPRS) is not national but deserves mention because the excessive funding it receives from the New York State Office of Mental Health makes it a powerful voice against prioritizing the most seriously ill. NYAPRS provides services and represents the business interests of those who provide peer support and other nonmedical rehabilitation services in New York. The executive director and other employees claim to have had a behavioral health issue in their past and use that to bestow peer status rather than provider status on the organization.[43] It has been a brilliant strategy. Marketing itself as a consumer organization as opposed to a trade association has given NYAPRS a seat in every local mental health policy battle, including those that involve the seriously ill. Political correctness has prevented NAMI and others from calling out NYAPRS for their hypoc-risy. Much of its advocacy has been directed at closing hospitals so that its member organizations can access the savings and oppose laws that would require its members to accept the most symptomatic.[44]

GUILDS

The guilds representing mental health workers are well-funded and can generate a lot of calls to Congress. It is in their financial interest to have more people identified as needing the services of their members and to ensure members don't have to serve the more difficult seriously ill popula-tion. However, associations with members who *have to* work with the most seriously ill do work to improve care for them. The American College of Emergency Physicians told Congress that the hospital shortage is causing emergency room overcrowding and the keeping (boarding) of patients in ERs, sometimes for days.[45] The American Psychiatric Nurses Association and American Association of Psychiatric Technicians address important issues like improving care and reducing workplace violence.[46]

American Psychiatric Association

The American Psychiatric Association (APA) represents psychiatrists and is a major driver of mental health policy. It has a well-staffed lobbying organization, chapters in all fifty states, and publishes various journals including *Psychiatric News* and the *Diagnostic and Statistical Manual* (*DSM*), which determines what gets a billing code. Historically APA was largely engaged in expanding the number of diagnoses and making it easier to qualify for each. But there is a subset of psychiatrists who do treat the seriously ill, and they are starting to redirect APA policy. Dr. Jeffrey Lieberman is a former president of the APA and a schizophrenia specialist. He wrote a terrific book, *Shrinks: The Untold Story of Psychiatry*, highly critical of the psychiatry of yore.[47] Past APA president Paul Summergrad continued the work of Lieberman to highlight serious mental illness and brought the APA out in full support of efforts to help the most seriously ill that were embedded in the Helping Families in Mental Health Crisis Act.[48] But serious mental illness is still only a part of APA's bailiwick, and many psychiatrists avoid focusing their practices on it.[49]

American Academy of Child and Adolescent Psychiatry

The American Academy of Child and Adolescent Psychiatry *2015 Annual Report* says it represents nine thousand child and adolescent psychiatrists. Many provide services to programs represented by the National Association for Children's Behavioral Health (NACBH), and like it, many may be dedicated to helping the seriously ill. But its financial interest is in expanding demand for its services by expanding the number of children defined as needing its help. Because it represents a warm and fuzzy clientele—sweet little kids—its opinion often carries great weight in Washington.

American Psychological Association

The American Psychological Association claims to represent "130,000 researchers, educators, clinicians, consultants and students." The most popular subjects for its members are addiction, bullying, marriage and divorce, personality, sexual abuse, and depression—not serious mental illness.[50] Some psychologists provide valuable services to people with the most serious mental illnesses, but the organization is in the forefront of medicalizing normality and expanding its reach into every area of behavior. Members define disparities in education, employment, and wealth as unmet mental health needs worthy of mental health funding, thereby diverting funds from serious mental illness.

1199 Service Employees International Union and affiliates

The 1199 Service Employees International Union (SEIU) East claims to be the largest local union in the world, representing nearly 400,000 members who "work in the homecare, hospital and nursing home industries, as well as pharmacies, freestanding clinics and other healthcare settings."[51] It has a mixed record. The union works to preserve all programs that employ its members, whether or not they serve the seriously ill. However, because a significant number work in hospitals, the union has lobbied to preserve hospitals. When Governor Cuomo proposed closing psychiatric hospitals in New York in spite of a shortage of four thousand beds, the SEIU and AFL-CIO–affiliated New York State Public Employees Federation (PEF) fought to stop it. But when Cuomo promised jobs to union members who worked at the hospitals slated for closing, the union dropped its objections.[52]

CELEBRITY-CENTRIC MENTAL HEALTH ORGANIZATIONS

Celebrity-centric mental health organizations disproportionately influence policy due to the fame of their founders.

One Mind for Research and the Kennedy Forum on Mental Health

One Mind for Research and the Kennedy Forum on Mental Health are recent initiatives of former congressman Patrick Kennedy, an in-demand speaker who talks openly about living with bipolar disorder. One Mind for Research is primarily involved in post-traumatic stress disorder, traumatic brain injury, and stigma education.[53] The Kennedy Forum aims to bring together various branches of the industry and considered rejecting legislative proposals that focused on serious mental illness because they might "divide our fragile community."[54] Thankfully, he thought better of it. Patrick Kennedy has recently become an important advocate for change and aggressively sided with the seriously ill. He called for ending provisions in Medicaid that discriminate against the seriously ill, making civil commitment easier, and has been on the right side of some of the important but politically incorrect issues that need to be addressed.[55]

Bring Change 2 Mind

Bring Change 2 Mind was founded by actress Glenn Close and her sister Jessie, who has bipolar disorder. It focuses on reducing stigma but does it in a much more honest and effective way than other efforts. Rather than teaching people there is stigma to mental illness, Bring Change 2 Mind teaches people with mental illness that there is not. Its public service announcements feature people with mental illness boldly announcing they have it, rather than the traditional approach of admonishing the public.

Carter Center

Former president Jimmy Carter and his wife, Rosalynn, created the $90 million Carter Center, which includes the Rosalynn Carter Symposium on Mental Health Policy. It "brings together national leaders in mental health to focus and coordinate their efforts on an issue of common concern."[56] None of the twenty-nine events to date have ever focused on the unique challenges and needs of people with serious mental illness.

Scientology and the Citizens Commission on Human Rights (CCHR)

The Citizen's Commission on Civil Rights (CCHR) was founded by the Church of Scientology to conduct antipsychiatry efforts. It believes that "psychiatry is torture" and has declared war on it.[57] Celebrities including John Travolta, Tom Cruise, Kirstie Alley, and other Scientologists have given the anti-treatment views a high profile. A Eugene, Oregon, nonprofit called MindFreedom has similar views on psychiatry as torture.[58]

GOOD GUYS: ADVOCATES FOR THE SERIOUSLY MENTALLY ILL

Treatment Advocacy Center

The Treatment Advocacy Center (TAC) in Arlington, Virginia, has a staff of twelve, including four attorneys. It was founded by Dr. E. Fuller Torrey, Jon Stanley, Mary Zdanowicz, Sharon Day, and this author among others in 1998 to address the most pressing issues affecting those with serious mental illnesses. It accepts no government or healthcare industry funding, and that independence has enabled it to produce invaluable reports on the shortage of hospital beds, inadequacy of civil commitment laws, incarceration, violence, police homicides, and other issues considered politically incorrect by many in the mental health industry. Its fact sheets are based on science, and it frequently exposes the pop psychology and pseudo-science promoted by SAMHSA and others. It has been relentless in educating the media about these issues, and legislators should turn to TAC for accurate analysis and ideas.

Mental Illness Policy Org.

Mental Illness Policy Org. (MIPO) in New York City was founded in 2010 by Treatment Advocacy Center cofounder and former NAMI board member DJ Jaffe, author of this book, to provide the media, policy makers, and advocates the easiest access to nonpartisan, science-based information on serious mental illness. It runs the most useful one-stop website on these issues and subsites focused on New York, California, SAMHSA, and federal initiatives. MIPO is an important resource for policy wonks and media needing well-sourced information on issues including violence and Assisted Outpatient Treatment. MIPO accepts no government or healthcare funding. It spreads information through op-eds and social media.

Clubhouse International

Clubhouse International is an exceptional trade association that grew out of New York City's stellar Fountain House program, run by Kenn Dudek. Clubhouses provide housing, rehabilitation, and activities for the most seriously ill. Unfortunately, many of their services are not reimbursable by Medicaid or Medicare, forcing clubhouses to raise a large percentage of their own funds. In addition, because the executive director and other staff may be professionals who are not necessarily "peers," support from SAMHSA and other funding streams is kept from them. Clubhouse International's agenda—creating more clubhouses—is perfectly aligned with the needs of the seriously ill and should be a goal of policy makers.

National Sheriffs' Association and Local Sheriffs

The National Sheriffs' Association (NSA) represents sheriffs and the institutional offices of sheriffs. To the extent that it focuses on mental illness, its aim is almost always to help the most seriously ill. In 2013, NSA passed a resolution proclaiming that,

> One of the most serious consequences of failing to treat severe mental illnesses is that there are more than twice as many mentally ill individuals in jails than any other facility, for longer periods of time than other incarcerated individuals, and more than one million people are admitted, with severe mental illnesses, to jails [and that] ... the consequences of nontreatment, including incarceration, suicide, homelessness, victimization and violence, can be prevented by having laws based on a "need for treatment" standard instead of a "dangerous" standard for those who refuse treatment.[59]

The resolution went on to support court-ordered treatment to those who can benefit from it.

The NSA often teams up with the Treatment Advocacy Center to issue reports highlighting the incarceration of people who are mentally ill, shootings of and by the mentally ill, inadequate civil commitment laws, and other issues.

Local sheriffs are also strong advocates for treatment. When a thirteen-hour standoff involving a man with untreated mental illness resulted in the loss of his deputy sheriff Eugene Gregory, Seminole County, Florida, sheriff (ret.) Don Eslinger promised his widow, Linda, that he would do something. He and the state sheriffs' association worked tirelessly to pass Assisted Outpatient Treatment (the Baker Act).[60] Local sheriffs including Muskegon County, Minnesota, sheriff Dean Roesler; Chicago sheriff Tom Dart; Summit County, Ohio, sheriff Drew Alexander; Harris County, Texas, sheriff Adrian Garcia; and others are also working to improve care.

International Association of Chiefs of Police and local police

The International Association of Chiefs of Police (IACP) and locals in New York, California, and other states are important public supporters of returning care of the most seriously ill to mental health departments. The IACP passed a resolution calling for greater use of Assisted Outpatient Treatment.[61] This was largely the work of New Windsor, New York, police chief (ret.) Michael Biasotti.[62] Police departments have also built on the work of Memphis Police major (ret.) Sam Cochran and set up Crisis Intervention Teams (CIT) to safely deescalate incidents involving those with serious mental illness.[63]

The mental health community criticizes law enforcement when their interactions with the mentally ill end in tragedy. But tragedies are the exceptions. Police and sheriffs attempt to deescalate the most serious incidents involving the most seriously ill at the time they are most dangerous. They are strong advocates for improving care and ending the revolving door. Unlike those in the mental health industry, they cannot simply look the other way when someone with serious mental illness needs help.

RESEARCH ORGANIZATIONS

The Brain and Behavior Research Foundation (BBR) championed by Steve and Connie Lieber; the Stanley Medical Research Institute (SMRI) founded by Ted, Vada, and Jon Stanley; the International Mental Health Research Organization (IMHRO) founded by the Staglin family; and the Broad Institute all research causes and treatments of serious mental illness and are terrific organizations worthy of support. However, they do not engage in policy advocacy.

The next chapter chronicles steps taken by mental health organizations to obfuscate the association between untreated serious mental illness and violence, and how those activities stymie attempts to reduce violence.

THE INDUSTRY IS IN DENIAL

Chapter 9

THE INDUSTRY FIGHTS EFFORTS TO REDUCE VIOLENCE

"Denial of a link between untreated serious mental illness and violence against self or others serves neither those with mental illness nor our larger society."
—Dr. Thomas Insel, former director of the National Institute of Mental Health (NIMH)

Violence is not associated with poor mental health or every mental illness. But as shown in appendix B, it is clearly associated with *serious* mental illness that is allowed to go *untreated*. The part of the mental health industry that's focused on improving mental health works to hide the relationship between untreated serious mental illness and violence for fear of causing stigma. This impedes attempts to reduce violence and increases its likelihood.

The most popular phrase in the mental health industry is "People with mental illness are no more violent than others." As commonly understood, this statement is false. It is based on studies of violence in the 18 percent of adults with any mental illness instead of the 4 percent with serious mental illness. When people ask, "Are the mentally ill more violent?" they are not thinking of treated coworkers on Zoloft or Prozac or those who have mild anxiety or ADHD. They are thinking of the seriously ill who are untreated and acting crazy. As former NIMH director Dr. Thomas Insel said, "We have to realize that part of having psychotic illness is you are not yourself and you do things you would not do without the illness and violence can be and often is part of this."[1]

SAMHSA created a widely distributed fact sheet to downplay the role of untreated serious mental illness in causing violence, and almost every nonprofit has adopted a form of SAMHSA's mental-illness-is-not-related-to-violence meme as policy.[2] When Representative Tim Murphy proposed legislation to reduce violence, the National Coalition for Mental Health Recovery (NCMHR), National Disability Rights Network (NDRN), Bazelon Center, and others issued a press release stating, "Rep. Murphy's bill is based on a false connection between mental illness and violence. Study after study shows that no such connection exists."[3] They repeat this after every tragedy.[4] Mental Health America (MHA) claimed, "Our toxic environment of racial and ethnic discrimination and conflict, abuse of women, children, elders, and the weaker members of our society, and the decline of community and family connections, are among the root causes of violence in the United States. Diagnosable mental health conditions are not."[5]

Everyone outside the mental health industry knows homeless, psychotic, screaming people are more likely than others to be violent and therefore avoids interacting with them to keep safe. Law enforcement knows. According to former attorney general Eric Holder, the FBI prevented up to 150 shootings and violent attacks by sending potential attackers to mental health treatment.[6] Those who run mental health programs simultaneously deny the link to violence while requiring their own homeless outreach workers to go out in pairs for safety. Nurses on psychiatric inpatient units work behind locked doors and wear "panic buttons." Nurses on cancer units do not. Police go on calls to address those with mental illness, not those with psoriasis. Yet the industry remains in denial.

The mainstream mental health industry simultaneously claims that mental illness does not cause people to become violent and that to reduce violence it should be given more money. Both claims cannot be true. If mental illness is not a cause of violence, then more treatment will not reduce it. Advocates even stymie research on the causes of violence for fear of what it might reveal.

THE INDUSTRY USES STATISTICAL TRICKS TO "PROVE" THE MENTALLY ILL ARE NOT MORE VIOLENT

One statistical trick the industry uses to "prove" that the mentally ill are not more violent than others is to quote studies of the treated. But those studies only show treatment works, not that violence is not associated with untreated serious mental illness. Another trick is to quote studies that exclude the violent. The widely quoted 1998 MacArthur Violence Risk Assessment Study was of those "in the community."[7] It therefore excluded many of those most likely to be violent: those who were in jails, prisons, long-term state hospitals, local hospitals, or forensic facilities, and those who were involuntarily hospitalized, committed suicide, lacked the capacity to consent to be studied, refused consent, were homeless or otherwise not "in the community."[8] Yet, even after excluding all those, a later analysis of the MacArthur data revealed that over half of the patients engaged in some form of threatening behavior within one year after discharge from the hospital.[9] Looking back, the original authors of the study subsequently noted "treatment in the community may *significantly reduce* the likelihood of subsequent patient violence."[10] (Emphasis added.)

THE INDUSTRY ATTRIBUTES INCREASED RATES OF VIOLENCE SOLELY TO SUBSTANCE ABUSE

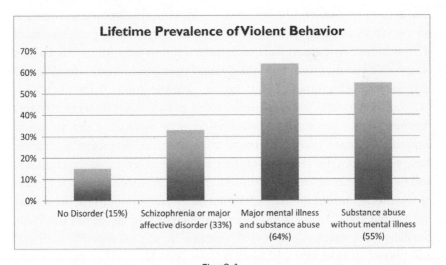

Fig. 9.1.

Data source: Jeffrey Swanson, "Mental Disorder, Substance Abuse, and Community Violence: An Epidemiological Approach," in John Monahan and Henry Steadman, eds., *Violence and Mental Disorder* (University of Chicago Press, 1994), pp. 101–36.

Another trick used by violence deniers is to attribute the increase in violence to substance abuse. But self-medicating with illegal substances is often a core component of having a serious mental illness, so eliminating those who abuse substances from studies is disingenuous. Further, one recent study found that the same genetic risk for illness may also increase the risk for substance abuse and for violence.[11] As the *New York Times* reported, the illnesses and substance abuse both increase violence, although substance abuse combined with mental illness does increase it even more.[12] That article cites a study by Dr. Jeffrey Swanson at Duke.[13] "When substance abusers were excluded, 33 percent of people with a serious mental illness reported past violent behavior, compared with 15 percent of people without such a disorder." The story went on to note that 55 percent of those with substance abuse and no mental illness were violent. When mental illness was combined with substance abuse, the violence rate shot up to 64 percent.

THE INDUSTRY DIVERTS ATTENTION FROM VIOLENCE WITH CLAIMS ABOUT VICTIMIZATION

The industry denies a link to violence by claiming that "people with mental illness are more likely to be victims of crime than to be perpetrators of it."[14] It is true that individuals with mental illness are more likely to be a victim of a violent crime than the general population.[15] But it is also true that they perpetrate more crime than the general public.[16] The claim that persons with mental illness are more likely to be victims than perpetrators may not be true because the studies relied on to make the claim are not of equivalently defined populations and use different criteria for victimization and perpetration. Perpetration studies are often of the treated mentally ill and exclude violence by those who abuse substances, thereby lowering rates of violence. Conversely, victimization studies can include those who were not treated and do abuse substances, thereby raising rates of victimization. Further, some studies define "victimization" loosely (anyone can claim it) and perpetration tightly (there must have been an arrest or police intervention). One study of equivalent populations showed that more mentally ill perpetrate injury-causing violence (8.7 percent) than are victims of injury-causing violence (7.5 percent).[17] A study in Wales and England found they are more likely to be murderers than murdered and that high rates of victimization were partly due to *being murdered by other people with mental illness*.[18] But even if persons with mental illness are more likely to be victims than perpetrators, it is largely irrelevant. The same treatments that reduce violence reduce victimization.

The industry's use of victimization to divert attention from efforts to reduce violence has been successful. When President Obama introduced his National Dialogue on Mental Health following the Sandy Hook shootings, his spokesman told reporters, "The vast majority of Americans with a mental health problem are not violent and, in fact, they are more likely to be the victims than perpetrators of the crimes."[19] This was repeated by numerous officials and is the de rigueur opening to many media reports.

The industry serves neither the needs of the ill nor the needs of the well by its refusal to admit that treatment reduces both violence and victimization and by playing one group off against the other.

THE INDUSTRY OPPOSES GUN RESTRICTIONS FOR PEOPLE WITH SERIOUS MENTAL ILLNESS

Between six thousand and nineteen thousand people with mental illness killed themselves with a gun in 2014.[20] You would think that to prevent these suicides, mental health industry advocates would favor keeping guns from people with mental illness or certainly those with serious mental illness who have been judged as a danger to self or others. You'd be wrong.

In the aftermath of high-profile mass shootings, the public, even the National Rifle Association (NRA!), unites around the reasonable and limited proposition that people with serious mental illnesses who are likely to become violent should not own assault weapons. The mental health industry disagrees and mobilizes to keep guns in the hands of the mentally ill. I was there when former American Psychiatric Association president Dr. Paul Applebaum made a March 2015 presentation at New York's Harlem Hospital on why staff should oppose gun restrictions for people with mental illness, and suggested audience members not talk about mental illness–related violence at cocktail parties for fear of causing stigma. The audience working at this urban hospital appeared dumbfounded by what seemed like a tone-deaf suggestion. After the shooting of former representative Gabrielle Giffords, NAMI legal director Ron Honberg told the *Wall*

Street Journal that NAMI opposed gun control legislation that included "the singling out of people with mental illness."[21] He made a similar claim after the shootings in Newtown.[22] When the Justice Department finalized regulations to prevent persons judged as a "danger to self or others" from owning guns, NAMI was there to object.[23]

The industry fought provisions of the Brady bill that help ensure that certain people with mental illness are included in the National Instant Criminal Background Check System (NICS), which would preclude them from buying guns. Recall that James Brady himself was shot by a symptomatic, untreated mentally ill John Hinckley. The CEO of MHA predictably claimed, "The fact is people with mental health conditions are no more likely to be violent than is the general population."[24] Former SAMHSA administrator Pam Hyde argued against gun control by noting that less than 25 percent of violence by the untreated seriously mentally ill involves guns.[25] Bazelon created a fatally flawed pseudo report on gun violence in order to help preserve the right of the seriously mentally ill to own guns and encourage the closing of psychiatric hospitals.[26] When President Obama issued an executive order clarifying that nothing in HIPAA prevented healthcare providers from disclosing to NICS names and addresses of people who have been involuntarily committed, and should be added to the no-carry list, NAMI and Bazelon objected.[27]

Facts are not on the side of those who want to preserve gun rights of persons with serious mental illness. A study in Connecticut found that adding more mental health records to the NICS created a 53 percent drop in the likelihood of a person who had been involuntarily hospitalized committing a violent crime.[28]

The mental health industry's defense of guns for the mentally ill continues at the state level. New York governor Andrew Cuomo proposed that therapists should report individuals with mental illness who they believe are dangerous and may own a gun to the no-carry list.[29] The industry predictably raised the "no more violent than others" argument. Harvey Rosenthal, a board member of Bazelon and head of NYAPRS, complained that reporting them "makes people not want to share or go to therapy" and "This approach will have the unintended consequence of deterring people from seeking care or trusting in and disclosing to their therapists."[30] Dr. Paul Applebaum parroted the claim in the *New York Times*.[31] In a March

11, 2014, e-mail to me, Dr. Applebaum later confirmed that he is unaware of research to support these statements. They are speculative. As I wrote for the *New York Times*,

> Therapists claim [the requirement to disclose to criminal justice that a patient is dangerous and may have a gun] will discourage future patients from coming in or being truthful. Maybe. But the overriding concern must be keeping the patient they are currently seeing alive and those around them safe—not some hypothetical future client. The far greater risk is to know someone has a serious mental illness, believe they are dangerous—despite their being under your treatment—and do nothing about it. . . . Therapists who object to informing authorities about patients who threaten others would have no problem if they were the target.[32]

It gets worse. New York State legislators amended Cuomo's original proposal to include a requirement that therapists' reports go to NICS via the county mental health director rather than going directly from the therapist to NICS. Legislators wanted to ensure that county mental health directors would be in the loop and made aware of potentially dangerous mentally ill individuals living in their communities so the directors could prioritize them for treatment. The New York State Conference of Local Community Mental Health Directors opposed the plan, preferring not to know about mentally ill individuals living in their counties who were dangerous and might own firearms.[33] They wanted to keep their own heads in the sand. The New York Coalition of Behavioral Health Agencies claimed the provision would cause an outbreak of stigma.[34]

The National Council for Behavioral Health, the Maryland Department of Health and Mental Hygiene, and the Missouri Department of Mental Health have all made the "mentally ill are no more violent than others" argument, but that didn't stop them from positioning a program they sell, Mental Health First Aid (MHFA), as a way to prevent gun violence.[35]

Dr. Jeffrey Swanson, a leading researcher on mental health and violence, observed,

> There may be times in the course of illness and treatment when we do know that risk is elevated. One of those times is the period surrounding

involuntary hospitalization. We think that if there are indicators of risk, that should be a time when firearms are removed. . . . There are lots of states when people are involuntarily detained for a 72-hour hold, never have a commitment hearing, and are not prohibited from firearms. People in that time frame, if guns were temporarily removed from them, that might have a big impact, particularly on suicide.[36]

Robert Davison, executive director of the Mental Health Association in Essex County, New Jersey, was one of the few mental health leaders who defied the industry. He said it best in the *New York Times*: "People with a history of violence and mental illness need treatment, not their guns returned to them."[37]

The next chapter exposes industry efforts to prevent the seriously ill from being treated until *after* they become a danger to self or others.

Chapter 10

THE INDUSTRY FIGHTS LIFE-SAVING INVOLUNTARY INTERVENTIONS

"The opposition to involuntary committal and treatment betrays profound misunderstanding of the principle of civil liberties. Medication can free victims from their illness—free them from the Bastille of their psychosis—and restore their dignity, their free will and the meaningful exercise of their liberties."

—Herschel Hardin, a former director of the British Columbia Civil Liberties Association

The objection to civil commitment is often rooted in the philosophy that mental illness does not exist. If it doesn't exist, then why would commitment be needed? This philosophy presupposes that all organs can become dysfunctional except the brain, which is always working perfectly. Leah Harris, a former leader of the National Coalition of Mental Health Recovery (NCMHR), bragged that she was "chipping away at what I call the 'anosognosic fallacy'... that some people 'lack insight into their illness.'"[1]

The annual Alternatives Conference, a gathering of the SAMHSA-funded peer industry, teaches people not that mental illness exists, but that hearing voices is normal. Susan, a horrified SAMHSA insider, told me,

Supporting those who view auditory hallucinations as philosophical experiences, while ignoring those who are terrorized by their auditory hallucinations is dangerous. People moved to action by auditory hallucinations or persecutory delusions are vulnerable and in need of assistance, while those who are comfortable with their benign hallucinations or delusions may not need federal assistance. Denying the former while promoting the latter is not a good public health policy; it doesn't protect the vulnerable and it doesn't protect the public.

As Contra Costa, California, judge Don Green testified, mental illness *is* real, and once that is accepted, then the justification for the occasional use of civil commitment becomes obvious:

> When a person is unable to understand the nature and consequences of their decisions because of their illness, that person is fundamentally deprived of the ability to exercise any civil rights. . . . We make a mockery of civil rights when we ignore people with severe mental illness, leaving them on the streets until they do something we characterize as a crime, then we lock them in our overcrowded jails and prisons.[2]

Darold Treffert understood what today's industry leaders do not:

> It is not "freedom" to be wandering the streets, severely mentally ill, deteriorating and getting warmth from a steam grate or food from a garbage can. That's abandonment. And it is not "liberty" to be in a padded jail cell instead of a hospital, hallucinating and delusional, without treatment because that is all the law will allow.[3]

Dr. Allen Frances reported on a conversation with Thomas Szasz, father of the "mental illness is a myth" movement, and found even he didn't buy into the current antipsychiatry fundamentalism:

> I posed to Tom Szasz a hypothetical in which his son was having a transient psychotic episode, was hearing voices commanding that he kill himself, felt compelled to act on this, and refused treatment. As a father, would you stand by your libertarian principles or protect your son from himself, even if this required coercion? Tom smiled ruefully and said: "I am a father first and protector of human rights second."[4]

Adam Gerhardstein, who has bipolar disorder and who once hit his mother during a manic rage, wrote about his own resulting involuntary commitment:

> For a long time, being strapped to that bed was the most traumatic experience of my life. But time has a way of rewriting history. With eight years of perspective, that trauma has morphed into gratitude. Without that intervention, I may have never been able to accomplish what I have

since—regain my health, build a successful career, marry a woman of gold, and make the dean's list in law school. Now, when I look back on my hospitalization, I am only haunted by what happened before I was involuntarily hospitalized.[5]

THE INDUSTRY OBSTRUCTS ACCESS TO ASSISTED OUTPATIENT TREATMENT

The mental health industry works to limit the use of Assisted Outpatient Treatment (AOT) and civil commitment by claiming that no one should be treated over objection until *after* the individual becomes a danger to self or others. That's ludicrous. Laws should prevent violence, not require it. Think seat belts. As shown in appendix D, AOT undeniably cuts homelessness, arrest, incarceration, and hospitalization rates in the 70 percent range among people with the most serious mental illnesses. It also cuts costs in half, while keeping the public and patients safer.

To disparage AOT, the industry ignores all recent studies in New York, California, Iowa, North Carolina, the District of Columbia, Ohio, Arizona, and New Jersey that show AOT works, and instead cite one old study of a *pilot* program at Bellevue Hospital in New York and one decades-old, flawed Rand study to prove it doesn't.[6] Quoting old studies to prove AOT doesn't work is akin to quoting studies of the Model T and concluding today's cars can't go more than forty miles per hour. The industry also works to trick legislators into ignoring all the relevant American research by citing a study on Community Treatment Orders (CTOs) in England. As Brian Stettin of the Treatment Advocacy Center documented, the study is irrelevant.[7] CTOs in England are used to release people from hospitals and don't involve a judge, court, or any legal procedure. There is little similarity between CTOs in England and AOT in the United States.

A more emotional argument used by anti-treatment advocates is to continually use the word "force" and say they are against it.[8] But AOT does not allow the use of force.[9] By opposing AOT, anti-treatment advocates are forcing patients into jails, prisons, and shelters, where they are subjected to force that is real.

The industry alleges that civil commitment violates civil rights. But it is courts, not the industry, that decide, and they have concluded that AOT does not violate rights.[10] Nonetheless, Peter Eliasberg, legal director of the

American Civil Liberties Union of Southern California said, "It's very clear that [AOT] infringes on people's civil liberties."[11] The SAMHSA-funded National Empowerment Center (NEC) told the *Boston Globe*, "Outpatient commitment is also a gross violation of human rights."[12] The director of the Pennsylvania Mental Health Consumers Association testified, "The mandated 'Assisted Outpatient Treatment' bill would promote the opposite of recovery."[13] The SAMHSA-funded Consumer Clearinghouse argues that "treatment administered against one's will is not treatment at all, but coercion and a violation of civil rights."[14] Repeating a falsehood does not make it true, and legislators need to understand that.

Federally funded Protection and Advocacy (PAIMI) firms in California, Colorado, Ohio, Kentucky, Washington, Wisconsin, Hawaii, Oregon, Rhode Island, and West Virginia are all raising the false flag of civil rights violations to justify their lobbying against implementing civil commitment reform.[15] PAIMI lawyers in New York knowingly created an unsound report that purported to show that AOT is not racially neutral.[16] An independent study showed they were totally wrong.[17] But the PAIMI community still regularly parades the flawed, self-serving, internally created faux study—and hides the independent study—to lobby against AOT. An attorney at the PAIMI in New Mexico wrote an op-ed repeating the ever-so-popular falsehood that New York "invested hundreds of millions of dollars in new appropriations" when it implemented AOT.[18] Not true. While the original bill enacting Kendra's Law did contain funds, much of it was for other voluntary health programs that were enacted as part of the same bill. They had nothing to do with Kendra's Law, which saves money.[19] SAMHSA, which has PAIMI oversight responsibilities, knows PAIMI is misusing the funds and illegally lobbying to fight this evidence-based form of treatment, but refuses to stop it.[20]

There is a big disconnect between those who purport to speak for the mentally ill and claim that AOT violates rights and those with serious mental illness who have actually experienced it.

- In New York, 80 percent of those who experienced AOT retroactively supported it.[21]
- Of patients who were coerced into taking medication or medicated over objection in a hospital, "60 percent retrospectively agreed with

having been coerced, 53 percent stating they were more likely to take medication voluntarily in the future."[22]

- A study in Arizona showed that far from driving people from care, "the percentage of patients who voluntarily maintained an active relationship with community treatment centers six months after commitment increased significantly after outpatient commitment was instituted."[23]

- A survey of the radical California Network of Mental Health Clients (CNMH) by the consumer-run "Well-Being Project" purporting that assisted interventions drive people from care really shows no such thing.[24]

Andrew Goldstein, who pushed Kendra Webdale to her death in front of a subway train in New York City and is incarcerated in upstate New York, has become a proponent of making Kendra's Law, the New York State AOT law named after his victim, even stronger.[25]

John Stuart Mill, the most vigorous defender of civil liberties, wrote, "It is, perhaps, hardly necessary to say that this doctrine [of unfettered civil liberties] is meant to apply only to human beings in the *maturity of their faculties*."[26] (Emphasis added.) He was wrong; the industry needs reminding.

Compelling people to take treatment they don't want sounds icky and seems to mock our most precious concept of civil liberty. But doing so carefully, correctly, and judicially can save the lives of people with and without mental illness, cut costs, and result in greater civil liberties for those we compel to accept treatment.

The following chapter documents how the industry makes it more difficult for people with serious mental illness to access a hospital bed, medications, and electroconvulsive therapy.

Chapter 11

INDUSTRY FIGHTS HOSPITALS, MEDICATIONS, AND ELECTROCONVULSIVE THERAPY

"Those who were hired to protect patients from snake pit conditions in the '70s are now working to prevent treatment. The result is that walking around naked and psychotic—in or outside a hospital—has moved from a condition to be deplored to a right that is being defended."

—Jay, hospital worker

THE INDUSTRY OPPOSES PSYCHIATRIC HOSPITALIZATION

Some seriously mentally ill need hospitalization but can't get it because the United States is short at least ninety-five thousand beds.[1] This is largely because the Institute for Mental Disease (IMD) Exclusion in Medicaid prevents states from receiving reimbursement for long-term hospital care of adults with serious mental illness. You would think the mental health industry would oppose this blatant form of discrimination as it only applies to the mentally ill. Wrong. The industry opposed congressional efforts led by Representative Eddie Bernice Johnson (D-TX) and Representative Tim Murphy to increase the number of beds, and is also fighting state-level efforts to increase beds.[2]

They are bringing suits to force states to empty hospitals, an activity that mental illness advocate Pete Earley contends could be creating a new era of disastrous deinstitutionalization.[3] Pennsylvania consumer leader Joe Rogers told an interviewer, "We don't need Haverford [psychiatric hospital]. We don't need Norristown [psychiatric hospital]. We don't need any of the state hospitals."[4] Georgia's Grady Hospital is so overcrowded that "psychiatric patients may wait days to be transferred to a bed, lying on gurneys without treatment."[5] But Bazelon legal director Ira Burnim argues, "Georgia is the primary example of a system where the problem is way too many hospital beds and too much money spent on hospitals." Advocates claim New York hospitals should be closed because California has only five hospitals and Texas eight, compared with New York's twenty-four. But in California, the mentally ill are almost four times as likely to be incarcerated as hospitalized. In Texas, it's eight times.[6]

The mental health industry views hospitals as a bank account, and it wants to make a withdrawal. It wants the money that comes from closing the hospitals and selling the land to go to them, a process they call "reinvestment." But community programs largely refuse to serve the seriously ill individuals who are being discharged from hospitals.[7] When New York governor Andrew Cuomo proposed closing psychiatric hospital beds, the state trade organizations, Mental Health America and the New York Association of Psychiatric Rehabilitation Services (NYAPRS) praised the closings.[8] NYAPRS hyperbolically wrote that the existence of hospitals is "essentially forcing people to remain institutionalized."[9] But the same two organizations oppose Kendra's Law, New York's assisted outpatient law that would require their members to serve the seriously ill.

As the chart in Fig. 11.1 shows, in 1981, almost two-thirds of state mental health agency controlled expenditures for mental health were devoted to psychiatric hospitals that by definition serve the most seriously ill, and one-third of spending went to those in the community. By 2012, it was reversed. Inpatient spending was only 23 percent of state-controlled spending, and community care represented 74 percent. The number of people treated in the community rose proportionately as did the number and percentage of persons with mental illness who are incarcerated. This chart belies the mental health industry claim that too much is spent on hospitals.

The industry would have us believe that psychiatrists send too many to hospitals too easily.[10] But Associate Professor of Law Amanda Pustilnik was right when she wrote,

Far from forcing people into treatment, psychiatrists every day face hard choices about who to force *out* of treatment: People who need and want help must be discharged due to lack of hospital space. People with major mental illnesses like psychosis and schizophrenia seek help at hospitals but are routinely turned away because the few available beds must be reserved for the handful who are truly dangerous. Getting out of psychiatric hospitals is occasionally hard for some people. Getting *into* them is hard for everyone.[11]

Data and Trends

State Mental Health Agency Controlled Expenditures for State Psychiatric Hospital Inpatient and Community-Based Services as a Percent of Total Expenditures: FY'81 to FY'12

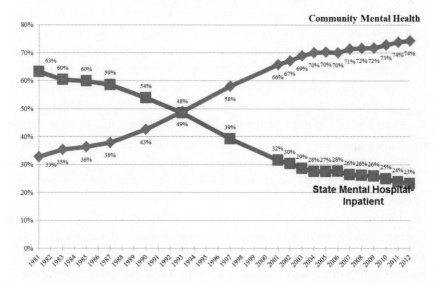

Fig. 11.1. This chart prepared by the trade association for state mental health commissioners shows how state mental health commissioners moved funds from hospitals that served the most seriously ill to community services for the less seriously ill.

Source: Joe Parks and Alan Q. Radke, eds., *The Vital Role of State Hospitals,* National Association of State Mental Health Program Directors (NASMHPD) (Alexandria, VA: NASMHPD, July 2014), http://www.nasmhpd.org/sites/default/files/The%20Vital%20Role%20of%20State%20Psychiatric%20HospitalsTechnical%20Report_July_2014(1).pdf (accessed July 14, 2016).

The industry argues that we shouldn't return to the days of yore when people were indiscriminately committed to wretched institutions. I agree. Everyone agrees. In fact, it is a strawman. The opposite is true. The lack of hospitals is the reason people are thrown into wretched institutions, specifically jails and prisons, a process called, "transinstitutionalization."

There is an inverse correlation between the number of hospital beds available and the number of mentally ill incarcerated.[12] Industry efforts to decrease the former are increasing the latter. As a result, sheriffs who run the jails are standing up for hospitals:

- In Minnesota, Muskegon County sheriff Dean Roesler noted that closing the state's psychiatric hospitals "created absolute chaos as far as the criminal justice system. . . . There is a failure in the mental health system."[13]
- In Illinois, Cook County sheriff Tom Dart told *60 Minutes*, "There is no person who could argue otherwise that the jails and prisons are not the new insane asylums. That's what we are. And the irony's so deep that you have a society that finds it wrong to have people warehoused in a state mental institution, but those very same people were OK if we warehouse 'em in a jail—you've got to be kidding me."[14]
- In Iowa, Wapello County sheriff Mark Miller noted that the state's plan to close psychiatric hospitals was staggering, observing that "the shortage of inpatient hospital units means that too many people with mental illness are stuck in jails like the one he runs in Ottumwa."[15]

In some states sheriffs are opening mental health wings in jails or forcing state psychiatric hospitals to increase their forensic capacity.[16] The mental health officials often accomplish this by taking beds from non-forensic populations and allocating them to those who come via the criminal justice system, further exacerbating the shortage.

Historically, hospitals controlled and medicated dangerous patients until the danger passed and the patient could be safely released. That's harder to do these days. "Advocates" now work to prevent hospitals from using violence-reducing restraints, seclusion, and involuntary medication.[17] As a result, hospitals now call the police when a patient becomes violent and send that person to jail. Patients "protected" by advocates are turned into prisoners.

Bob had schizoaffective disorder and stayed well and hospital-free on medications but did poorly when off. Despite this, his treatment provider took a dim view of medicine and took him off. As a result, he was "evicted from his apartment, banned from an area grocery store, repeatedly hospitalized, and arrested twice—the first time for assaulting a male nurse at Rutherford Hospital, the last for breaking and entering into a stranger's home" and is now incarcerated.[18]

THE INDUSTRY IS BIASED AGAINST MEDICATIONS

As discussed in chapter 6, side effects notwithstanding, medications remain the single best way to ameliorate symptoms and prevent many people with serious mental illness from becoming homeless, suicidal, arrested, violent, and incarcerated. Some won't take them, and they don't work on everyone, but when they do, no other treatment does as well. The industry ignores this. Rather than admit to the importance of medications for those with serious mental illness, it focuses on the problems with them and tries to limit their use.

Scientology and its Citizens' Commission on Human Rights (CCHR) are two leading anti-medication advocates. They may be outside the mainstream, but not by much. Directors of the SAMHSA-funded National Empowerment Center and the SAMHSA-funded Center for Psychiatric Rehabilitation both sit on the board of the Foundation for Excellence in Mental Health Care (sic) that funded MindFreedom, an organization that claims that "the long term effectiveness of psychiatric medications has not been demonstrated."[19] The National Empowerment Center website lists multiple resources on how to go off medications and none about the benefits.[20] In 2003, CCHR and other organizations succeeded in having dire "Black Box" warnings put on antidepressants. A 2014 study found that these "decreased antidepressant use, and there were simultaneous increases in suicide attempts among young people."[21]

Robert Whitaker has developed a cult-like following within the SAMHSA-funded antipsychiatry community by writing books and giving speeches focused on the side effects of medication that barely mention their efficacy.[22] Whitaker's work has been widely criticized by medical experts.[23] Anti-medication advocates claim the following:

- People who went off medicines did better than those who stayed on. The advocates failed to consider that those who stayed on may have stayed on because they were sicker. To them, the fact that people on, say, chemotherapy are sicker than those not on chemotherapy is proof that chemotherapy doesn't work.
- Because medications change brain structure, they are harmful. But medication-related changes in brain structure may explain *why they are effective*. They also fail to acknowledge that some brain structure changes appear in people with mental illness who are never medicated.[24]
- Schizophrenia medications reduce life expectancy. But research shows that those on appropriate doses of antipsychotics live longer than those who are not.[25]

If anti-medication advocates differentiated more forcefully between the worried well, who may not need medications, and the seriously mentally ill who often do, their arguments would ring closer to the truth.

Sheila, an activist with schizophrenia, attended a conference where Whitaker was speaking and remembers his message that healing can be done without meds. "I thought this was very dangerous rhetoric spoken to a roomful of consumers of mental health services needing to take medications."

When a SAMHSA staffer tried to stop a SAMHSA-funded Alternatives Conference from teaching people how to go off medications and from having a speaker at a plenary session teach the evils of medications, she herself was reported to have been stopped by then SAMHSA administrator Pam Hyde, who greenlighted the anti-medication programming.[26]

THE INDUSTRY FIGHTS THE USE OF ELECTROCONVULSIVE THERAPY

As described in chapter 6, electroconvulsive therapy (ECT) can be a very beneficial treatment for the most seriously ill, especially individuals who have not been helped by other treatments. But parts of the mental health industry, siding with Scientology's Citizens Commission on Human Rights (CCHR) work to limit access to it. They circulate the negative Hollywood portrayal of it that appeared in *One Flew Over the Cuckoo Nest* and position

Peer pressured to stop taking medications

Iris Loomknitter, an advocate for people with serious mental illness who lives near LaCrosse, Wisconsin, and has several different mental health diagnoses, sent me a note complaining about the anti-medication bullying by SAMHSA-funded consumers:

> There is too much prejudice against those of us who take psychiatric medications: It needs to stop! For example, when some people say that our psychiatric medications "turn people in to zombies," it hurts we who take the psychiatric medications! Call it "stigma" if you want to. I call it prejudice. It is spreading cruel, ignorant lies! It is a form of fear mongering.
>
> I have experienced this: anti-medication people who tried to frighten or convince me to not take my life-saving psychiatric medications. However those same anti-medication people could not "handle" my past suicidal, extremely needy, severely depressed or mixed bipolar episodes. They expected me to use my will power and/or ineffective "natural remedies," which did nothing to help me. When nothing they offered helped me, they turned on me and shamed and blamed me, calling me horrible names like "energy drain" and "energy sucking!" I am not suicidal now, because I am on the right psychiatric medications.
>
> Yes, anti-medication people have freedom of speech, but I also have the freedom of speech to warn people against them and to write against their counter-productive beliefs. Anti-medication people tend to take any negative side effects of prescription, pharmaceutical psychiatric medications and try to convince very sick people to avoid and to not take any medications at all! My psychiatric medications don't make me a "zombie!" Comments like that HURT!

that as reality today. They refuse to use the medical term "electroconvulsive therapy" and substitute the loaded word "shock," often combining it with "force." They note that the results of ECT may not last, without explaining that neither do the results of medications if you stop taking them, or that sometimes ECT *does* result in permanent remission.

In 2015 and 2016, when the FDA wanted to make ECT more widely available, the National Coalition for Mental Health Recovery and many of its SAMHSA-funded member organizations circulated a petition ginned up by a radical anti-treatment group to protest. The petition claimed, "Psychiatric labels are not actual medical diagnoses," "Most psychiatric drugs are ineffective," and "There is no situation that qualifies as an 'emergency.'"[27] Mental Health America (MHA) ignores the science on the efficacy and instead provides information on the "controversy" that CCHR and anti-psychiatrists purport exists.[28] As a result of industry and Scientology challenges to the use of ECT, it is hard to access. In the state of New York, few state psychiatric hospitals even have the device. If a patient at a hospital without an ECT machine needs ECT, she would have to be discharged from the hospital, transportation arranged to the hospital with the equipment, someone would have to sit with the patient, get her admitted to the new hospital, and then transport her back to the original hospital to be readmitted. This would have to be done for every course of the treatment. As a result of impediments like that to the use of ECT, it is rarely available to people without financial resources but is often used by the wealthy who have more choices. Kitty Dukakis, wife of 1988 Democratic presidential candidate Michael Dukakis, wrote *Healing Power of Electroconvulsive Therapy*, based on her experience with it. Actress Carrie Fisher wrote *Shockaholic* describing her experience and how she wished she had tried it earlier. Talk show host Dick Cavett told *People* magazine his ECT treatment was "miraculous."[29] Roland Kohloff, former lead timpanist of the New York Philharmonic orchestra told the *New York Times*, "What I think it did was to act like a Roto-Rooter on the depression."[30] It is mind-boggling that the same peer groups that claim consumers should have "choice" in which treatments they choose work to make sure consumers can't choose ECT.

Not only does the mental health industry impede access to effective treatments, but it also encourages the use of ineffective treatments. How they do that is discussed in the next chapter.

DIVERTING FUNDS TO WHAT DOESN'T WORK

Chapter 12

THE INDUSTRY DIVERTS FUNDS TO PROGRAMS THAT LACK EVIDENCE AND DON'T HELP

"'Evidence-based' is too often an ill-gotten branding based on weak evidence generated by promoters of treatments who want us to ignore their conflicts of interest."

—James Coyne, research critic

The mental health industry diverts funds from programs that have evidence they help people with serious mental illness to programs that don't have evidence. To be considered "evidence-based," a program should be (a) *independently* proven to (b) improve a *meaningful* outcome in (c) people with *serious* mental illness. The mental health industry champions programs that do not meet these three criteria. This makes treating the seriously mentally ill more difficult. SAMHSA's National Registry of Evidence-Based Programs and Practices (NREPP) has taken the endorsement of non-evidence-based programs to harmful heights.

Historically, nonprofits pretended that their non-evidence-based programs were evidence-based. But when Representative Tim Murphy inserted a provision in a bill that would require programs to be evidence-based before receiving SAMHSA and CMHS funds, the industry went apocalyptic. The Children's Mental Health Network sent an e-mail alert urging members to stop the bill:

> Note to family and youth organizations currently funded by SAMHSA—
> Did you know that if the Murphy bill were to pass as is currently written none of you would be eligible for grant funding? Unfortunately, your

organizations do not meet the narrow definition of "evidence-based" as written in the bill.[1]

John Grohol of PsychCentral complained to his followers,

It appears that grants will only be given to those utilizing evidence-based practices and must focus on people with "serious" mental illness. Everything from here on out is to be data-driven. So any of those SAMHSA programs that helped people in things that don't have science behind them, or can't quantify their results? Gone.[2]

Nonprofits claim that their non-evidence-based programs work by quoting studies conducted by those who run or sell the programs, a conflict of interest. These self-reports rarely focus on those with serious mental illness and often measure process rather than progress. Suicide programs will measure the number of calls, not any reduction in the number of people who committed suicide. Referral programs measure referrals made, not whether treatment was obtained. Self-studies often measure multiple unimportant soft outcomes including "sense of empowerment" and report an uptick in any single unimportant outcome, no matter how minor the uptick or meaningless the metric, as "proof" the program is "evidence-based," even if the majority of measures were insignificant, negative, or if people in the program wound up homeless or incarcerated. Those served do not need to have a mental illness. Walter Stawicki, whose mentally ill son, Ian, killed five people at a Seattle café, proposed the following "study" to me: "Show people pictures of cute kittens. If they smile, then you've proved pictures of cats are evidence-based to improve mental health."

The voter initiative that created California's Mental Health Services Act now generates over $1.7 billion annually for mental health programs and requires programs that receive the funds to be evidence-based. Hannah Dreier of the Associated Press documented some of the non-evidence-based programs that managed to qualify:[3]

- $8 million to community centers that provide "art classes, equine therapy, tai-chi and zumba to the general public"
- $250,000 to build a "stronger sense of community among blacks"

- $1 million for a horseback-riding program for underachieving students
- $50,000 for a sweat lodge and drumming circle for Native Americans
- $500,000 to take kids on a wilderness adventure
- $500,000 for meals for homebound seniors

Twenty percent of the funds are legislatively required to go to programs that "prevent mental illness from becoming severe and disabling." Instead, they are going to yoga, line dancing, Soul Chi (soulful movement), a hip-hop carwash, family activity nights, creative learning circles, school programs to reduce dating violence, bullying, and sexual harassment, outings for the elderly, homework clubs, tuition, market research, and employment offices.[4] Joy Torres, a California advocate, submitted testimony to the Mental Health Services Oversight and Accountability Commission (MHSOAC) berating it for codifying a regulation that allows any program that is popular, even in the absence of research, to be declared "evidence-based" and eligible for funding.[5] Mental Illness Policy Org. documented numerous non-evidence-based programs being funded.[6] A favorite was gardens for those of Hmong ancestry.[7]

The state and county mental health planning boards that distribute government funds are populated with industry insiders who drive funding to their own favored programs. No evidence needed. California county planning boards are among the worst. Each year they distribute over $200 million in state Mental Health Services Act (MHSA) Prevention and Early Intervention (PEI) funds mainly to programs that do not serve the seriously mentally ill or lack evidence they improve meaningful outcomes.[8] County behavioral health directors rubberstamp the non-evidence-based distributions.[9] Thirty-four county mental health directors used the funds to buy themselves iPads.[10]

A California oversight commission is supposed to monitor county planning board expenditures to ensure they go to evidence-based programs. But it is populated with industry insiders. They sent at least $23 million in funds to their own programs.[11]

California mental health industry insiders' grip on funds is so tight that even after the Associated Press exposé; an investigation by the California State Auditor report that found that "the State has little current assurance that [mental health] funds ... have been used effectively and appropriately"; two Little Hoover Commission reports that found essentially the same thing; and documentation compiled by Mental Illness Policy Org. and California advocates Rose King, Teresa Pasquini, Jennifer Hoff, Kathy Day, and Joy Torres; there is still virtually no public outcry over the waste of funds.[12] Those who should be leading the outcry are profiting. The fox is guarding the henhouse.

THE INDUSTRY CREATED A NEW ILLNESS—"AT RISK"— AND DIVERTS FUNDS TO IT

The industry created a new illness—"at risk"—and built an expensive industry of "early intervention" around it funded with mental health dollars. "At risk" means that one day, perhaps, maybe, the person might develop some sort of issue that could be broadly classified as having to do with behavioral health. Mental health funds go to determining how to predict who has "at risk" and how to identify and prevent it. The industry sets the bar low, defining bad grades, too much energy, a bad marriage, poverty, poor education, being unemployed, coming from a one-parent or bad-parent household, racism, and, most recently, bullying and cyberbullying as evidence of suffering from "at risk." It argues that those factors predict who will develop serious mental illness. Nonsense. Two issues may be associated, but that does not mean one causes the other. A much more likely scenario is that mental illness is the cause of poverty, bad grades, lack of employment, or problems with parents, not the other way around. Those may be problems that need addressing, but they are not mental illnesses.

Most of the money that should be helping the seriously ill is wasted on people, often children, who will never develop a mental illness. Dr. Thomas Insel noted, "The majority of 'high-risk' individuals never go on to develop a psychotic disorder."[13] One study found "only about one third of patients at high risk for psychosis based on current clinical criteria convert to a psychotic disorder within a 2.5-year follow-up period."[14] That means that two-thirds of the money the mental health industry is spending on "at risk" is wasted.

Outreach to find those at risk is often conducted at schools and malls and other venues where the most seriously ill are least likely to be found, rather than at the exits to psychiatric hospitals, homeless shelters, jails, and prisons, where people actually at risk really are. Ron Manderscheid, executive director of the powerful National Association of County Behavioral Health & Developmental Disability Directors (NACBHDD), wrote an article subtitled, "Poverty causes mental illness. How can we defeat this trap?" arguing that for mental health officials "to do less [than defeating poverty] is to fail to accept our responsibility for wellbeing of the whole person, a basic requirement of social justice."[15] So much for delivering treatment to people with serious mental illness.

THE INDUSTRY DIVERTS MONEY TO PROGRAMS IT CLAIMS PREVENT MENTAL ILLNESS

Serious mental illness cannot be prevented. But prevention is SAMHSA's number one strategic initiative, "Prevention Works" is part of its motto, and a "National Prevention Week" is held annually.[16] Advocates parade the word "prevention" in front of legislators—along with spreadsheets showing the alleged savings—in order to increase their own funding. The National Coalition for Mental Health Recovery (NCMHR) claims we can prevent mental illness.[17] So does MHA.[18] The American Mental Health Counselors Association urged Vice President Biden to "immediately implement . . . programs to . . . prevent mental illness," advice that was echoed by the NACBHDD.[19] California alone spends $200 million a year on "prevention and early intervention."[20]

Advocates got President Carter to include funding to prevent mental illness in his Mental Health System Act.[21] President Clinton declared in his 1999 State of the Union speech, "We must step up our efforts to treat and prevent mental illness."[22] Representative Paul Tonko (D-NY) claimed a bill he cosponsored supported "prevention . . . of mental illness."[23]

To support the false idea that serious mental illness can be prevented, the industry often quotes a 1994 Institute of Medicine (IOM) report.[24] But the report said "the nation is spending billions of dollars on programs whose effectiveness is not known." Specifically,

> To date, the definitions [of prevention] have been so broad and flexible that almost everything has been labeled prevention at one time

or another. Some have defined prevention as "increasing the ability to overcome frustration, stress, problems, enhancement of resilience and resourcefulness" versus preventing serious mental illness. ... Prevention programs that currently exist are service programs and demonstrations that have not incorporated rigorous research methodologies. Even those that have an evaluation component usually have not used rigorous standards for assessment of effectiveness.

To justify conducting advertising and PR campaigns aimed at preventing mental illness, the industry says it comports with the IOM-defined "universal prevention" activity, which is prevention "targeted to the general public or a whole population group that has not been identified on the basis of individual risk."[25] Universal prevention campaigns have helped prevent the spread of contagious illnesses. For example, advertising campaigns have cut the incidence of flu and sexually transmitted diseases by convincing the public to get a flu shot and use condoms. But serious mental illness is not contagious, and universal prevention campaigns cannot prevent it. The report unequivocally stated that "universal and selective interventions to prevent the onset of schizophrenia are not warranted at this time. Much more risk factor research is needed."[26]

Advocates sometimes cite the 2009 update to the 1994 IOM report to justify diverting funds to prevention.[27] But that report focuses only on youth and specifically excludes "some rare but often severe disorders; for example, schizophrenia, bipolar disorders." It also says, "Studies to date [on schizophrenia and bipolar disorder] have not been large or numerous enough to capture these rare disorders with any hope of accuracy."

We can't prevent serious mental illness, but we can and should prevent the mental health industry from diverting funds by claiming it can.

THE INDUSTRY ENCOURAGES HIRING "PEERS" TO REPLACE PROFESSIONALS

Peer support for those with mental illness is championed by almost all in the mental health industry, and their overblown claims of its benefits are regularly repeated by the media and politicians.[28] Being among peers can make some people feel better. So can any social activity. Yes, you can learn coping strategies from peers that you won't learn from doctors. This is true for all illnesses. But for the mental health industry, peer support is a revenue stream that has risen to mythical status and is usually proposed as the first "solution" whenever mental illness is mentioned. As described in chapter 6, there is no evidence that peer support improves meaningful outcomes for people with serious mental illness.

The National Association of State Mental Health Program Directors encourages states to expand peer support.[29] CMHS funds peer supporters, peer travel, peer conferences, peer webinars, and peer support organizations and coerces states to use mental health block grants for peer support.[30] SAMHSA and CMHS encourage establishing "peer-run respite centers" that intentionally and explicitly turn the most seriously ill away.[31] CMHS is headed by a peer and focuses on little else. SAMHSA claims that peer support "play[s] an *invaluable* role in recovery . . . [and provides] *important* resources to assist people along their journeys of recovery and wellness."[32] (Emphasis added.) Yet, that's not what SAMHSA's own research review shows: "The literature [on peer support] that does exist tends to be descriptive and lacks experimental rigor."[33]

Major mental health groups use reports by their own employees who run the peer programs as "evidence" that the programs work. These so-called "studies" rarely include control groups or meet minimum scientific requirements. Most do not show that peer support improves meaningful outcomes, like homelessness, arrests, violence, hospitalizations, or suicides, for the seriously ill, because they only report on soft measures, like "hopefulness," "sense of empowerment," and "wellness." CMHS's seventy-six-page publication *Consumer-Operated Services: The Evidence* lists multiple studies on what peer support is, its history, its popularity, its importance, how to expand its usage, and what its future will be.[34] But despite its title, the publication includes no good evidence that peer support improves meaningful outcomes in people with serious mental illness. Dr. Pippa Abston, a pediatrician and former member of the board of directors of NAMI Alabama, reviewed the National Empowerment Center's repository of studies on peer support and found the studies don't claim a reduction in homelessness, suicides, arrests, incarcerations, or other hard measures, and many of the studies were methodologically flawed—for example, by not having a control group or studying too small a population to draw a meaningful conclusion.[35]

The industry claims a report from the Institute of Medicine proves peer support works for mental illness, but it did not.[36] Some claim a study of peer support on veterans proves peer support works, but they must not have read it. "This study adds to the evidence suggesting no short-term incremental benefit (or harm) from peer services beyond usual care."[37]

The industry promotes peer support by using public relations to circumvent lack of evidence. It arranges for local newspapers to report glowingly on peer support, and circulates the published stories as further "proof" peer support is effective.

Peer support seems to have become a jobs creation program. People at the top are acting little different than featherbedding union leaders when they pressure state agencies to hire peers. Whether it is helping people sign up for the Affordable Care Act, investigating abuse in the mental health system, training police to handle people with mental illness better, speaking at public forums, or counseling those with mental illness, the industry insists that peers be hired to do it without any evidence they are better than professionals or non-peers. Political correctness is preventing the rest of the industry from protesting. Over the past ten years, California has spent hundreds of millions of dollars on "Full Service Partnership" (FSP) case management teams. The industry got the oversight commission to put a peer on each team, despite the fact there is no evidence of improved outcomes. It did drive up costs, thereby ensuring fewer received access to the case management services. The industry opposed Assisted Outpatient Treatment (AOT) in San Francisco, but when the county supervisors enacted it, the industry insisted the "care team" include a person with mental illness.[38] It basically argues that AOT doesn't work, but if money is going to support AOT, it wants in. Consumer leaders encourage states to implement unproven programs like Mental Health First Aid (MHFA) and Wellness Recovery Action Plan (WRAP) because the models encourage hiring peers to teach them. When President Obama allocated $15 million to MHFA, the industry probably broke out the champagne.[39]

Peer support, like all treatments, can and sometimes does cause negative outcomes. A basic tenet is that it requires people, even those who are psychotic, to self-direct their own care. That doesn't always end well. The peer movement runs from being mildly anti-medication to rabidly so, and that bias is often transmitted to those who receive the peer support. Mary Gibson-Leek, a consumer, cried "foul."

I am a client of a county mental health clinic. I believe that the quality of my care and the privacy of my treatment are threatened by heavy-hitting, ego-centered, and power-driven members of consumer, survivor, or ex-consumer organizations. I have experienced firsthand the wrath of the extremists who linger within the mental health system so that they can bring it down, take control, and receive government dollars to pretend that they are providing my treatment. They call it "alternative treatment," which is meant to eventually replace all forms of professionalism in the field. They are careful to say that they are working "in conjunction with, not as a replacement for" the mental health system—but in the underground, they joke that once they infiltrate, they will rule.[40]

The real danger of the SAMHSA-funded peer movement is that it works to make it more difficult to treat those with serious mental illness. Peer movement leaders use their funding to bus consumers to hearings to oppose policies that disproportionately help the most seriously ill. Many states that have tried to preserve hospitals, implement AOT, and make electroconvulsive therapy (ECT) easier to access have found their efforts stymied by hearings stuffed with peer program–led consumers who have been paid a stipend to attend and oppose the efforts. The peers are given matching T-shirts emblazoned with a motto and talking points to read at public expense.

That is not to suggest that those who run peer support programs are bad people. They are just not advocates for the seriously ill. There is no denying that getting hired as a peer support worker can increase the self-esteem of those being hired, an important factor. And the paycheck is nice. Likewise talking to anyone, including someone who has been through what you have been through, does have rewards. But that doesn't trump the fact that peer support fails to improve outcomes as much as housing, case management, medications, and visits to doctors do. And while peer support may be a useful ancillary service for some, systemically, the funds that go to it are too often used for political lobbying to prevent care of the sickest. The importance of this cannot be overstated.

There isn't anyone who doesn't wish serious mental illness could be treated simply by talking to someone else with it. But that's not the world we live in.

THE INDUSTRY DRIVES FUNDS FROM SERIOUS PTSD
TO WHAT IT CALLS "TRAUMA"

Post-traumatic stress disorder (PTSD) symptoms are often mild, manageable, treatable, and fade over time.[41] But mild PTSD is being reclassified as severe, and the definition of PTSD is becoming meaningless. Dr. Jeffrey Lieberman, former president of the American Psychiatric Association (APA), wrote in *Shrinks: The Untold Story* that after World War I, "shell shock," the forerunner of today's PTSD, was identified by "profuse sweating, muscle tension, tremulousness, cramps, nausea, vomiting, diarrhea, and involuntary defecation and urination," and that "other symptoms of shell shock read like a blizzard of neurological dysfunction: bizarre gaits, paralysis, stammering, deafness, muteness, shaking, seizure-like fits, hallucinations, night terrors and twitching." Contrast that to today. Thanks to the APA's changes to the *Diagnostic and Statistical Manual* (*DSM*), nightmares, angst, flashbacks, and a claim you have it are almost all that's needed to qualify.[42] Mild angst versus significant functional impairment is enough to get the diagnosis. Separately, in 2010, the US Department of Veterans Affairs (VA) was pressured into awarding PTSD disability benefits to those who never saw battle but merely feared hostile activity. As Dr. Sally Satel wrote,

> The very notion that one can sustain an enduring mental disorder based on anxious anticipation of a traumatic event that never materializes is a radical departure from the clinical—and common-sense—understanding that disabling stress disorders are caused by traumatic events that actually do happen to people.[43]

The VA spends $3.3 billion annually addressing post-traumatic stress disorder, yet "no PTSD outcome measures are used consistently to know if these treatments are working or not."[44]

Making PTSD easier to qualify for wasn't enough for SAMHSA and those it funds. As discussed in chapter 7, SAMHSA declared "trauma" in and of itself an illness and "trauma-informed care" something needed by everyone. Ron Manderscheid, the executive director of the National Association of County Behavioral Health and Developmental Disability Directors (NACBHDD) jumped on board, claiming, "The majority of mental illnesses are due to personal trauma rather than brain disease."[45]

The "trauma" of natural storms like Hurricane Sandy is now "causing" mental illnesses, according to "experts."[46] Two years after Hurricane Sandy, MHA claimed that 700,000 people were still suffering from mental illness caused by the storm. When the World Trade Center was attacked, 3,000 died, triggering $137 million in FEMA funds being distributed to 200 New York mental health agencies to address supposed trauma in 1.5 million people.[47] Only 10 percent of those served were direct victims or even family members of victims; 90 percent were not. Crisis workers who were supposed to be doing outreach to the homeless seriously mentally ill were called off the job to do outreach to those who watched the trade center fall on TV and—as is normal—felt awful about it. But feeling awful about something you should feel awful about is not a mental illness; it is normality.

Trauma and "trauma-informed care" can now be anything or its exact opposite. The 2008 director of the National Coalition for Mental Health Recovery (NCMHR) claimed trauma-informed care is needed for all the trauma caused by *getting* treatment.[48] Alternatively, the 2014 executive director claims it is needed for the trauma caused by *not getting* treatment.[49] She also said what doctors call "schizophrenia" is really trauma. The National Association of State Mental Health Program Directors (NASMHPD) promotes trauma-informed care for people who "may or may not have a diagnosis of mental health or substance use disorders."[50]

The industry even calls for trauma-informed care to reduce the "trauma caused by seclusion and restraint."[51] What hypocrisy! Industry bias against medications and opposition to treating people before they are dangerous is what is causing people to be put in seclusions and restraints.[52] MHA teaches kids how to get over the trauma of seeing school shootings reported on TV, but refuses to support steps to treat the seriously ill over objection before they shoot.[53]

One Nation Under Therapy by Christina Hoff Sommers and Dr. Sally Satel documented the financial forces causing an explosion in PTSD. These include the ability to get over $2,000 tax-free for life from the VA if you falsely contend you have it and the ability to make harassment, accident, and almost every other legal case more compelling and lucrative by claiming it caused PTSD. The authors exposed how the mental health industry promotes the idea that what used to be normal adversity now makes us all frail, brittle, emotional wrecks. Simultaneously, individuals who claim to be strong and resilient are denigrated as being unwilling to express the trauma the therapists know they suffered. The very failure to acknowledge having PTSD is used by the therapy industry as evidence of the severity of their trauma.

It is comforting to have an explanation for what is so far unexplainable, so some people blame trauma for causing their mental illness. But it is likely the illness that causes the trauma.[54] Persons with serious mental illnesses are more likely to be homeless, live in shelters, and interact with drug dealers and therefore more likely to be raped, beaten, victimized, and experience other very real traumas than the general public.[55]

THE INDUSTRY TOUTS TALK

Talk may be a useful treatment for mental illnesses including minor depression or anxiety, and may be a useful adjunctive treatment for serious mental illness. But the mental health industry makes the evidence-free claim that talk is an alternative to medications for the seriously ill.

One talk "treatment" highly touted by antipsychiatrists is the Finnish "Open Dialogue" approach. Open Dialogue is a social network–based approach to treatment whereby a treatment team regularly engages in "open dialogue" with the patient and the family and social network of the patient. A key laudable tenet of the model is, "The social network of the patient should be invited to take part in the meetings from the outset and for as long as necessary." Another tenet states, "The treatment should be adapted to the needs of the individual patient and their family."[56]

Proponents claim it delivers huge medication-free success rates. Canadian advocate Marvin Ross and others have questioned the results. He found that many in it were in fact on medications.[57] There are only a few studies on Open Dialogue. They involved only a tiny group of people. The inventors of the program conducted all of them. Even proponents of the intervention recognize there have been no randomized control studies.[58]

Dr. Alex Langford in Oxford investigated the claims being made for Open Dialogue and found the results were overstated and generated by a flawed methodology:[59] "The evidence which suggests that Open Dialogue works better than any other treatment is slim to none." However, even if the claims of medication-free or medication-reduced successes turn out to be true, Open Dialogue requires the involvement of family members. That means it could not be implemented for many consumers in the United States who don't want their families involved or are too psychotic to consent. Dr. Langford explained:

> I do have reservations that this is suitable for all patients. Especially where I work in London, perhaps more so than in Lapland, we see an awful lot of extremely psychotic people. People whose mental states are an acute and serious risk to themselves or others, people whose experiences are plainly so extreme that to deny their pathological nature and take immediate action would be irresponsible. ... Another issue would be that we see a lot of people who are so psychotic that they cannot engage in a series of meetings, either because they are unable or unwilling to talk, often with marked hostility or confusion. Also, many of our patients either lack any semblance of social network or possess one that actually contributes to their illness. Many would simply refuse to consent to the process.[60]

It might be easier to implement Open Dialogue in the United States if HIPAA laws were amended to allow family participation with or without client approval. But those who promote Open Dialogue also fight creating exemptions in HIPAA. Perhaps the ultimate evaluation of Open Dialogue is that it remains largely confined to northern Finland and has not spread to other parts of the country, to say nothing of Sweden, Denmark, or elsewhere in Europe.

THE INDUSTRY DIVERTS SUICIDE FUNDS TO PROGRAMS THAT DON'T REDUCE SUICIDE

The mental health industry spends tens of millions of dollars to create, publish, and air public service announcements (PSAs) to reduce suicide.[61] But they don't work. As the largest and most sound review, "Suicide Prevention Strategies: A Systematic Review," published in the *Journal of the American Medical Association*, found, "Public education and awareness campaigns, largely about depression, have no detectable effect on primary outcomes of decreasing suicidal acts or on intermediate measures, such as more treatment seeking or increased antidepressant use."[62]

Time magazine reported on a 2009 *Psychiatric Services* review of two hundred suicide awareness programs. It found that they only "contributed to modest improvement in public knowledge of and attitudes toward depression or suicide" but could not find that they actually decreased suicidal behavior. A study in 2010 found that suicide billboards had *negative* effects on adolescents, making them "less likely to endorse help-seeking strategies."[63]

Industry-sponsored suicide initiatives are targeted to where suicide isn't, rather than where it is. Acting SAMHSA administrator Kana Enomoto told a 2016 budget committee that in 2014 there were 43,000 completed suicides of which 5,500 involved people under the age of twenty-four. Congressional mandates targeted $54 million in suicide prevention funds to that age group and only $2 million to address the 37,500 completed suicides by people over twenty-four.[64] Much of the suicide spending goes to colleges. But college students are less likely than other same-aged non-college students to have serious thoughts of suicide (6.5 percent vs. 8.4 percent), make suicide plans (1.5 percent vs. 2.4 percent), or attempt suicide (0.8 percent vs. 1.8 percent).[65] The college-targeted PR programs are no more effective than the campaigns that target the general public.[66]

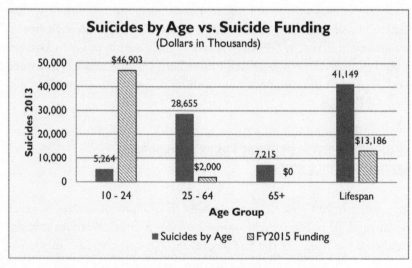

Fig. 12.1. The bulk of 2015 suicide funds
did not go where they were needed most.

Data source: US Department of Health and Human Services (HHS), "Fiscal Year 2017, SAMHSA, Justification of Estimates for Appropriations Committees," p. 87, http://www.samhsa.gov/sites/default/files/samhsa-fy-2017-congressional-justification.pdf (accessed September 25, 2016).

The industry justifies targeting students with the claim that suicide is "the second leading cause of death among persons aged ten to fourteen and fifteen to twenty-four."[67] True. But few people in that age group die of any cause. They are the least likely to commit suicide. In 2014, the highest suicide rate (19.3 percent) was among people eighty-five and older. The second-highest rate (19.1 percent) was for those forty-five to sixty-four.[68] Further, age may not be the most efficient way to allocate funds. Targeting interventions based on diagnosis and history of hospitalization is smarter. A recent study found that within ninety days after psychiatric hospital discharge, suicide rates for depressive disorder (235.1 per 100,000), bipolar disorder (216.0 per 100,000), and schizophrenia (168.3 per 100,000) were substantially higher than the US general population (14.2 per 100,000).[69]

Why are mass market media campaigns so popular in spite of little evidence they work and mounting evidence they don't? Money. It is easy and profitable for a mental health provider to write a brochure, staff a telephone support line, or produce a PSA, rather than try to reduce suicide. And the media campaigns increase the provider's visibility and sense of self-importance. As one researcher concluded,

> The conflict between political convenience and scientific adequacy in suicide prevention is usually resolved in favor of the former. Thus, strategies targeting the general population instead of high-risk groups (psychiatric patients recently discharged from hospital, suicide attempters, etc.) may be chosen ... especially if the desired outcomes also include a number of conditions frequently associated with suicidal behaviours (such as poor quality of life, social isolation, unemployment and substance misuse).[70]

The former executive director of the American Association of Suicidology (AAS), Lanny Berman, told *Time* magazine, "The bottom line is that the people most at risk are people who don't get into treatment, and a public health approach [education] shifts attention from high-risk patients to large populations of folks. I don't know that public awareness campaigns work for the people you most want to reach, the people who are already suicidal."[71] Individuals at the highest risk of suicide include those who have previously attempted suicide, first-degree relatives of those who completed suicide, and persons with serious mental illness—not the general public.[72]

These individuals are likely known, by name, to the mental health system as a result of their suicide attempt or family history. Another high-risk group is prisoners. Suicide in jail is three times more common than in the general population.[73] These are the high-risk groups the industry should be targeting, but is not.

While the lifetime risk for suicide in people with schizophrenia is only 5 percent, we do know how to predict and prevent those particular suicides. The biggest risk factors are "number of prior suicide attempts, depressive symptoms, active hallucinations and delusions, and the presence of insight . . . a family history of suicide, and comorbid substance misuse."[74] The only consistent protective factor for suicide is treatment.[75] As far as we know, no mental health providers are proposing to use suicide funds to treat the seriously ill. But there is evidence they should: clozaril, lithium, and possibly electroconvulsive therapy (ECT) decrease the incidence of suicide among individuals with severe psychiatric disorders.[76] Assisted Outpatient Treatment reduced suicide attempts and physical harm to self by 55 percent.[77] Easier access to hospitals, something the industry fights, would also help.

> July 7, 2016: Marine and Army National Guard veteran Brandon Ketchum took his own life less than one day after being denied treatment at the Iowa City VA Medical Center, where he had requested admittance for "serious mental issues."[78]

Another very effective suicide prevention strategy is means removal: putting locks on guns, medicine cabinets, and drawers containing knives.[79] However, mental health industry groups are unlikely to give up funds they can use to create billboards featuring their logos in order to reduce suicide.[80]

Perhaps the biggest problem is that those doling out and receiving the funds refuse to measure the number of suicides to see if the funds are having an impact. As long as the government gives out suicide funds without requiring accountability, it is unlikely those funds will reduce suicides.

THE INDUSTRY FOCUSES ON CHILDREN WITHOUT MENTAL ILLNESS, RATHER THAN ADULTS WITH MENTAL ILLNESS

Some children have serious mental illness that does need treatment, but "the propensity of experts to pathologize and medicalize healthy children en masse has gotten way out of hand."[81] The mental health industry champions putting more mental health workers in schools, arguing that "half of all mental illness begins before age fourteen."[82] As described in chapter 5, that may be untrue for "all" mental illness and is certainly untrue for serious mental illness. Serious mental illnesses usually begin in the late teens to midtwenties. Most "problems" in children go away with nothing more than time, yet we are routinely labeling children as ill. Children may have social services needs and require intensive support to get better grades, but needing social services is not the same as having a mental illness. The "age fourteen" claim is used by the industry to justify funding school art classes, tutoring, film classes, "early intervention," and sports with mental health funds that should go to help children who really have a mental illness. I don't agree with Robert Whitaker on much, but he was right when he wrote,

> Not too long ago, goof-offs, cutups, bullies, nerds, shy kids, teachers pets, and any number of recognizable types filled the schoolyard, and all were considered more or less normal. . . . But today, children diagnosed with mental disorders—most notably, ADHD, depression and bipolar illness—help populate the schoolyard.[83]

How popular is giving children a diagnosis? Today, 20 percent of all teenage boys are diagnosed with ADHD, half before the age of six.[84] Those under nineteen in the United States are seventy-two times more likely to walk out of a hospital with a bipolar diagnosis than those discharged from hospitals in the United Kingdom.[85] It's less likely an epidemic of illness than an epidemic of overdiagnosing to satisfy the self-interest of providers. Regulators in New York discovered that "over 90% of evaluators [used to evaluate children] in New York City . . . provide direct services to children they previously evaluated."[86]

The focus on children without mental illness over adults with it has been aided by the media. Andrea, a mom cum advocate with a seriously ill daughter, said, "If our mental health commissioner puts a new social worker in our grade school, our PTA will give her an award and put her picture in the paper. If she tries to open a new group home for the seriously mentally ill in our community, the PTA will run her out of town and put her picture in the paper."

While the suicide campaigns, peer support, trauma programs, and efforts targeting children without mental illness take funds from those with serious mental illness, the stigma campaigns described in the following chapter are perhaps the most damaging.

Chapter 13

THE INDUSTRY DIVERTS FUNDS TO IRRELEVANT STIGMA PROGRAMS

"[W]alking the streets of San Francisco and seeing untreated, seriously mentally ill people would convince most observers that the biggest problem of the mentally ill is not stigma. Yet millions of tax dollars are spent on anti-stigma campaigns."
—Fred Martin, mental illness advocate

Mental health industry advocates spend innumerable hours teaching the public "there is stigma to mental illness." But stigma is a "mark of shame," "token of disgrace," or a "discreditable characteristic." Advocates should know better than anyone that serious mental illnesses are no-fault biologically based brain disorders, so there is no mark of shame or disgrace to having one. It is true that some people are uneducated and misinformed, and they are prejudiced against and discriminate against those with mental illness. We should fight that prejudice and discrimination the same way we fight prejudice and discrimination directed against African Americans, gays, and other minority groups: by changing laws, not teaching there is stigma. Over fifty years ago, a major federal task force explained stigma in a way that would be politically incorrect today:

> Mental illness is different from physical illness in the one fundamental aspect that it tends to disturb and repel others rather than evoke their sympathy and desire to help. ... The reason the public does not react desirably is that the mentally ill lack appeal. They eventually become a nuisance to other people and are generally treated as such.[1]

Stephen Seager, author of *Behind the Gates of Gomorrah*, came to a similar conclusion following similar logic:

> Stigma is a Greek word which means a "dot, puncture, brand or mark." What is the mark? It's the often bizarre, psychotic, violent behavior of those so afflicted. This is what marks the serious mentally ill. This is what causes the public aversion. This is what we should be spending money to correct. People will never tolerate bizarre, violent, psychotic behavior. Never have. Never will. To think otherwise is tragically naive.

If we want to reduce the lack of appeal, eliminate the mark, then we must change the laws so they facilitate treatment. Instead, mental health advocates have raised stigma to deity status. It is as if mental illness doesn't exist, and stigma itself is the illness. It is difficult to find a mental health nonprofit that doesn't solicit stigma funds or a government agency that doesn't dole them out. Sadly, thousands of advocates who should be fighting against discriminatory laws and prejudicial policies have been diverted to this quite tangential issue. And fear of losing their government stigma money prevents these "stigma-busters" from speaking up on policy issues. The industry claims that stigma is the major impediment to care, but as seen in chapter 6, that is clearly not true for the seriously mentally ill.

THE INDUSTRY "FIGHTS STIGMA" BY SHUNNING AND HIDING THE SERIOUSLY ILL

The mental health industry fights stigma by hiding the most seriously ill. Stigma-busters create presentations designed to communicate that people with mental illness are high-functioning, successful executives, "just like you and me." The public service announcements (PSAs) never show the homeless, psychotic, incarcerated, or untreated. Advocates feel that would cause stigma. TV host Dr. Phil aired a show featuring an obviously mentally ill and highly symptomatic Shelley Duvall, an actress in *The Shining*.[2] Ms. Duvall made bizarre claims that Robin Williams is still alive and is a "shape-shifter" and that the Sheriff of Nottingham and Robin Hood were both threatening her. Rather than thanking Dr. Phil for letting the public see what serious mental illness looks like, the Internet blew up with stigma-busters shaming Dr. Phil for letting the public see the dark side of mental illness. What these advocates don't understand is that trying to gain support for mental illness by only showing the highest functioning is like trying to raise money for starving children by only showing the well-fed. The 1961 Joint Commission on Mental Health and Mental Illness identified the folly of this approach by calling for public education campaigns "to overcome society's many-sided pattern of rejecting the mentally ill, by making it clear that the [seriously] mentally ill are singularly lacking appeal, why this is so, and the need to consciously solve the rejection problem."[3] Today, those who lack appeal are simply kept in the closet.

Stigma is perhaps the most unifying ideology and common income line in the mental health industry. It's also a weapon used to oppose anything the industry doesn't like and drive funds to anything they do. The industry has used the battle cry of "STIGMA!" to oppose Assisted Outpatient Treatment, civil commitment reform, gun restrictions, expanding access to hospital care, and even getting the right diagnosis.[4] The industry's message has reached high places, with President Obama declaring, "We've got to get rid of that stigma."[5]

THE INDUSTRY "FIGHTS STIGMA" BY MUZZLING THE MEDIA

As part of their attempts to reduce stigma, NAMI and others insist reporters avoid using the term "suffering" when describing people with mental illness.[6] Yet many people with serious mental illness do suffer, and we shouldn't be hiding that from the public. Trying to "normalize" the illness makes it less likely, not more likely, that the public will provide help. When someone with untreated serious mental illness commits a violent act, rather than using that as a teachable moment the industry tries to quash media coverage because it believes it is the coverage, not the act, that creates stigma:

- After the Sandy Hook shootings, the Bazelon Center for Mental Health Law said, "The media coverage and policy debate often turns to scapegoating, stereotyping and discriminating against people with mental illnesses (even when it is unclear whether the perpetrator had a mental illness), wrongly branding Americans with mental illnesses as dangerous and violent."[7]

- Another industry leader wrote in the *New York Times*, "This kind of coverage can only add to the discrimination and prejudice associated with mental health conditions and drive people away from seeking treatment."[8]
- After the Navy Yard shooting, when *60 Minutes* reported on how to help those who do become violent, NAMI and Bazelon went on the attack.[9]

But it is not media reporting on violence that causes stigma. It is violence by the minority that tars the nonviolent majority. "Probably nothing contributes more to the stigmatization of mental illness than the commission of violent crimes by persons who are clearly severely mentally ill."[10] Researcher Henry Steadman wrote as long as there is violence, "it is futile and inappropriate to badger the news and entertainment media with appeals to help destigmatize the mentally ill."[11] No mental health stigma PSA, radio spot, or presentation to a high school class will trump the bullet of a mass shooter. A board member of the National Council for Community Behavioral Healthcare acknowledged, "It only takes one or two well-publicized allegations of crime to further ingrain the stigma against people with mental illness."[12] The surgeon general rhetorically asked, "Why is stigma so strong despite better public understanding of mental illness?" He answered his own question: "The answer appears to be fear of violence: people with mental illness, especially those with psychosis, are perceived to be more violent than in the past."[13] The best way to reduce stigma is to reduce violence, and the best way to do that is to provide treatment for the seriously ill.[14]

CONCENTRATING ON STIGMA INCREASES STIGMA

Even if one accepts that stigma is a reason people with mental illness don't access care, then belaboring it will make them less likely to get care. The mental health industry recognizes repeated media mentions of "mental illness" and "violence" in the same sentence reinforces the public's association of the two, but it doesn't recognize that mentioning "mental illness" and "stigma" in a single sentence does the same.[15]

Fighting stigma requires teaching those with mental illness that there is none. Glenn Close's Bring Change 2 Mind campaign gets it right. Her PSAs feature people with mental illness wearing shirts boldly emblazoned with the name of their illness: "schizophrenia," "bipolar," and others. It encourages those with mental illness to fight prejudice and discrimination by being open about their illness. Kevin Earley, a young man with serious mental illness wrote, "If you are afraid to tell your story, then the stigma wins."[16] A former NAMI consumer board member told me, "The most stigmatizing thing we do is talk about stigma."

What bothers me most is that stigma has become the black hole of advocacy, stealing thousands of advocates away from fighting to change our laws and policies.

The following chapter describes major federal initiatives and legislation affecting the seriously mentally ill, including those that make treating people with serious illness more difficult.

FAILING THE SERIOUSLY MENTALLY ILL

Chapter 14

FEDERAL POLICIES THAT FAIL
THE SERIOUSLY ILL

"The prevention of mental illnesses and the promotion of mental health were little more than attractive slogans. . . . Given that neither the etiology nor the pathology of mental illnesses was understood, how could strategies be developed that would prevent such disorders and promote health? The absence of any data demonstrating the effectiveness of preventive and promotion strategies did not, however, act as a deterrent."
—Gerald Grob, author and mental illness historian

W hen developing legislation, the policy pattern rarely changes. "Psychiatrists and other interested parties first [get] the attention of lawmakers by focusing on state hospitals and the plight of the most seriously mentally ill."[1] A presidential or congressional task force or panel is then convened. Inevitably, a bait and switch takes place as "testimony shifts to preventing mental diseases and eventually to promoting mental health." Many of the government actions discussed in this chapter followed that pattern. The 21st Century Cures Act discussed at the end of this chapter amends some of the federal laws discussed below.

1946–1949: NATIONAL MENTAL HEALTH ACT OF 1946
CREATING THE NATIONAL INSTITUTE OF MENTAL HEALTH (NIMH)

The National Mental Health Act of 1946 created the National Advisory Mental Health Council that led to the 1949 founding of the National

Institute of Mental Health (NIMH).[2] NIMH was originally supposed to be called a National "Neuropsychiatric" Institute and focus on "diseases of the nervous system which affect mental health," but there evolved a "growing conviction that psychological and social change were inseparable. ... The mental health of ordinary citizens would become a consequential public policy issue in its own right."[3]

Mental health industry insiders, rather than those concerned about serious mental illness, became NIMH administrators causing serious mental illness to play fourth fiddle.[4] Dr. Jeffrey Lieberman wrote that "from 1949 to 1964, the message coming out of the largest research institution in American psychiatry was not, 'We will find answers to mental illness in the brain.' The message was: 'If we improve society, then we can eradicate mental illness.'"[5] Dr. Torrey wrote, "By 1969, NIMH had virtually abandoned treatment of mental illness as its primary mission in favor of promoting mental health."[6] It wasn't until Dr. Thomas Insel took the helm in 2002 that NIMH started focusing on serious mental illnesses.

1955–1960: MENTAL HEALTH STUDY ACT OF 1955 AND *ACTION FOR MENTAL HEALTH,* THE REPORT OF THE JOINT COMMISSION ON MENTAL ILLNESS AND HEALTH

The Mental Health Study Act of 1955 (Public Law 182-84) called for an "objective, thorough, and nationwide analysis and reevaluation of the human and economic problems of mental illness."

The result was the 1960 *Action for Mental Health* report, the last federal action somewhat focused on the seriously mentally ill.[7] It noted that "the mental hygiene movement has diverted attention from the core problem of major mental illness. It is our purpose to redirect attention to the possibilities of improving the mental health of the mentally ill" and warned against the chimera of prevention:

> Hardly a year passes without some new claim, for example, that the cause or cure of schizophrenia has been found. The early promises of each of these discoveries are uniformly unfulfilled. ... The one constant in each new method of psychiatric treatment appears to be the enthusiasm of its proponents.

Finally, it made the important observation that people with mental illness "disturb and repel others rather than evoke their sympathy and desire to help" and called for solutions to address that.

1961–1963: JOHN F. KENNEDY'S INTERAGENCY COMMITTEE ON MENTAL HEALTH AND THE MENTAL HEALTH RETARDATION FACILITIES CONSTRUCTION ACT ESTABLISHING COMMUNITY MENTAL HEALTH CENTERS (CMHCS)

Improving treatment for people with serious mental illness and developmental disabilities was important to President John Kennedy, as his sister Rose suffered from both. He created a cabinet-level Interagency Committee on Mental Health, but as Dr. E. Fuller Torrey studiously documented in *American Psychosis*, the president was led astray by the mental health industry. The committee sold the president on a plan it claimed would eliminate psychiatric hospitals, prevent mental illness, and serve the most seriously ill. It was wrong on all counts.

The committee's work led Congress to create 789 Community Mental Health Centers (CMHCs).[8] However, the CMHCs refused to ensure that seriously mentally ill individuals leaving hospitals entered CMHCs and instead served all others. "Most outpatients [in CMHCs] . . . had no prior inpatient experience."[9] Torrey found, "Patients who had been discharged from state mental hospitals . . . made up only 3.6% to 6.5% of all CMHC patients. Moreover, the longer a CMHC was in business, the fewer state hospital patients it saw."[10] "The belief that many individuals—including those with severe and persistent mental illnesses—could be treated in outpatient clinics was an article of faith even though there was virtually no supporting data."[11]

The legislation "encouraged the closing of state mental hospitals without any realistic plan regarding what would happen to the discharged patients, especially those who refused to take medication they needed to remain well. . . . It focused resources on prevention when nobody understood enough about mental illnesses to know how to prevent them."[12]

The centers drifted "toward a social service model offering counseling and crisis intervention for predictable problems of living. One result [was] neglect of the mentally ill, especially chronic and deinstitutionalized patients."[13] The centers fought the wars on poverty, racism, bad grades, and inequality, but not the war on serious mental illness.

The industry continues to claim the concept was good but the CMHCs were underfunded. They are wrong. About $133 billion (in 2010 dollars) was spent to build the facilities, at least one of which included a swimming pool.[14] Then, as now, the problem was not lack of funding; it was that those who received the funds simply refused to serve the seriously ill and promised they could do the impossible: prevent serious mental illness.

In 1981, direct federal funding of the CMHC program was largely ended and the money given to states as part of the Alcohol, Drug Abuse, and Mental Health Administration (ADAMHA) block grants, which became SAMHSA-administered mental health block grants in 1992.[15]

1965: MEDICAID AND MEDICARE

Medicaid

Medicaid (Title 19 of the Social Security Act) is a federal healthcare program for the poor that reimburses states about 50 percent of the cost of care for people enrolled in it. It is an important source of revenue for useful outpatient programs and provides $30 billion to help the mentally ill.[16] It has two major problems. Until the 21st Century Cures Act passed, it prohibited same-day billing for mental health and physical health services, making it likely that people would receive one and not the other. Further, an obscure provision, the "Institutions for Mental Disease (IMD) Exclusion," largely prohibits Medicaid from reimbursing states for adults with mental illness between ages twenty-two and sixty-four who receive long-term care in a psychiatric hospital or facilities with more than sixteen beds.[17] It causes states to pay 100 percent of the cost of care for the seriously ill who need long-term hospital care, compared to 50 percent for those treated in the community. So states simply lock the front door of the hospital and open the back to make patients' Medicaid reimbursable.

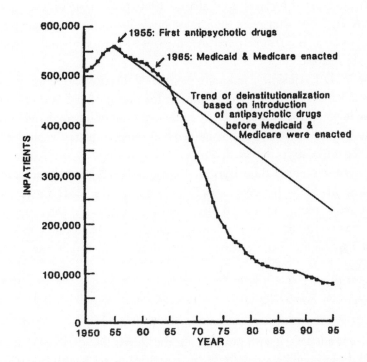

1955: First antipsychotic drugs

1965: Medicaid & Medicare enacted

Trend of deinstitutionalization
based on introduction
of antipsychotic drugs
before Medicaid &
Medicare were enacted

Number of Inpatients in Public Mental Health Hospitals

Fig. 14.1. The advent of antipsychotics started deinstitutionalization, but the rate of deinstitutionalization increased dramatically after Medicaid and Medicare were enacted, which created a financial incentive to kick the seriously mentally ill out of hospitals.

Source: E. Fuller Torrey, *Nowhere to Go: The Tragic Odyssey of the Homeless Mentally Ill* (New York: Harper & Row, 1988).

In spite of common lore, it is Medicaid, more than the advent of antipsychotics and tranquilizers, or the construction of community mental health centers, that caused and continues to cause deinstitutionalization.[18] "The overall effect of the exclusion ... has been to create incentives for states to move patients out of state hospitals, which has contributed to homelessness and inappropriate incarceration."[19]

Those kicked out have been "transinstitutionalized," moved to jails and nursing homes. "Nursing and old-age homes contained 19% and 25% of all institutionalized persons in 1950 and 1960, ranking second to mental hospitals. By 1970, they were the largest single institutional category containing 44% of all institutionalized persons, whereas mental hospitals contain only 20%."[20]

The IMD Exclusion is federally sanctioned discrimination against the seriously mentally ill. It singles them out for inferior Medicaid coverage. Because it encourages states to move individuals out of hospitals, Medicaid ends up paying anyway; hence, the original purpose of the exclusion, to reduce federal costs, is defeated.

Congresswoman Eddie Bernice Johnson (D-TX), a former psychiatric nurse, regularly introduces a bill to eliminate the IMD Exclusion.[21] It is the most important mental illness bill Congress could pass. President Trump has mentioned plans to block grant the Medicaid funds to states, but details have not been released so its effect on the IMD Exclusion is not known.

Medicare

Medicare is a federal health program for the elderly and disabled that pays $17 billion in benefits annually for those with mental health issues.[22] By requiring non-elderly disabled individuals to be on Social Security Disability Insurance (SSDI) for two years before receiving Medicare benefits, many seriously mentally ill individuals who need medical benefits immediately or do not have a work history are excluded. Medicare also includes a cruel 190-day lifetime cap on psychiatric hospitalization.[23]

A third problem with Medicare is mental illness–related waste and fraud. In 2015, Dr. E. Fuller Torrey and Mental Illness Policy Org. collected examples of $4–8 billion in fraud, waste, and excess profit, most of which was paid for by Medicare.[24]

1956 AND SUBSEQUENT YEARS:
SOCIAL SECURITY DISABILITY INSURANCE (SSDI)

Social Security Disability Insurance (SSDI) is the country's most expansive and expensive mental health program, paying over $50 billion in benefits to the mentally disabled.[25] SSDI benefits go to people with serious mental illness, those with minor mental health issues, certain children, and those who pretend to have mental illness. The original definition of disability in SSDI was strict. It required an individual to have "an impairment of mind or body which *continuously* renders it *impossible* for the disabled person to follow *any* substantial gainful occupation" and would last the person's entire life.[26] Today, qualifying for benefits is easier.[27] In 1988, only 11 percent of those receiving SSDI had mental disability, but by 2014, that figure grew to 31 percent.[28] Of the over 3.2 million individuals receiving SSDI for mental disability, only 510,000 (14 percent) have schizophrenia or other psychotic disorders.[29] Two-thirds of children who get SSDI survivor benefits get them as a result of mental disability.[30]

Legislation passed in 1996 made it harder for the seriously mentally ill who also abuse substances to collect benefits.[31] Recent budget cutbacks have slowed down approval of applications for social security and created long wait periods before benefits are received.

Like all programs, SSDI suffers from fraud. Back when Ronald Reagan was president, he ordered the Social Security Administration to review claims for fraud, and as a result one million people were kicked off, many for allegedly faking mental disabilities.[32] The mental health industry pushed back hard. Reagan's Health and Human Services secretary Margaret Heckler stopped the reviews and increased the "percentage of beneficiaries . . . exempt from normal periodic review."[33] There have been no serious attempts to rein in SSDI mental illness–related fraud since then. Recently, 130 New York police and fire fighters were arrested for swindling benefits by claiming they had "trauma" and "depression" caused by working at the World Trade Center in the aftermath of the September 11, 2001, attack.[34]

1972: SUPPLEMENTAL SECURITY INCOME (SSI)

Supplemental Security Income (SSI) provides income to the poor who are disabled, which includes many seriously mentally ill.[35] "By 2009, 41 percent of SSI recipients under age 65 (and about half of children) qualified for SSI on the basis of a mental illness."[36] One problem with SSI is that it creates a disincentive for parents to provide housing because it cuts benefits by one-third to mentally ill individuals who live at home. There is a questionable workaround.[37]

1978: PRESIDENT CARTER'S COMMISSION ON MENTAL HEALTH AND THE MENTAL HEALTH SYSTEMS ACT

Rosalynn Carter was interested in mental illness, and when her husband was elected president, she transmitted that enthusiasm to him. President Carter established a presidential mental health commission, and as happened with Kennedy, the mental health industry prevented it from focusing on the most seriously ill.[38] Gerald Grob, a mental illness historian, examined the commission's work in detail and found why it went off course:

> The twenty commissioners came from diverse backgrounds, and their interests revolved around the mental health of minorities and underserved groups rather than the specific needs of persons with severe and persistent mental illnesses. Indeed, some believed that mental health problems could be resolved only by dealing with such broad social problems as unemployment, discrimination, and poverty.[39]

Carter, following the commission's lead, proposed Congress fund the "prevention" of mental illness.[40] Congress toyed with Carter's proposal and in 1980 passed Ted Kennedy's Mental Health Systems Act, loosely based on it.[41] It gave more money to the mental health industry primarily by increasing funding for CMHCs. It also funded rape prevention and control but included virtually nothing for the seriously mentally ill. The law had a short shelf life. Reagan's 1981 budget block granted the CMHC funds to states and let them do what they would with the funds. Rosalynn Carter described Reagan's action as "one of the greatest disappointments of my life."[42] The Carters went on to found the Carter Center, which, among other issues, focuses on mental health, but is as devoid of concern for the seriously mentally ill as their previous efforts.

1980: CIVIL RIGHTS OF INSTITUTIONALIZED PERSONS ACT (CRIPA)

The Civil Rights of Institutionalized Persons Act (CRIPA) authorizes the Department of Justice (DOJ) to protect the civil rights of institutionalized mentally ill when a state is responsible for a pattern of "egregious or flagrant conditions which deprive such persons of any rights, privileges, or immunities . . . [or causes them to] suffer grievous harm."[43] The attorney general cannot intervene in individual cases or those involving the noninstitutionalized. Historically, CRIPA cases tended to focus on improving conditions for the incarcerated.[44] But recently, DOJ is weaponizing the Supreme Court's Olmstead decision, discussed in the next chapter, to encourage states to empty institutions without ensuring the discharges are appropriate and the deinstitutionalized have an appropriate place to go. DOJ is under pressure to involve more people from the federally funded disability community in its decision making.[45] Doing so would likely change the focus of the program from protecting civil rights toward "freeing" people from care.

1985: FDA REGULATES DIRECT TO CONSUMER ADVERTISING OF PHARMACEUTICALS

Direct to Consumer (DTC) advertising of pharmaceuticals is a $5 billion dollar industry that is banned in every country except the United States and New Zealand.[46] The United States regulates it rather than prohibits it. DTC advertising theoretically helps consumers make more informed decisions, but disease-mongering by pharmaceutical companies also encourages people who are mostly well to think they are ill. About 8 percent of people aged twelve and over who take antidepressants have no current depressive symptoms.[47] These medications are often paid for by Medicare and other publicly funded programs.

1986: EMERGENCY MEDICAL TREATMENT AND LABOR ACT (EMTALA)

This act was intended to ensure that people who needed emergency room care were not turned away because of an inability to pay.[48] It generally requires emergency rooms to examine anyone who requests an examination and prohibits ERs from refusing to treat emergency medical conditions. But enforcement of EMTALA is only triggered by a complaint. Perhaps a lawyer could improve services for the seriously mentally ill by bringing an EMTALA suit on behalf of those with mental illness who have been turned away by ERs.

1986: PROTECTION AND ADVOCACY FOR INDIVIDUALS WITH MENTAL ILLNESS ACT OF 1986

In 1985, after holding hearings exposing horrific neglect and physical abuse of people with serious mental illness in psychiatric hospitals, Congress passed the Protection and Advocacy for Individuals with Mental Illness Act of 1986 (PAIMI or P&A).[49] The legislation and subsequent amendments created fifty state-chosen, independently run, federally funded public interest law firms that often go by the name of "Disability Rights [Name of State]" with the authority to investigate patient neglect, abuse, and civil rights violations in institutions and community programs.

The PAIMI programs have largely ignored their federal mandate, and the results have been a disaster. As Rael Jean Isaac and Virginia Armat documented in *Madness in the Streets*, ending the PAIMI program would save money and improve care for the seriously mentally ill. The program has been taken over by mental health lawyers working to close institutions and defend the "right" of the psychotic who wants to refuse treatment that can restore his sanity. Any federal or state treatment policy PAIMIs don't like on a philosophical ground becomes "abuse" or a "civil rights violation" and networks of federally funded lawyers are mobilized to fight it regardless of the merits of the claim.

In an exceedingly important article, Amanda Peters, writing in *Oregon Law Review*, found that PAIMIs "have taken on additional and legally impermissible responsibilities that Congress never envisioned or authorized."[50] Patient advocates have violated congressional mandates against lobbying and lobbied against laws that would benefit mental health consumers. SAMHSA's own investigation of PAIMIs, which SAMHSA ignored, found the following:[51]

- There has been a "steady decline in [PAIMI] cases related to abuse and neglect."
- PAIMIs decided to serve a population far more expansive than the one mandated by Congress.
- PAIMIs expanded the definitions of neglect and abuse beyond that which Congress intended.
- PAIMIs stopped focusing on the institutionalized.
- PAIMIs work to close psychiatric institutions in spite of noting that "as public psychiatric institutions close, more individuals with psychiatric disability are found in nursing homes and jails."
- Thirty percent of state PAIMIs work to reduce stigma even though it is not the focus of the legislation.
- PAIMIs worked to prevent the enactment of state laws creating outpatient commitment systems.
- SAMHSA's Center for Mental Health Services fails to monitor PAIMI compliance with the enabling legislation.

PAIMIs do provide valuable advocacy services to some individuals with serious mental illness, but that is totally eclipsed by their major systemic impact, which has been to make treatment more difficult by suing, threatening to sue, cajoling, and bullying hospitals, doctors, and state mental health directors who attempt to deliver care to the most seriously ill.

1990–2014: AMERICANS WITH DISABILITIES ACT, AMENDMENTS, AND OLMSTEAD INTERPRETATION

The Americans with Disabilities Act (ADA) of 1990 and ADA Amendments Act of 2008 prohibit discrimination against the disabled in employment, government services, public accommodations, telecommunications, and transportation.[52] Disability was originally defined as a mental or physical impairment that *substantially* limits at least one major life activity. Advocates had the bill amended in 2008 to define a wider range of activities as "major life activities" and to allow for people with mental impairments to qualify for protection even if the impairment is not severe or permanent, and is successfully ameliorated with treatment. As a result, ADA likely benefits more people with mental health "issues" than individuals with serious mental illness.

The Title I provisions of ADA prohibiting discrimination in employment are largely irrelevant to many people with serious mental illnesses, because the treatments are not yet good enough to allow most to work.

The Title II provisions requiring states to provide services in the "most integrated setting appropriate to the needs of the individual" are important and should have benefitted people with serious mental illness. However, as described in chapter 15, through Olmstead lawsuits, federally funded PAIMI lawyers and DOJ CRIPA lawyers have misused those provisions to force states to empty group homes, nursing homes, and hospitals of individuals with serious mental illness and put them into less restrictive independent living where many are isolated and receive nowhere near the support they need.

1991: NIMH REPORT *CARING FOR PEOPLE WITH SEVERE MENTAL DISORDERS: A NATIONAL PLAN OF RESEARCH TO IMPROVE SERVICES*

This largely ignored report focused on the most severely mentally ill and described a laundry list of clinical and services research needed to improve care.[53]

1992: ALCOHOL, DRUG ABUSE, MENTAL HEALTH ADMINISTRATION (ADAMHA) REORGANIZATION ACT

The ADAMHA Reorganization Act created SAMHSA within the Department of Health and Human Services (HHS), and replaced direct federal funding of Community Mental Health Centers (CMHC) with block grants to be distributed directly to states by the newly formed Center for Mental Health Services (CMHS) located within SAMHSA.[54] Committee chair Henry Waxman told Congress that the object in creating SAMHSA was to "target funds to populations most in need."[55] Twenty years later, SAMHSA administrator Pam Hyde told Congress the same thing at the same time her agency was issuing multiyear strategic plans that failed to even mention "schizophrenia."[56] As described in chapter 7, SAMHSA and

CMHS have never focused on the people most in need. Fixing SAMHSA and CMHS should be a major goal of Congress. The 21st Century Cures Act of 2016 discussed later took a step in that direction.

1993: PRESIDENT CLINTON'S TASK FORCE ON NATIONAL HEALTH CARE REFORM

In 1993, President Clinton created a President's Task Force on National Health Care Reform and appointed First Lady Hillary Clinton to head it. Tipper Gore, wife of Vice President Al Gore, who had a degree in psychology, suffered from depression, and had strong connections to Mental Health America (MHA), served as an advisor on mental health policy.[57]

The mental health industry convinced the task force to include "a wide range of mental health services" in its national healthcare plan and to reject "arbitrary or special limits on amount and duration of mental health services."[58] By insisting on all services for everyone, not just treatment for the seriously mentally ill, the industry bloated the cost and increased projected premiums $275 a year per person. This "became a major barrier to the Clinton administration's acceptance of the idea."[59] Hillary Clinton refused to solve the problem by focusing on serious mental illness only and instead stepped back from including any mental health coverage.[60] The healthcare bill that emerged didn't pass Congress. But even if it had, it would have done little for anyone with mental illness because of the industry's attempted money grab.

1996: MENTAL HEALTH PARITY ACT OF 1996

Senators Pete Domenici (R-NM), Paul Wellstone (D-MN), and Ted Kennedy (D-MA) all had relatives with serious mental illness and wanted insurers to offer parity coverage for it. Pete Domenici's daughter Clare had schizophrenia, Paul Wellstone had a brother with schizophrenia, and Ted Kennedy had a mentally ill and developmentally disabled sister, Rosemary. These leaders understood the difference between poor mental health and severe mental illness and in 1992 passed a bill requiring government to calculate the cost of "medical treatment for severe mental illness commensurate with other illnesses" and defined "severe mental illness" narrowly.[61] The resulting report found that,

> [F]or an additional annual cost of $6.5 billion—representing approximately a 10% increase over current total direct costs of mental health care—the nation can provide coverage for adults and children with severe mental disorders commensurate with coverage for other disorders. . . . The annual savings in indirect costs and general medical services would amount to approximately $8.7 billion. . . . [This] would represent an estimated net economic benefit for the nation of $2.2 billion annually.[62]

The Mental Health Parity Act (MHPA) was attached to other legislation making its way through Congress.[63] It did not mandate mental health coverage. It did prevent businesses with over fifty employees, and that provided mental health coverage to their employees, from imposing caps on mental illness coverage more restrictive than those applied to physical illnesses (subject to certain exceptions).[64]

Because the law affected only employer-based policies, it did not help the seriously mentally ill who were too disabled by their illness to have ever worked. It did help seriously mentally ill children who were on the health plans of their parents, but since serious mental illness tends to strike in the teens and early twenties, individuals affected would quickly age out of that coverage.

The law passed because the sponsors ignored the mental health industry and focused narrowly on serious mental illness. Wellstone and Domenici's efforts were heroic and laid the groundwork for more comprehensive legislation later.

HEALTH INSURANCE PORTABILITY AND ACCOUNTABILITY ACT OF 1996 (HIPAA) AND THE FAMILY EDUCATIONAL RIGHTS AND PRIVACY ACT OF 1974 (FERPA) AS AMENDED THROUGH 2001

The Health Insurance Portability and Accountability Act of 1996 (HIPAA) required the Department of Health and Human Services (HHS) to draw up regulations to protect patients' medical information.[65] The resultant regulations often prevent proper treatment of those with mental illness who are over eighteen—or fourteen in some states—because the regulations largely prohibit doctors, hospitals, and treatment programs ("covered entities") from disclosing medical information to their families, even when those families provide housing, case management, and support to their mentally ill loved ones and need the information to prevent their deterioration.[66] Parents refer to this as the "HIPAA Handcuffs." As a result:

- When a mentally ill family member goes missing, his family can't find him because HIPAA prevents hospitals and shelters from disclosing who is in their facilities.
- When a hospital releases a person with mental illness to a family's care, the hospital can't inform the parents first, tell them the diagnosis, or even determine if a family exists and is willing to accept the patient.
- When a family member is given a prescription or a follow-up appointment, the parents can't be told and therefore can't ensure prescriptions are filled or arrange transportation to the appointment.

HIPAA is silent on whether doctors can *receive* information from family members, but many healthcare providers falsely claim they can't. This leads doctors to try treatments that have previously failed. A common situation is for a patient to tell the doctor she will take medications when the family knows she won't. As a result, rather than putting the patient on a long-acting injectable, which could be easily monitored, the doctor puts the patient on pills that cannot be easily monitored. The patient stops taking the pills and deteriorates. Patients can waive their right to keep the information confidential, but psychotic patients often will not sign the waiver and doctors rarely ask them to.

The same problems exist as a result of the Family Educational Rights and Privacy Act of 1974 (FERPA), which largely limits what healthcare information educational institutions can disclose about enrolled students, even to parents who are paying their tuition.[67] James Holmes was identified by school authorities as being potentially dangerous before he shot and killed twelve people at a theater in Aurora, Colorado, but FERPA kept his parents oblivious. The report on the mass shootings by Seung-Hui Cho, who killed thirty-two at Virginia Tech on April 16, 2007, detailed how HIPAA and FERPA may have played a role in the tragedy.[68] Rachel Pruchno, author of *Surrounded by Madness*, wrote in an editorial, "I've been dealing with the mental health system since my daughter was 12. . . . Once she turned eighteen, however, I went from valued member of the health care team to its pariah."[69] The mental health industry successfully fought off provisions in the original version of the 2013 Helping Families in Mental Health Crisis Act that would have fixed these problems. The 21st Century Cures Act passed in 2016 does require regulators to clarify HIPAA provisions and educate the public, but it is not likely that those provisions will lead to meaningful reform. Ideas for remedying HIPAA and FERPA are in appendix E.

1999: THE SURGEON GENERAL'S REPORT ON MENTAL HEALTH

Mental Health: A Report of the Surgeon General (1999) was as widely hailed as it was disastrous.[70] It represented the ascendency of the "mental health is whatever you want it to be" mentality. The report declared it a problem that in "years past the mental health field often focused principally on mental illness in order to serve individuals who were most severely affected." It declared that mental health and mental illness are "points on a continuum" and made no attempt to prioritize one over the other. Mental health issues like anxiety and want of marriage counseling were given greater weight than treating people with schizophrenia, because they are more common. Non-evidence-based programs including self-help, peer support, consumer-operated services, and stigma busting were extolled.

Most damaging, the report urged a movement toward a discredited "public health" approach focused on "health promotion [and] disease prevention."[71] Treating people with serious mental illness did not make the list. The single chapter on adults with mental illness concluded, "Good mental health enables individuals to cope with adversity" and "Stressful life events . . . can disrupt the balance adults seek in life."

2000: NATIONAL COUNCIL ON DISABILITIES: *FROM PRIVILEGES TO RIGHTS: PEOPLE LABELED WITH PSYCHIATRIC DISABILITIES SPEAK FOR THEMSELVES*

The National Council on Disability (NCD) is an independent federal agency mandated to make recommendations to the president and Congress on disability issues. Its report *From Privileges to Rights* was perhaps the worst on mental illness ever written.[72] Antipsychiatrists served as members of the commission and staffers. Commissioner Rae Unzicker was also national coordinator of the radical National Association of Psychiatric Survivors (NAPS), which does not even believe mental illness exists.[73] She was also "the inspiration and driving force behind the National Association for Rights Protection and Advocacy (NARPA)," which has the goal of the "abolition of all forced [sic] treatment."[74] Antipsychiatrist Judi Chamberlin was a drafter of the report.

NCD scheduled hearings in the same cities at the same time that radical antipsychiatrists were holding meetings, to ensure its report would be dominated by "mental illness is a myth" doctrine.[75] The report uses the term people "*labeled* with psychiatric disabilities" over one hundred times, rather than simply saying "people with mental illness." NCD continues to impede mental health reform today.[76]

2003 MEDICARE PRESCRIPTION DRUG, IMPROVEMENT, AND MODERNIZATION ACT

This act created prescription drug coverage under Medicare, but it prevents consumers from importing medicines from places like Canada where they are cheaper, and prevented the government from negotiating for lower prices from pharmaceutical companies.[77] This drives up the cost of treatment.

2003: PRESIDENT BUSH'S NEW FREEDOM COMMISSION ON MENTAL HEALTH AND ITS FINAL REPORT, *ACHIEVING THE PROMISE: TRANSFORMING MENTAL HEALTH CARE IN AMERICA*

In 2002, President George W. Bush created the President's New Freedom Commission on Mental Health.[78] Michael Hogan was named chairman and Dan Fisher a commissioner. Hogan had been a state mental health commissioner who endorses the idea that the goal of the mental health system should be to "create hope filled, humanized environments and relationships in which people can grow."[79] Fisher was the codirector of the SAMHSA-funded National Empowerment Center, which, as far as we know, does not recognize that "mental illness" exists.

> The commission did not take on the most difficult cases. . . . Instead it focused on "consumers"—the politically correct word for psychiatric patients—who are willing and able to make use of treatments, programs, and opportunities. . . . [T]hey did not hear from the sickest silent minority that is languishing in back bedrooms, jail cells, and homeless shelters. They are too paranoid, oblivious, or lost in madness to attend hearings, never mind testify.[80]

The commission's final report, *Achieving the Promise: Transforming Mental Health Care in America*, offered nothing for those who have anosognosia, were institutionalized, psychotic, schizophrenic, or prone to violence.[81] The main goal was "transformation." The system "must focus on increasing consumers' ability to successfully cope with life's challenges, on facilitating recovery, and on building resilience not just managing symptoms." The report's "nineteen recommendations are a hodgepodge of boilerplate and evasion," not to mention platitudes.[82] It endorsed the public health approach of ensuring "Americans understand that mental health is essential to overall health." The second goal was to ensure that "mental health care is consumer and family driven," thereby leaving out those who can't drive their own care. It endorsed the "recovery model" over the medical model, called for a "national campaign to reduce stigma," and endorsed funding everything remotely related to mental anything.

In 2003, hundreds of thousands of Americans were sleeping on street grates or behind bars because they suffered from serious mental illness. As

National Review editor Rich Lowry wrote, the commission "was an opportunity to address this neglect, but it, disgracefully, took a pass."[83]

2004: INDIVIDUALS WITH DISABILITIES EDUCATION ACT (IDEA)

The 2004 Individuals with Disabilities Education Act (IDEA) "ensures that all children with disabilities have available to them a free appropriate public education that emphasizes special education."[84] It requires schools to provide eligible students with an "Individualized Education Plan (IEP)" to address their special needs. The IEP plan often includes tutoring, smaller classes, or classes with a higher teacher-to-student ratio—everything a parent would want. IDEA has helped many students. But because it is limited to those under twenty-one years old, it is not really a program that helps large numbers of seriously mentally ill adults.

2008: MENTAL HEALTH PARITY AND ADDICTION EQUITY ACT (MHPAEA) OF 2008

The Mental Health Parity and Addiction Equity Act (MHPAEA) of 2008 plugged holes in the Mental Health Parity Act of 1996 (MHPA) and was championed by Senators Kennedy and Domenici, after cocreator Senator Wellstone died in a plane crash.[85] MHPAEA "requires group health plans and health insurance issuers to ensure that financial requirements (such as co-pays and deductibles) and treatment limitations (such as visit limits) applicable to mental health or substance use disorder benefits are no more restrictive than the limitations applied to substantially medical and surgical benefits."[86]

Like MHPA, MHPAEA applied only to large group health plans and therefore left out many of the most seriously mentally ill, who could not work, although it did help children of the covered. As of July 1, 2014, it required individual and small group plans to cover mental illness at the same level as medical and surgical care, but many people have found that the insurance industry is not complying.

2005–2013: STATE CUTS TO MENTAL HEALTH BUDGETS

Forty-one states cut their mental health budgets a total of $5 billion between 2008 and 2013.[87] California, Illinois, Nevada, and South Carolina made the deepest cuts. These cuts affected housing, assertive community treatment, access to psychiatric medications, and crisis services.[88] They also affect the number of hospital beds, making deinstitutionalization a problem of the present, not just the past. "The number of state psychiatric beds decreased by 14% from 2005 to 2010, from 50,509 to 43,318. Thirteen states closed 25% or more of their beds."[89] At the same time that states closed hospitals and programs that served the seriously mentally ill, they expanded stigma campaigns and "wellness centers" for all others. Deinstitutionalization is alive and well.

2010: AFFORDABLE CARE ACT (ACA)

The Affordable Care Act (ACA, aka "Obamacare") made insurance more affordable to many and allowed parents to keep a child on their coverage until age twenty-six.[90] It also created a pilot program allowing the use of Medicaid for private hospital care for certain mentally ill, but that program was brought to an end.[91] ACA also eliminates the incremental Medicaid payments hospitals with a disproportionate share of the indigent (Disproportionate Share Hospitals, or DSHs) receive. "In 2010, thirty-seven states received a total of $2.8 billion in DSH funds, representing 27 percent of all state hospital revenues.... Due to these ACA-mandated cuts in DSH payments, hospitals could see reductions of close to $22 billion between 2014 and 2021."[92] Because these payments are used for both inpatient and outpatient care, cuts in DSH will affect both. President Trump has said he will repeal and replace the ACA, but has not yet provided details on his plan.

2013: OBAMA/BIDEN NATIONAL DIALOGUE ON MENTAL HEALTH

In the wake of the Newtown, Connecticut, shootings, President Obama called for a "National Conversation on Mental Health," not mental illness.[93] The usual suspects and platitudes were paraded in front of the press and more government websites like *mentalhealth.gov* created. In the plus column, the president did implement gun control regulations to prevent purchases by certain mentally ill.[94]

2013–2016: THE HELPING FAMILIES IN MENTAL HEALTH CRISIS ACT, MENTAL HEALTH AND SAFE COMMUNITIES ACT, AND MENTAL HEALTH REFORM ACT AS INCORPORATED IN THE 21ST CENTURY CURES ACT

After the 2012 shootings at the Sandy Hook Elementary School in Newtown, Connecticut, Representative Tim Murphy (R-PA), the only practicing psychologist in Congress, used his position as chairman of the Oversight and Investigations Subcommittee of the House Energy and Commerce Committee to conduct an investigation of the nation's mental health system and propose remedies. The 2013 Helping Families in Mental Health Crisis Act (H.R. 3717) introduced by Representatives Murphy and Eddie Bernice Johnson (D-TX) garnered 178 cosponsors but did not pass due to intense lobbying of Democrats by the mental health industry who objected to provisions shifting resources toward science and the seriously ill.[95] In July 2016, Representative Murphy shepherded a watered-down, but still very useful version (H.R. 2646) to an almost unanimous 142-2 vote in the House, thereby bringing pressure on the Senate to pass a similar bill.[96] Senator John Cornyn (R-TX) championed some of the most important provisions of H.R. 2646 in his Mental Health and Safe Communities Act (S. 2002) and added his own important provisions. Senators Chris Murphy (D-CT), Lamar Alexander (R-TN), and Bill Cassidy (R-LA) included some of the provisions in the Mental Health Reform Act (S. 2680). Versions of all these bills were incorporated in the 21st Century Cures Act (H.R. 34) that passed both houses and that President Obama signed on December 13, 2016.[97]

The mental health provisions of the 21st Century Cures Act are very important despite the compromises that were made. The law creates an assistant secretary of Mental Health and Substance Use Disorders to run SAMHSA and to try to focus SAMHSA, CMHS, and other federal departments on using evidence-based practices to help the most seriously mentally ill. The success of that attempt will depend on whether President

Trump nominates an assistant secretary who understands serious mental illness and is committed to focusing the mental health resources of the federal government on it.[98]

The 21st Century Cures Act increases funding through 2022 for pilot Assisted Outpatient Treatment (AOT) programs and makes AOT available to nonviolent offenders. It provides funding for mental health courts, assertive community treatment, forensic case managers, and training for police on how to deescalate interventions with the seriously ill. It provides for the collection and dissemination of data on the number and types of crimes committed by mentally ill individuals, the involvement of mental illness in deadly incidents involving law enforcement officers, and the costs of imprisoning the seriously ill, which hopefully will force Congress to address these issues. It requires regulators to look at HIPAA, a process that will likely result in clarification that healthcare providers may *receive* information from families, even when they can't *disclose* information to families. It clarifies that Medicaid can reimburse for mental health and physical health services that are received on the same day, strengthens parity provisions, and takes steps to increase the number of mental health workers so more people who need treatment can access it. There is a lot it didn't do.[99] But it is the most important reform bill in decades. Representative Murphy deserves the credit for that, and he has promised more to come.

The following chapter describes how various Supreme Court decisions also made it more difficult for the seriously mentally ill to receive treatment.

Chapter 15

COURT DECISIONS THAT FAILED THE SERIOUSLY ILL

"Here is the Kafkaesque irony: Far from respecting civil liberties, legal obstacles to treatment limit or destroy the liberty of the person."

—Herschel Hardin, a former director of the British Columbia Civil Liberties Association

INTRODUCTION

People with serious mental illness need their rights protected, but the ACLU, Bazelon, and federally funded Disability Rights (PAIMI) attorneys have placed dangerous roadblocks between patients and treatment. They defend the right to be psychotic, rather than the right to treatment. Parents of the seriously ill must often hire a lawyer instead of a doctor.

The role of the federally funded protection and advocacy attorneys in preventing the seriously ill from receiving life-saving care is hard to overstate. They use federal funds to attack hospitals, doctors, programs, and state mental health departments that try to deliver care to the seriously ill. They get salaries if their suits are unsuccessful, complemented by large publicly funded payouts if they succeed. Those sued or threatened by these groups may not have the resources to defend themselves, and because the suits often free them from the obligation to provide care, they sometimes don't want to defend against them. This chapter discusses some of the core legal concepts guiding and preventing treatment of the seriously mentally ill and the court cases that gave rise to them.

CIVIL COMMITMENT

The decision to involuntarily commit someone should not and cannot be made lightly. Almost all states allow police and clinicians to initiate short-term commitments lasting up to seventy-two hours to handle obviously imminent emergencies.[1] Due to their emergency nature, these commitments do not allow time for or require extensive due process protection.

The government can remove freedom to prevent someone from becoming a danger to others (police powers) and to protect those who can't protect themselves (*parens patriae* powers). Police powers are often used in reaction to a crime, while *parens patriae* powers are often used to help adults with dementia or children who can't help themselves. All states allow commitment—restrictions placed—on those who are a danger to self or others.[2] But states and courts vary in their interpretation of what constitutes dangerousness and when it occurs. Must someone be "imminently" or "overtly" dangerous, or does danger occur earlier, for example, when cognitive impairment causes someone to eat trash from a Dumpster? Does someone become dangerous when he declares he wants to kill himself or others, or only after he develops a plan or attempts it? When someone buys a gun and bullets, or only after the person pulls the trigger? Must the danger involve physical harm to another person? What about trashing a house? Starting fires? What burden of proof must the state meet to establish dangerousness? These questions have all been the subjects of court decisions. In each case, the mental health bar encouraged the courts to place procedural hurdles in the way of treatment.

To supplement a narrowly defined danger to self or others standard, some states added "gravely disabled" and "need for treatment" standards. "Gravely disabled" generally means that "due to mental illness, the person is substantially unable to provide for his or her basic needs for food, clothing, shelter, health, or safety." "Need for treatment" generally means that "due to a mental disability, the person is in need of treatment to prevent deterioration" that will lead to danger to self or others. Technically, these are just expanded definitions of dangerousness as opposed to discrete standards. Consideration should be given to also using a "lack of capacity" standard that would allow treatment for those who "as a result of mental illness are unable to fully understand or lack judgment to make an informed decision regarding his or her need for treatment, care, or supervision."

Wisconsin's well-thought-out, albeit lengthy, "Fifth Standard" generally permits "the commitment of an individual who, due to mental illness, is unable to understand the advantages, disadvantages, or alternatives to a particular treatment or is unable or unwilling to apply them to his or her situation and requires such treatment to prevent severe mental, emotional, or physical harm."[3]

> It does not require that the alleged mentally ill person pose a substantial direct risk of harm to self by his or her actions. Nor does it rely upon the provision of grave disability to authorize commitment. Rather, the new standard focuses on whether the person's "acts or omissions" lead to a "substantial probability" that, if left untreated, the illness would result in the "loss of the individual's ability to function independently in the community or loss of cognitive or volitional control." Thus, this new Fifth Standard of Dangerousness explicitly places its emphasis on whether the alleged person is able to maintain living within the community instead of relying upon serious overt acts of violence or extreme neglect of personal self-care to provide for commitment.[4]

O'Connor v. Donaldson (1975) was one of the most important Supreme Court decisions concerning involuntary commitment but is frequently misrepresented.[5] It did establish that a finding of dangerousness is needed to commit some individuals. But not all. The court held that

> a State cannot constitutionally confine, without more, a nondangerous individual who is capable of surviving safely in freedom by himself or with the help of willing and responsible family members or friends.

The mental health bar shorthands the court's holding to mean "the state cannot confine a nondangerous individual" and ignore that it applies only to those "capable of surviving safely in freedom." They ignore the court's specific refusal to rule on "whether the State may compulsorily confine a nondangerous, mentally ill individual *for the purpose of treatment*." (Emphasis added.) The decision specifically recognized an individual can be released if there are "willing and responsible family members or friends" to help someone be "capable of surviving safely in freedom." Hospitals take advantage of that language to empty their beds. They often ask parents, in front of the ill relative, if they are willing to take them home. Parents are thereby pressured to say yes or risk the wrath of their child. Unfortunately, in concurring with the decision, Justice Warren Burger specifically rejected the notion that mental patients have a right to treatment, something at least one lower court had held that they did.

Kansas v. Hendricks **(1997)** is a more recent decision addressing involuntary commitment that could one day prove helpful for getting treatment to the most seriously mentally ill.[6] Kansas convicted Leroy Hendricks of pedophilia, and *after he served his sentence,* the state civilly committed him under its Sexually Violent Predator (SVP) Act.[7] The SVP Act allowed for indefinite civil commitment of those who have a "mental abnormality" or a "personality disorder," and are "likely to engage in repeat acts of sexual violence if not treated for their mental abnormality or personality disorder." Hendricks claimed his sentence had been served and additional commitment was double jeopardy. The Supreme Court upheld the act and his continued commitment by recognizing that "involuntary confinement . . . is not punishment" and that it had "never held that the Constitution prevents a State from civilly detaining those for whom no treatment is available, but who nevertheless pose a danger to others."

The decision may ultimately benefit people with serious mental illness if there are pro bono lawyers who will bring a suit on the issue.[8] It allows civil commitment for those with a "mental abnormality" or a "personality disorder," which are likely easier to find than a "mental illness." It also allows commitment of those "likely" to engage in the specified act, which is less restrictive than the "imminent" danger that is often used in the commitment of the mentally ill. It seems reasonable that the decision could apply to people who are likely to repeat dangerous acts other than pedophilia or rape. Since the court allowed inpatient commitment to prevent an act that is "likely," it seems reasonable that it would also allow placement in Assisted Outpatient Treatment, which is less restrictive than the commitment Hendricks received. On the other hand, its allowance of "indefinite" commitment versus time-limited commitment could lead to abuse.

Subsequent to the *Kansas v. Hendricks* decision, many states have adopted legislation similar to Kansas's SVP Act. They have made extensive use of it, thereby filling state psychiatric hospitals with SVPs, leaving fewer beds for the seriously mentally ill.

FREEDOM FROM RESTRAINTS AND A LIMITED RIGHT TO TREATMENT

Youngberg v. Romeo **(1982)** held that the due process clause entitles involuntarily committed patients to "reasonably safe conditions of confinement, freedom from unreasonable bodily restraints, and such minimally adequate [treatment] as reasonably may be required by these interests."[9] Some have argued that the decision creates a right to receive some treatment—at least that needed to keep someone safe and free of restraints. It also established that "whether respondent's constitutional rights have been violated must be determined by balancing these liberty interests against the relevant state interests. The proper standard for determining whether the State has adequately protected such rights is whether professional judgment, in fact, was exercised. And in determining what is 'reasonable,' courts must show deference to the judgment exercised by a qualified professional, whose decision is presumptively valid."

MEDICATION OVER OBJECTION OF THE CRIMINALLY INVOLVED

The Supreme Court has ruled on when those awaiting trial, being tried, or are imprisoned can be treated over objection.

Washington v. Harper **(1990)** established that the state can treat a prison inmate who has a serious mental illness with antipsychotic drugs against his will if he is dangerous to himself or others and the treatment is in his medical interest.[10] Sufficient due process exists as long as a committee of professionals not currently involved in the inmate's diagnosis and treatment reviews the decision.

Prison inmate Walter Harper claimed that his due process rights were violated when antipsychotic medication was administered over his objection without a full judicial hearing. The Supreme Court upheld the administrative hearing procedure because "requiring judicial hearings will divert scarce prison resources, both money and staff's time, from the care and treatment of mentally ill inmates." Harper also alleged that medication could not be administered over his objection unless a judge found him incompetent to make his own medical decisions. The court upheld the state's criteria for administering involuntary medication, which required mentally ill inmates to be "gravely disabled" or pose a "likelihood of serious harm" to himself, others, or property. The court recognized prison officials' interest in maintaining a safe environment to protect corrections officers and prison staff, as well as the obligation to provide for the medical needs of its prisoners.

Riggins v. Nevada **(1992)** went the other way.[11] It established that involuntarily medicating a prisoner *during the period of his trial* violated due process rights. David Riggins was mentally ill, on trial for murder, and given Mellaril over objection to help reduce psychosis and make him competent for trial. He complained that its effect on him would deny him due process and a fair trial because he had the right to show jurors his true mental state when he offered his insanity defense. The court agreed. The decision creates a hurdle for involuntarily medicating prisoners being held for trial, but it is hard to understand how a fair trial can occur if the jury can't witness the person in an unmedicated state.

Sell v. United States **(2003)** established when the government could medicate a nondangerous person charged with a serious crime to make that person competent to stand trial.[12] The Supreme Court rejected the lower court's holding that medication can be forced solely to make a patient competent to stand trial, deciding that it can only be done "if the treatment is medically appropriate, is substantially unlikely to have side effects that may undermine the fairness of the trial, and, taking account of less intrusive alternatives, is necessary significantly to further important governmental trial-related interests."

LEAST RESTRICTIVE SETTING

Olmstead v. L. C. **(1999)** established that the American's with Disabilities Act (ADA) has an "integration mandate" that requires states to place people with mental disabilities in the "least restrictive settings . . . *appropriate* to the individual . . . taking into account the resources available."[13] (Emphasis in original.) The decision requires the state's "treatment professionals" to determine that community placement is appropriate and not opposed by the affected individual.

Olmstead is being weaponized by PAIMI lawyers and the Department of Justice CRIPA lawyers to force states to sign consent agreements stipulating that they will empty hospitals, adult homes, and nursing homes of people with serious mental illness and place them in less restrictive set-tings.[14] That is sometimes a good idea, but sometimes the least restrictive setting is not the most beneficial and may be dangerous. Mental health lawyers have worked vigorously to ensure the criterion of "least restrictive setting" is met, while ignoring whether it is "appropriate to the individual." Massachusetts-based mental illness attorney Mary Zdanowicz wrote,

> There are several aspects of the Court's opinion that have been lost in translation by disability advocates. The Court emphasized the word "appropriate" integrated setting. In Olmstead, the state's professional [who was determining what is appropriate] were physicians. In recent state settlement agreements, the "professional" need not have medical or specialized training in mental illness. The Court did not elaborate on the phrase "essential eligibility requirements." In practice ... all that is needed is that the person accept community placement, regardless of whether they have the capacity to make an informed decision about the proposed placement or not.[15]

Olmstead could be turbocharging another round of inappropriate dein-stitutionalization and leading to individuals being moved from congregate housing with intensive onsite supports and a social network to indepen-dent living largely devoid of human contact.[16] But some see opportunities to use Olmstead to facilitate Assisted Outpatient Treatment.[17]

DUE PROCESS

Due process protections are an important foundation of liberty, but over-zealous attorneys try to make them as burdensome as possible so they become a barrier to treatment. The attorneys established due process pro-tections based upon criminal procedure that require the state to go to court, present witnesses, meet a high burden of proof, and comply with strict rules of evidence. This often prohibits the court from considering critical information, such as how well patients previously did on or off medica-tions, because in criminal procedure, past behavior is not "proof" they did something currently. Patients are free to not speak (self-incriminate), which prevents judges from hearing their psychotic thoughts. During the long and cumbersome proceedings, the individual continues to suffer, and states often decide to simply discharge the patient without treatment.

Addington v. Texas **(1979)** raised the burden of proof required to involuntarily commit someone with serious mental illness from "preponderance of the evidence," the burden of proof used in civil cases, to the more difficult to meet "clear and convincing evidence."[18] This "protection" makes it less likely that the seriously ill will get treatment.

Zinermon v. Burch **(1990)** made it more difficult for hospitals to admit voluntary patients.[19] It essentially requires hospitals to assume a Catch-22: patients with mental illness who ask for voluntary treatment should be presumed to lack the capacity to consent to treatment. Darrel Burch was mentally ill and transported to a hospital. "While allegedly medicated and disoriented, [he] signed forms requesting admission." Long after release, he sued the hospital for admitting him, claiming the hospital "knew or should have known that Plaintiff was incapable of voluntary, knowing, understanding and informed consent to admission and treatment." The court ruled on a technical issue but generally agreed that the hospital should make a capacity determination before providing treatment.[20] This places an additional burden on voluntary admissions, but hospitals work around it by asking voluntary patients a few preadmission questions to document the patient has capacity. However, theoretically those who fail to pass the competency exam must be admitted under cumbersome involuntary commitment procedures, complete with lawyers, even when they don't object to admission.

NOT GUILTY BY REASON OF INSANITY

In reaction to John Hinckley being found "Not Guilty by Reason of Insanity (NGRI)" of shooting President Reagan, states have made it more difficult for a defendant to mount an NGRI defense.[21] It is attempted in less than 1 percent of felony cases and is rarely successful.

Historically, many states based an NGRI finding on the common-law M'Naghten Rule, established in Britain and used in the United States, which provided that someone is insane (inculpable) if (a) the person had such a severe defect or disease of the mind he didn't understand what he was doing (cognitive standard), *or* (b) the illness was so severe the person didn't know the difference between right and wrong (moral capacity). That has changed.

Clark v. Arizona **(2006)** allowed states to use a single prong of the M'Naghten Rule.[22] The case centered on Eric Clark, who shot and killed a space alien and then ran away. Actually, it was a police officer, Jeffrey Moritz, not a space alien, but Eric was so delusional due to his untreated schizophrenia he didn't know the difference. Arizona law allowed an insanity defense only for those who met the second part of the M'Naghten Rule, requiring the lack of understanding of the difference between right and wrong. The Arizona court held that because Clark ran away, he knew what he did was wrong, and therefore had moral capacity and could not be found NGRI under state law. Clark argued to the Supreme Court that Arizona needed the cognitive prong of the M'Naghten Rule, allowing him to be found NGRI because he didn't understand what he was doing. The Supreme Court allowed Arizona's law to stand. Eric Clark was sentenced to twenty-five years to life in jail.

The M'Naghten standard doesn't go far enough, because it doesn't recognize what we've learned about serious mental illness since the 1800s, when it was formulated. We now know some people with serious mental illness do understand what they are doing and do understand that it is wrong but lack *volition*, meaning they are unable to stop themselves. For example, mentally ill Mark Becker killed his beloved football coach in Iowa because he "knew" he was Satan. He knew it was wrong to kill, but also "knew" he needed to kill Satan to protect everyone else. He was found guilty. In chapter 16 on solutions we propose an alternative to an NGRI plea.

DEATH PENALTY

In *Ford v. Wainwright* **(1986)** the Supreme Court ruled that executing the mentally ill violates the Eighth Amendment prohibition against cruel and unusual punishment.[23] "For centuries, no jurisdiction has countenanced the execution of the insane, yet this Court has never decided whether the Constitution forbids the practice. Today we keep faith with our common-law heritage in holding that it does."

Panetti v. Quarterman **(2007)** determined what constitutes a mental illness sufficient to proscribe execution.[24] A lower court ruled that Eric

Panetti, a man with a long history of serious mental illness convicted for killing his parents-in-law in Texas, could be executed if he was aware he had committed the murders, aware he was going to be executed, and aware of why he was going to be executed. The Supreme Court rejected that, noting that people with mental illness may have "awareness" but need a "rational understanding." The Supreme Court found that the lower court "improperly treated a prisoner's delusional belief system 'as irrelevant.'"[25]

GUN POSSESSION (SECOND AMENDMENT)

In *District of Columbia v. Heller* **(2008)** the Supreme Court ruled that individuals have a right to possess firearms but specifically stated, "[N]othing in our opinion should be taken to cast doubt on longstanding prohibitions on the possession of firearms by . . . the mentally ill."[26]

SIGNIFICANT LOWER COURT DECISIONS

Absent further direction from the Supreme Court, decisions by the thirteen Courts of Appeal set precedents to be followed in their jurisdictions. Following are some important lower court decisions.

Medication over Objection of Hospitalized Patients

The Supreme Court has ruled on when those involved in the criminal justice system can be treated over objection, but has *not* ruled on the necessary standards and due process protections required to allow medication over objection for patients who have been involuntarily committed to a hospital and are not criminally involved. Lower courts have. In California's *Riese v. St. Mary's*, New York's *Rivers v. Katz*, Massachusetts's *Rogers v. Okin*, and New Jersey's *Rennie v. Klein*, it was largely established that dangerous involuntarily committed patients retain the right to refuse treatment.[27]

Under these decisions, if someone is involuntarily committed (dangerous) and objects to treatment, a hearing is required to see if he or she lacks capacity and can therefore be medicated over objection. During the untreated period—after they have been involuntarily committed but before the hearing is held to see if they lack capacity—people with serious mental illness sometimes lash out at their nurses and doctors. So the hospitals call the police and send people who need treatment to jail. Many hospitals, when forced to hold someone who is dangerous (i.e., who meets the commitment standard) but whom they are not allowed to treat (i.e., who has not yet been found to lack capacity), simply declare that the person is no longer dangerous and release him or her.

Utah's *Jurasek v. Utah State Hospital* (1998) is a slight outlier because Utah's grave disability commitment standard has lack of capacity built into it.[28] It precludes commitment unless the patient meets all the criteria, including "lacks the ability to engage in a rational decision making process." To determine if someone lacks that capacity, the Utah State Hospital was convening an independent medical review board consisting of a psychiatrist, psychologist, and the hospital program administrator, in lieu of going to court. Jurasek objected that violated his due process rights, but the court disagreed.

The court affirmed the right of the hospital to medicate a gravely disabled individual when it is in the patient's medical interest. The decision is significant because overt immediate dangerousness was not required, and by endorsing the use of an independent hospital committee that was not involved in the treatment of the patient to make the treatment decision, the court allowed the hospital to cut the delay between when an involuntary commitment begins and the patient can be treated. The Utah court basically took Supreme Court decisions that had been geared to prisoners, including *Washington v. Harper* and *Riggins v. Nevada*, and applied them to individuals who had been involuntarily committed. All states should do this.

Right to Treatment

Wyatt v. Stickney (1971) for a short time established that institutionalized patients have a "constitutional right to receive such individual treatment as will give each of them a realistic opportunity to be cured or to improve his or her mental condition."[29] This ostensibly would have benefitted people with mental illness by establishing a "right to treatment." But how the case came about was a good example of the disingenuousness of the mental health bar.

In 1960, Morton Birnbaum wrote a seminal law journal article asserting that the mentally ill had a "right to treatment" while hospitalized; otherwise they were essentially being incarcerated without having committed a crime.[30] Years later, laid-off employees at Bryce Hospital in Alabama wanted their jobs back. Lawyers for the laid-off employees thought they could use Birnbaum's argument that the institutionalized mentally ill had a right to treatment to force the state to hire them back to provide the treatment. However, as Rael Jean Isaac and Virginia Armat described in *Madness in the Streets*, the mental health bar, led by Bruce Ennis, believed institutions were a form of oppression and joined the case because,

> There was "advance information" that the judge "would not only say there is something in the abstract called the 'right to treatment,' but that he would set standards so high that the State of Alabama literally would not be able to meet them." This meant the state "was going to have to discharge many of the residents in its institutions." Winning "the right to treatment" would thus serve, said Ennis, "as the best method for deinstitutionalizing thousands of persons."[31]

It worked for a while. Institutionalized patients gained a right to treatment, so states simply closed hospitals to avoid the obligation to provide the treatment. Similar suits were then brought in Louisiana, Minnesota, and Ohio. However, any "right to treatment" was largely obviated by Justice Burger's 1975 concurrence in *O'Connor v. Donaldson*, where he rejected the notion that patients have a right to treatment.

Dangerousness

Lessard v. Schmidt **(1972)** had the effect of narrowing the definition of dangerousness to cases where "there is an extreme likelihood that if the person is not confined he will do immediate harm to himself or others," which can be evidenced by "a finding of a recent overt act, attempt or threat to do substantial harm to oneself or another."[32] It also required that commitment proceedings provide the mentally ill with the same protections provided to suspected criminals, including the right to counsel, to remain silent, to exclude hearsay evidence and the requirement of the state to prove its case by proof "beyond a reasonable doubt" versus by a "preponderance of evidence." In making civil commitment procedures comport with criminal procedures, the court made treatment much more difficult. For example, the best predictor of future behavior by someone with mental illness is past behavior. Under criminal procedure, that past behavior is generally not admissible.

In justification of making commitment more difficult, the court noted that too many people were hospitalized: "In 1963, 679,000 persons were confined in mental institutions in the United States; only 250,000 persons were incarcerated." Partially as a result of this bad decision, and others like it, today the numbers are reversed. Now 1,100,000 with any mental illness are in jails and prisons and less than 50,000 in state hospitals.

Assisted Outpatient Treatment

Protection and Advocacy, ACLU, and Bazelon-inspired challenges to Assisted Outpatient Treatment (AOT) have not reached the Supreme Court. But New York courts have decided that AOT is an appropriate use of the states' police powers and *parens patriae* powers and therefore does not violate civil rights.[33] The courts noted that AOT does not entail confinement as treatment takes place in the community. And since it is only available to those with certain narrowly defined histories, including previously becoming dangerous, homeless, hospitalized, arrested, or incarcerated, it is appropriately narrowly targeted and there are important state interests at stake.

Protection and Advocacy funds, supplemented by state funds, continue flowing to anti-treatment Disability Rights attorneys. People with a serious mental illness are being denied necessary care as a result of hurdles put in place by these mental health lawyers working in conjunction with the Bazelon Center and the ACLU. Many of these groups would be forced to stop their anti-treatment advocacy if the federal government and states would stop funding them.

In the next chapter we propose solutions.

WHERE DO WE GO?

Chapter 16

SOLUTIONS

"Reasonable people adapt themselves to the world. Unreasonable people expect the world to adapt to them. All progress was therefore made by unreasonable people."
—George Bernard Shaw

The problems are fixable, and solving them is affordable. However, we need politicians willing to base policy on science rather than on mythology spread by the mental health industry and its advocates. We must target resources on people most likely, not least likely, to become tragedies. Congress and state legislators must be made to understand that throwing money at mental health is not the same as delivering treatment to people with serious mental illness.

INTRODUCTION: CUT, CONSOLIDATE, AND COORDINATE PROGRAMS

Cut

Cut what's wasteful so the resources can go to what's useful. Programs to cut could include peer support programs, stigma programs, suicide advertising, and programs that claim to predict or prevent mental illness. Cut all mental health programs listed in SAMHSA's NREPP database that don't improve meaningful outcomes for people with serious mental illness like Wellness Recovery Action Plans (WRAP) and Mental Health First Aid (MHFA). Cut outreach programs that refuse to go to the exits of jails, prisons, shelters, hospitals, and homes where the seriously ill are. Cut social service programs that masquerade as mental health programs and let them compete with other social service programs for funds. Jobs programs can be funded by labor departments; tutoring and after-school programs by education departments; anger management by criminal justice; and wellness centers and parenting classes by health departments.

Consolidate and coordinate funding

Step two in an ideal world would be to conglomerate existing mental health funds. There are over one hundred discrete federal programs funding mental health services supplemented by multiple state, county, and local funding streams. Congress regularly allocates discrete funding for specific subpopulations, including mentally ill children, mentally ill elderly, mentally ill veterans, mentally ill homeless, mentally ill gays, mentally ill moms, and other groups. There are also disease-specific funds. This balkanization of mental health funding prevents funding from helping those who need it most. Medicaid supports hospitalization of people under twenty-two and over sixty-four, but not adults between those ages who are the ones most likely to need hospitalization. Suicide funds go to populations least likely to commit suicide. Legislators feel compassionate when they target subpopulations, but it forces localities to spit out endless applications, maintain patient-level micro-ledgers, and to hire officials to fill out forms rather than doctors to provide care.

A smart but radical approach would combine all the multiple funding streams into a single department, within a single low level of government that would be responsible for all things mental illness in that locality. The department would be responsible for everything: housing, treatment, education, job training, case management, inpatient treatment, outpatient treatment, voluntary treatment, and involuntary treatment. It should even have responsibility for—be billed for—the cost of arresting, trying, and incarcerating those with mental illness in order to create an incentive to reduce those costs.

Drs. John Talbott and Steven Sharfstein proposed the federal government establish a new social security program just for individuals with serious mental illness that would consolidate the multiple task-specific federal funds and pass them on as capitated payments to states to use prospectively, rather than as reimbursement for past services.[1] The new program would allow states to use the funds for treatment, housing, and supports regardless of which federal program provided the original funds.

Following are perhaps more doable ideas.

TARGET THE SICKEST

Use the federal definition of "serious mental illness" and require research, services, and benefits programs to prioritize those who meet the definition

Federal and state governments should use an existing definition of "serious mental illness" in adults and require that a large-stated percentage of their mental health funds serve the population defined. Existing definitions are described in appendix A. Some oppose prioritizing serious mental illness, arguing that we would never let cancer get to stage four before treating it. But cancer does become serious if left untreated. Leaving anxiety untreated does not cause it to become schizophrenia or bipolar disorder.

Incorporate "mental illness" in the nomenclature of bureaucracies

Federal and state agencies should stop shunning the term "mental illness." State departments for the "insane" were renamed "mental illness" departments, then "mental health" departments, then "behavioral health" departments, and now "wellness" departments. With each iteration, their focus moved away from the seriously mentally ill. They should go back to "mental illness." Congress should change the name of the Substance Abuse and Mental Health Services Administration (SAMHSA) to Substance Abuse and Mental *Illness* Services Administration (SAMISA); the Center for Mental Health Services (CMHS) to Center for Mental *Illness* Services (CMIS), and rechristen the National Institute of Mental Health (NIMH) the National Institute of Mental *Illness* (NIMI) so everyone understands the core mission. "Mental illness" is not a pejorative unfit for polite company. It is a useful term designating those who need our help the most.

Put criminal justice leaders on all mental illness policy committees

There should be significant criminal justice representation on all mental health policy boards and commissions. When someone with mental illness is incarcerated, that is a "success" for the mental health department: one less person it has to treat. The policies embraced by the mental health industry, like closing psychiatric hospitals, making involuntary treatment difficult, and diverting funds to the non–seriously mentally ill increase homelessness, arrest, violence, incarceration, and burden on police. Police and sheriffs should be at the table so they can reject these policies when the mental health advocates propose them.

REORIENT FEDERAL PROGRAMS

Preserve hospitals by eliminating the IMD Exclusion

As described in chapter 6, there is a dangerous nationwide shortage of psychiatric hospital beds largely due to the Institutes for Mental Disease (IMD) Exclusion prohibiting Medicaid from reimbursing states for adults with mental illness between ages twenty-two and sixty-four who need long-term care in psychiatric institutions. Homelessness and inappropriate incarceration and suicide are the result. Language to eliminate this federally sanctioned discrimination can be found in H.R. 2757, introduced by Representative Eddie Bernice Johnson.[2] This is the most important change Congress can make.

Eliminate Medicare's 190-day cap on hospitalization and focus its spending on serious mental illness

Medicare imposes a 190-day lifetime cap on psychiatric hospitalization.[3] The cap causes states to discharge elderly and disabled adult mentally ill from hospitals into squalid nursing homes simply to shift the cost of care to Medicare. The discriminatory cap should be eliminated.

Eliminate or radically reform SAMHSA and CMHS

As documented in chapter 7, it would be difficult to improve services for the seriously mentally ill without eliminating or radically reforming SAMHSA and CMHS. They are the major barriers to prioritizing and treating the most seriously mentally ill and to implementing evidence-based practices. The 21st Century Cures Act attempts to reform SAMHSA by establishing the position of assistant secretary and requiring the appointee to focus on serious mental illness. If that approach doesn't work, then legislation should be introduced to eliminate SAMHSA and transfer NREPP to NIMH; the Youth Violence Prevention and its Criminal and Juvenile Justice efforts to DOJ; suicide prevention and Programs of Regional and National Significance and all the data collection programs to CDC; and the Disaster Response programs to Homeland Security. If SAMHSA and CMHS can't be eliminated, legislation should require them to:

- Focus on serious mental illness using one of the definitions in appendix A.
- Distribute funds based on measurable and meaningful outcomes like reducing homelessness, arrest, violence, incarceration, suicide, and hospitalization.
- Be headed by medical doctors with demonstrated expertise at helping the most seriously mentally ill.
- Stop distributing funds to antipsychiatry groups and organizations that work to prevent treatment of the seriously mentally ill or do not believe mental illness exists.[4]
- Stop requiring states to use mental health block grants on non-evidence-based practices and programs that do not serve people with serious mental illness.[5]

Focus PAIMI on helping the seriously mentally ill get into treatment rather than out of treatment

As described in chapter 8, the threat of anti-treatment suits from federally funded PAIMI organizations ("Disability Rights [Name of State]"), facilitated by the National Disability Rights Network (NDRN), is a major impediment to state and federal legislators who want to help the most seriously ill.[6] The PAIMI program should be eliminated. Funds and responsibility for any important work PAIMI does can be transferred to the Civil Rights of Institutionalized Persons Act (CRIPA) division within DOJ. CRIPA largely covers the same areas PAIMI does but without the anti-treatment bias and could be mildly expanded to allow it to represent individuals. It should also be required to ensure that people with serious mental illness are not excluded from mental health programs.

Free parent-caregivers from HIPAA handcuffs and FERPA restraints

Regulations issued to carry out the Health Insurance Portability and Accountability Act (HIPAA) and, for those in school, the Family Educational Rights and Privacy Act (FERPA) largely prohibit doctors, hospitals, and treatment programs from disclosing medical information about people with mental illness to their families, even when those families are the ones providing housing, case management, transportation, and support for their mentally ill loved ones.[7] Because families can't be told the diagnosis of their family members, what medicines they should be taking, and when their next doctor's appointments are, they are powerless to see that prescriptions get refilled or to arrange transportation to doctors.

HIPAA and FERPA are laws, not constitutional rights. HIPAA and FERPA regulations should be amended so parents who provide care and support for mentally ill relatives out of love get the same information that paid providers receive. Appendix E contains suggestions.

Enable consumers to import medications from out of the country and Medicare to negotiate for lower prices

Eliminating the provisions in the Medicare Prescription Drug, Improvement, and Modernization Act of 2003 that prevent consumers from importing medicines from countries with lower prices and prevent the government from negotiating prices with pharmaceutical companies would lower prices of medicines and enable more people to receive them.[8]

OPTIMIZE RESEARCH

Invest in basic and treatment research focused on serious mental illness

The government must provide more funding for basic research on the causes of and treatments for serious mental illness. When he was the director of NIMH, Dr. Thomas Insel properly reoriented the NIMH research port-folio toward serious mental illness and specific underlying biology rather than the more amorphous collection of symptoms described in the all-encompassing *Diagnostic and Statistical Manual* (*DSM*).[9] His replacement, Dr. Joshua Gordon, should continue Insel's work. Some criticized this approach, suggesting that biological research takes too long to bear fruit and that research should therefore focus on services. But services research is often little more than combining the known standard ingredients of medications, early intervention, supported housing, case management, psy-chotherapy, and—for a dose of political correctness—peer support, mixing them in different proportions, targeting them to different subgroups, giving it a brand name, and claiming to have created a new model that improves outcomes when compared to models that don't offer all that. These new models are then placed on a shelf, and no one benefits from them.

Individuals who want to contribute to high-quality research focused on serious mental illness should donate to nonprofits like the Stanley Medical Research Institute (SMRI), the Brain and Behavior Research Foundation (BBR), the International Mental Health Research Organiza-tion (IMHRO), and the Broad Institute.

Improve the quality of research

Research by pharmaceutical companies on new medications is becoming unreliable because the companies have a financial incentive to report posi-tive results and hide adverse side effects. One possibly problematic solu-tion might be to require pharmaceutical companies to pay the FDA or another independent agency to conduct the research with the pharmaceu-tical company blinded to the progress and results.[10] Pharmaceutical com-panies could also be required to make the full anonymized data sets on their research available for public scrutiny. This would allow one pharmaceutical company to criticize the work of another, which would hopefully result in the emergence of truth.

But it's not just pharmaceutical companies that are reporting bad results. Dr. Thomas Insel noted, "As much as 80 percent of the science from academic labs, even science published in the best journals, cannot be replicated."[11] Many of those studies rely on multiple regression analysis, an after-the-fact attempt to find if two previously recorded outcomes are correlated. For example, an after-the-fact study of airline passengers might find that those who wear diamonds traveled more than those who don't, leading to a study and headline reporting "Diamonds Proven to Cause Air Travel." Of course, individuals who wear diamonds are likely wealthier than other travelers. If an experimental design study tested the result, it would likely find that the cause of the increased travel was increased wealth, not bigger diamonds. University of Michigan psychology professor Richard Nisbett has made misuse of regression analysis his cause celebre, going so far as to propose putting a warning on articles, stating, "These data are based on multiple regression analysis" as a way of signaling "you probably shouldn't read the article because you're quite likely to get non-information or misinformation."[12]

Another problem is that science journals will only publish studies with profound positive or unique findings, forcing academics to game their results to get published. If the research as originally designed doesn't show good results, no problem: "Data can be tortured until they confess."[13] The poor results may be retroactively analyzed—"data-mined"—to tease out a good result ("P-Hacking").[14] Studies analyze multiple, unimportant outcomes, like sense of hopefulness, happiness, or well-being and ignore meaningful outcomes like reductions in homelessness, arrest, violence, incarceration, and hospitalization. Mathematical contortions are imposed at will. If researchers find just a tiny improvement in any one meaningless outcome, or in any subset of the total group, they hide the null results and successfully label their intervention an "evidence-based program" due to the one single slightly significant result in the newly defined subgroup. Additionally, the pernicious effect of political correctness causes researchers to emphasize findings that portray mental health in a positive light, deemphasize findings that highlight problems caused by people with serious mental illness, and skew their abstracts accordingly.

There is a whole group of scientists, "neurocritics," who are working to solve these problems.[15] Among the solutions they propose are having studies "pre-registered," with the methods, data analysis techniques, and outcomes that are to be measured publicly disclosed before the study begins.[16] If the research is government-funded, a mechanism should be established so the findings on the pre-registered questions are published even when null. Full underlying data sets could be made anonymous and publicly available so others can analyze them for bias.[17] The Center for Open Science (COS) created Transparency and Open Promotion (TOP) Guidelines that numerous journals and organizations have agreed to abide by.[18] Another fascinating idea is to hide the results of the studies from the reviewers and editors who choose what the scientific journals publish. This would force them to choose studies based solely on the scientific rigor rather than how well the results were gamed.[19]

There is no way to control what the mass media reports, but it would be helpful if it was more skeptical of the success stories, feel-good programs, pop psychology, pseudo-science, self-reports, and multiple regression studies the mental health industry encourages it to report on. Newspapers regularly run glowing anecdotal stories on interventions without questioning what they are being told.[20] This wide distribution of junk science is causing policy makers who rely on it to waste millions.

JUDICIAL REFORMS

Allow treatment before tragedy

Charles Krauthammer wrote, "Today you can intervene to help the homeless mentally ill only if you can prove that they are dangerous to themselves or to others. That standard is not just unfeeling, it is uncivilized. The standard should not be dangerousness but helplessness. Society has an obligation to save people from degradation, not just death."[21] We should prevent tragedy, not require it. Every state should implement the following civil commitment reforms.

Enact, fund, and use Assisted Outpatient Treatment (AOT)

As described in chapter 6 and appendix D, for the small group who cannot or will not comply with voluntary treatment, and have a history of becoming homeless, arrested, or violent as a result, there is no more proven, humane, or cost-efficient intervention than Assisted Outpatient Treatment (AOT). In addition to involuntarily committing the patient to accept community treatment, the court order can involuntarily commit the mental health system to provide it, thereby ending the industry's addiction to cherry-picking the easiest to treat.

The Treatment Advocacy Center created a model AOT bill and helps legislators looking to implement it.[22] New York's Kendra's Law is another good model.[23] All AOT legislation should *require* mental health authorities to receive reports from family members about seriously ill loved ones who may qualify for AOT and to investigate and file petitions when appropriate. If that provision is not included, AOT will be on the books but rarely used. From a political standpoint, increasing the use of AOT is more likely to occur when advocates from the criminal justice community speak out. The International Association of Chiefs of Police, National Sheriffs' Association, and Department of Justice have all endorsed AOT. So has the United States Conference of Catholic Bishops.

Screen civilly committed patients and mentally ill prisoners who are about to be released

States should require all people with serious mental illness who are being discharged from jails and prisons or who are coming to the end of an involuntary inpatient commitment to be evaluated and connected to outpatient services, including AOT if appropriate. These are the highest-risk patients. They have already been ruled criminal or were a danger to self or others. They are the ones who are most likely to become a tragedy without treatment.

Enact other civil commitment reforms

Every state should also:[24]

- Allow individuals to be moved between AOT and inpatient commitment as appropriate without excessive procedural hurdles. AOT is often useful when individuals are no longer at imminent risk, and inpatient commitment is needed when they are. The two systems should work together seamlessly while ensuring adequate due process protections.
- Determine if an individual lacks capacity—i.e., can be treated over objection—at the same time the decision on involuntary commitment is being made.[25] Some have suggested limiting commitment to those who meet both the commitment standard and the lack of capacity standard.[26] This would ensure that those who are committed can also be treated. Utah does this.
- Interpret the "dangerousness standard" more broadly than "imminently" dangerous. Assisted treatment should be available when an individual:
  - ° Is gravely disabled, which means that the person is substantially unable, except for reasons of indigence, to provide for any basic needs, such as food, clothing, shelter, health, or safety, or
  - ° Is likely to substantially deteriorate if not provided with timely treatment, or
  - ° Lacks capacity, which means that as a result of the brain disorder the person is unable to fully understand or lacks judgment to make an informed decision regarding the person's need for treatment, care, or supervision. Wisconsin's "Fifth Standard" is a useful model.[27]
- Consider past history in making determinations about involuntary commitment and/or court-ordered treatment, since past history is often a sound way to anticipate the future course of illness. A person who deteriorated and became homeless and dangerous off treatment in the past is likely to become homeless and dangerous if he or she again goes off treatment. California recently amended its civil commitment law to allow consideration of past history.[28]

- Provide an independent administrative and/or quasi-judicial review of all involuntary commitment and/or court-ordered treatment determinations. Individuals being considered for commitment should be given free representation by someone knowledgeable about brain disorders and the opportunity to submit evidence in opposition to commitment. However, due process is faster and more affordable when conducted by an administrative or quasi-judicial body rather than in a full trial.
- Vest specific treatment decisions with medical professionals working in conjunction with the individual, family, and other involved parties, rather than requiring courts to rule on strictly medical issues.
- Set the legal standard to justify emergency commitments for initial twenty-four to seventy-two hours at "information and belief" and for periods beyond that at "preponderance of evidence" if possible, and "clear and convincing evidence" if not.
- Subject involuntary commitments and/or court-ordered treatment decisions to periodic administrative review to ascertain whether circumstances justify continuation.
- Require private and public health insurance plans to cover the costs of involuntary inpatient and outpatient commitment and/or court-ordered treatment.[29]

Train law enforcement

Police step in after one condition has been met: the mental health system failed. So police and sheriffs have become front-line mental health workers and therefore need training. Crisis Intervention Teams (CIT) are teams of senior officers within police departments who receive special training on how to deescalate interactions with the seriously mentally ill and connect them to treatment. But they only work in nonemergency situations where the initial responding officers can stand back, call the specially trained team, and wait for it to arrive. Chief (ret.) Michael Biasotti, newly appointed to the CMHS advisory board, believes police interact with the mentally ill so frequently that *all* officers should be trained as part of their basic training at the police academies, before they join their forces. Many police departments are too small to have dedicated teams and all police go on mental health calls, so it is better to have all of them trained than not. Portland, Oregon, and New Windsor, New York, are training all their officers. The highly respected major (ret.) Sam Cochran, the inventor of CIT training, works through the CIT Center at the University of Memphis and CIT International to help communities implement CIT training, and NAMI also has an initiative to assist with training.[30]

Create and expand mental health courts

States and localities should establish mental health courts.[31] If agreed to by the defense and prosecution, cases involving people with serious mental illness are referred from the criminal court to the mental health court.[32] Mental health court judges can order a psychiatric evaluation and, if appropriate, order the individual to accept court-ordered treatment in lieu of determining guilt or innocence. Mental health courts are similar to AOT in that they provide mandated and monitored treatment. But AOT provides the treatment *before* a crime has been committed while mental health courts can only do it *after* a crime has been committed. The individual must continually reappear before the court so the judge can ensure continued compliance. Mental health courts work. Fewer mentally ill individuals are rearrested, booked, and use substances, and they serve fewer days in jail.[33] Seventy-nine percent stay out of trouble and "graduate" (have charges dropped). The Bureau of Justice Assistance at DOJ and the National Center for State Courts help localities create the courts.[34]

Implement a "Guilty and Mentally Ill (GAMI)" plea

"Guilty" and "Not Guilty by Reason of Insanity (NGRI)" are often inadequate solutions for people who committed crimes because of mental illness. Some are guilty *and* mentally ill. Jurors are reluctant to find people with mental illness NGRI because that sends the person to a hospital until sanity is restored, after which he or she will be theoretically released, free to go off medications and create mayhem again. As a practical matter, few judges are willing to accept responsibility for releasing those found NGRI, so even when sanity is restored they are kept committed. Another injustice. After John Hinckley was found NGRI for the attempted assassination of President Ronald Reagan, states made using the insanity plea more difficult.[35] Some states replaced it with "guilty because of mental illness (GBMI)." Individuals found GBMI go to a hospital until their sanity is restored and then to jail to finish out their sentence. This forces individuals who had no culpability for their actions to go to jail at the exact time it's not needed—when they've regained their sanity.

States should enact "Guilty *and* Mentally Ill" (GAMI) legislation. If the cause of the crime was lack of treatment, then the person should be sentenced to mandatory long-term mental illness treatment—including medications—so the person doesn't become a criminal again. The sentence to "treatment years" would be as long as, or longer than the *maximum* sentence that would be imposed had the person been found guilty. The treatment could take place in an inpatient setting on a locked ward or on an outpatient basis. Over time, it would most likely be both. The sentenced patient could be moved from inpatient care to outpatient care when doing well and instantly back to inpatient care with no further court hearings needed if he or she started to deteriorate. In either case, the individual would be closely monitored by a psychiatric probation officer to see that the person stays on violence-preventing medications.[36] If this change were adopted, incarceration would be reduced, safety ensured, and money saved.

Initiate Psychiatric Parole and Probation (Forensic AOT)

Many mentally ill prisoners could be released if they were put in mandated and monitored community treatment similar to Assisted Outpatient Treatment or that used by mental health courts. This can be accomplished by establishing Psychiatric Parole and Psychiatric Probation programs.

Establish Secure Congregate Therapeutic House Arrest Facilities

The Greenburger Center for Social and Criminal Justice is developing a new model to take mentally ill who won't get better in prison and put them in a place where they will improve, while still providing tight security. Hope House, to be located in Bronx, New York, will be an alternative to incarceration that places mentally ill people accused of felony-level crimes in a small therapeutic, locked group home or congregate setting with on-premises support for up to two years.[37] The diversion would have to be agreed to by the mentally ill person who committed the crime, the district attorney, and the court. An unsecured surety bond would be issued for each patient/prisoner to facilitate the return to prison should he or she elope.

TREAT THE SERIOUSLY ILL

Fund programs that have actual evidence they work

The government should only fund programs that meet a strict definition of "evidence-based," which is one that has (a) *independent* proof that it (b) improves a *meaningful* outcome in (c) people with *serious* mental illness. As seen in chapter 12, much of what is funded does not meet those three criteria. The studies are not independent, the outcomes being measured are not meaningful, and the people being treated do not have serious mental illness.

The term "evidence" as used by SAMHSA, CMHS, and the mental health industry often means self-reports on meaningless metrics like "sense of hopefulness," or process measures like how many people clicked on a website. Meaningful metrics include reductions in homelessness, arrests, incarcerations, hospitalizations, and suicides. But care must be taken to ensure that programs don't improve those rates by refusing to accept the most seriously ill.

Ensure access to doctors, medications, and electroconvulsive therapy (ECT) for the most seriously mentally ill

As shown in appendix B, arrest, crime, and homelessness among the seriously mentally ill are almost always associated with lack of treatment. Access to constantly titrated medications (the right medications at the right dose) is the *sine qua non* for turning people who think the FBI planted a transmitter in their head into those who are able to survive safely in the community. Access to doctors—on demand when a crisis occurs, not two months later "by appointment only"—is key. There aren't enough psychiatrists working with the seriously mentally ill, so they are forced to limit appointments to seven minutes, and appointments with them have to be scheduled long in advance. This prevents them from taking an appropriate history, thoughtfully titrating medications, or being available off-hours and at the last minute to handle emergencies. Half of psychiatrists don't take insurance. Half of US counties don't have a psychiatrist. Compensating for the shortage of psychiatrists can be achieved by offering telepsychiatry to those in underserved areas, giving nurse practitioners and psychologists licenses to prescribe or refill medications if working under psychiatrists, requiring psychiatrists who receive publicly funded training to accept public insurance for a certain period, and raising reimbursement rates and allowances for training so more doctors accept insurance and enter the specialty.[38]

There must also be programs that get medications to those who can't afford the copays or need transportation or have trouble with the paperwork. Electroconvulsive therapy (ECT) must also be made available to those who can benefit from it, which means ensuring that more hospitals have the machines and doctors well trained in how to use them.

Create supported housing and group homes

The seriously mentally ill already live in the communities, but they should be living in housing rather than on the streets. For many, housing is the most important service after access to doctors and medications. Supported housing combines housing with an appropriate level of case management services to keep patients functioning.[39] Group homes with on-premises support are terrific, but "not in my backyard" (NIMBY) activity makes them difficult to site, and the IMD Exclusion limits them to sixteen beds. To avoid this problem, the industry is moving away from establishing group housing to handing out housing vouchers and placing clients in "scatter-site" apartments that do not have 24/7 on-premises support. This less intensive form of supported housing works for some, but fails for others.

The industry is also moving toward the "Housing First" model. Housing First is based on the idea that people should be given permanent housing rather than treatment first. It sometimes works. But while actively psychotic, some people with mental illness would not be able to maintain the housing and a landlord is not likely to accept them.

The government is also balkanizing housing by allocating it to multiple subcategories including people "at risk" of becoming homeless, veterans, GLBTs, families, teens, pregnant moms, domestic abuse victims, and others. Sometimes the government takes housing away from one group, so it can announce "new" housing for another. Whenever housing or services are available for people with mental illness and anyone else, it is usually the "anyone else," not the mentally ill, who benefit. Stephen Eide of New York's Manhattan Institute came out with a thoughtful proposal that cited both the unmet need and the potential savings, and concluded two-thirds of supported housing should go to the seriously ill, specifically those with schizophrenia and bipolar disorder.[40]

Localities have to create more housing and stop pressuring patients to "graduate" from congregate settings such as nursing homes, adult homes, group homes, and hospitals with appropriate support and move into lower levels of support. States do this to save money. They are also under pressure from federally funded mental health lawyers who use Olmstead to encourage this. They have a misguided belief that "less restrictive" is always better and everyone can provide for themselves. This forced migration from congregate housing with 24/7 support to independent living with a drive-by caseworker visiting twice a week for less than an hour causes some seriously ill to lose their social networks and become isolated, alone, and forced to fend for themselves.

Establish Intensive Case Management (ICM) and Assertive Community Treatment (ACT) teams

Individuals with serious mental illness need intensive, time-consuming *professional* support to prevent them from becoming victimized by their own disordered thinking. Assertive Community Treatment (ACT) teams and Intensive Case Management (ICM) services described in chapter 6 provide this special service.

These programs are well regarded, but many states call their ordinary case management programs ACT or ICM without maintaining fidelity to the models. Unfortunately, the models are also becoming needlessly expensive because the SAMHSA-funded peer community insists that peers be hired in addition to the professionals, thereby driving up costs without any known increase in efficacy. States should establish true ICM and ACT teams and ensure that they maintain fidelity to the model and are assigned to the most seriously ill.

Open clubhouses

Clubhouses, like the world-famous Fountain House run by Kenn Dudek in New York, are professionally run programs with a physical location that provide comprehensive one-stop support for the most seriously mentally ill, who are known at the clubhouse as "members." The clubhouse offers a long-term versus time-limited commitment to members by keeping them enrolled even if they become symptomatic, high-needs, hospitalized, incarcerated—or recover. Clubhouses help members rehabilitate by requiring them to cook, clean, answer phones, pay bills, shop, and do whatever else is needed to maintain the clubhouse community. Members share in decision making for the clubhouse. Staff attempts to arrange for paid, supported, subsidized jobs for members with local businesses and assistance in accessing education. The clubhouse provides or arranges for crisis intervention services, social and recreational events, and help in finding and maintaining housing when they don't provide it directly. The Clubhouse Model is stellar, and every community should have at least one.

SAMHSA does not encourage states to use block grants to fund clubhouses, and many of the important services they provide are not reimbursable through Medicaid or Medicare, forcing the executive directors to spend much of their time raising money rather than serving the ill. In addition, because their services are often provided communally, allocating the cost of the social worker who arranged the service is difficult because public and private insurance programs require services to be billed patient by patient. Medicaid should establish a robust "blended rate" for clubhouses, insurance programs should reimburse for them, and localities should establish them. Clubhouse International helps those wishing to establish clubhouses.[41]

The people who run the mental health industry are not bad people. But their goal is no longer to help those with serious mental illness. Congress and state legislators have to replace industry-driven mission creep with real mission control. In the last chapter we discuss how likely that is to happen.

Chapter 17

THE FUTURE

"Never believe that a few caring people can't change the world. For, indeed, that's all who ever have."

—Margaret Mead

When asked if things are getting better, I'd like to say yes. They are for my sister-in-law, Lynn, who found a good group home and is now once more trying her hand at independent supported living. But for most of the seriously mentally ill, it is not getting better. Homelessness, arrest, violence, incarceration, shootings by police, shootings of police, tragedies, and expenditures are all climbing. More people without serious mental illness are getting services while fewer with it are. Programs that help the most seriously ill are ignored while those that don't help have millions of dollars poured into them.

Will things get better? I think it depends on how many tragedies there are and how many innocents are killed. Tragedies let the public see behind the curtain and get a glimpse of a worst-case scenario of what can happen when someone with serious mental illness is allowed to go untreated. Major reforms like Kendra's Law, Laura's Law, and the Helping Families in Mental Health Act came about as a result of public pressure in reaction to violence. Progress occurs in spite of the mental health industry, not because of it.

Tragedies present a teachable moment. But even in the aftermath of tragedies, reform is difficult. The media self-righteously declares a moratorium on mentioning the name of the perpetrator, in the mistaken belief that it was a desire for notoriety, rather than a brain disorder that caused the tragedy. It presents the public with a black-and-white comic strip, "forces of evil" view by sanctimoniously substituting the words "the killer" for the mentally ill perpetrators' real name. The public is prevented from learning that this is not a monster, but a young man with serious mental illness who was allowed to go untreated. In many cases, the media even blames the family. "Why didn't the parents do anything?"

In the aftermath of tragedy, mental health advocates try to stop reform. Rather than propose solutions, they turn up efforts to divert attention away from violence. They declare that smart solutions proposed by law enforcement and families of the most seriously ill are "knee-jerk" reactions.

Democrats (disclosure: I am one) buy into this mental health industry narrative and react to the tragedies with time-worn proposals for more of the same: throw money at inconsequential sideshows. They call for more outreach programs to identify the mentally ill. But identification is not the problem. Families beg for treatment for people already known to be seriously ill and cannot get it. Democrats have been taught by the mental health industry and advocates that hospitals are not needed, everyone recovers, and spewing forth psychotic delusional thoughts is a right to be protected. Democrats have been taught that to even admit to violence is "stigmatizing."

Yet, there is hope. And it's coming from surprising quarters. Republicans have generally not been supportive of programs that help the needy, but they have been supportive of cutting costs, ending government waste, and restoring law and order, and are starting to be concerned about massive use of incarceration. It is largely Republicans who have embraced providing better treatment for the most seriously ill and reorienting existing programs toward them, rather than toward the least ill. In the last few years, Representative Tim Murphy and Senators John Cornyn and Bill Cassidy all proposed legislation containing smart ways to help the most seriously ill. Some argue that other Republicans are only interested in mental health policy as a way to divert attention from gun control. Maybe. But while that may be an impure motivation, it has led to proposals that address core problems faced by the most seriously ill and the public.

Further support for better care comes from the criminal justice community. Police and sheriffs are sick and tired of being forced to run a shadow mental health system. They want the mental health industry to accept responsibility for treating the most seriously ill. They are working to return care of the seriously ill to the state and local mental health departments. Sheriff Tom Dart in Chicago, Chief (ret.) Michael Biasotti in New Windsor, New York, and Judge Steve Leifman in Florida are some of those in the criminal justice community seeking reform. But while many others in criminal justice know something is wrong, they do not know enough about the internal workings of the mental health system to fix it. Mental illness advocates who want to improve care must bring criminal justice into their conversations.

Another perpetual area of hope is in research. If we find a cure, game over. Before leaving the National Institute of Mental Health (NIMH), Dr. Thomas Insel focused it on searching for causes and cures and hopefully the next NIMH director will stay on that path. Private charities focused on mental illness research are starting to gain financial support from millionaires with seriously ill family members. But the brain hides its secrets. It can't be cut open except after it has stopped working, so brain research has moved at a snail's pace. No major new treatments have been introduced in decades.

PRESIDENT DONALD TRUMP

The election of Donald Trump could, counterintuitively for some, bode well. It is true that his proposals to end the Affordable Care Act and block grant Medicaid funds to the states could be disastrous, but not enough is known about those plans to judge them yet. On the plus side, his policy platform called for freeing parents of the seriously mentally ill from HIPAA Handcuffs, reforming the mental health system, and using mental health resources to reduce violence.[1] He has said he will "drain the swamp" in Washington, and no swamp is more fetid than the one at SAMHSA and CMHS. He could keep his campaign promise by appointing an assistant secretary of Mental Health and Substance Use Disorders who is committed to reforming them.

WHAT'S MISSING?

The major impediment to reform is the lack of a national grassroots organization advocating exclusively on behalf of the most seriously mentally ill.

Organizations like Mental Illness Policy Org. and the Treatment Advocacy Center that do advocate for the most seriously ill are not grassroots membership organizations and so have not generated the massive number of calls and visits to legislators needed to effect change. NAMI National used to advocate exclusively for the seriously ill, but it has moved on to all mental health, and no organization has filled the void.

This is the greatest need: a well-funded grassroots organization, free of pharmaceutical and government funding, that advocates exclusively for the most seriously ill, a place where families of the most seriously ill can gather and organize to improve the system at the state and federal levels.

There are hundreds of thousands of heroic moms, dads, sisters, brothers, and children around the country who desperately seek help for seriously mentally ill loved ones and cannot get it. Who will help them?

SERIOUS MENTAL ILLNESS DEFINED

Two major federal efforts and many lesser efforts did a good job of defining serious mental illness in adults and calculating its prevalence. They all concluded that adults with schizophrenia and bipolar disorder constitute the bulk of those with serious mental illness, and serious mental illness is relatively rare, affecting less than 6 percent of the population. We use the definition established when SAMHSA's Center for Mental Health Services (CMHS) was created, because it is used in the annual National Survey on Drug Use and Health (NSDUH), is based on sound science, and there is a large amount of data on it.[1] That definition defined serious mental illnesses in adults as,

> "[T]hose mental illnesses that met the criteria of [latest edition of] *DSM* and ... resulted in *functional impairment* which *substantially* interferes with or limits one or more *major* life activities."[2] (Emphasis added.)

To calculate how many adults over eighteen in each state had serious mental illness, CMHS had to define "functional impairment."[3] CMHS noted that "90% [of those meeting the criteria for serious mental illness] either have a severe disorder like schizophrenia or bipolar disorder, or a disorder and work impairment, or a disorder and report being suicidal." Its latest estimate is that 4 percent of the population over eighteen has serious mental illness.[4] However, CMHS fails to focus on those individuals and regularly takes steps to include millions more.[5]

A separate major effort to define serious mental illness and calculate its prevalence took place in 1993 when the Senate Committee on Appropriations asked that the National Advisory Mental Health Council report on how much it would cost to provide insurance coverage for people with "severe mental illness" commensurate with the coverage of other illnesses.[6] Congress itself defined "severe mental illness" for the Advisory Council:

> Severe mental illness is defined through diagnosis, disability, and dura-tion, and includes disorders with psychotic symptoms such as schizo-phrenia, schizoaffective disorder, manic depressive disorder, autism, as well as severe forms of other disorders such as major depression, panic disorder, and obsessive compulsive disorder.[7]

In this effort, Congress relied largely on diagnosis and symptoms, rather than functional impairment, to define severe mental illness. This may have left out some individuals, but not many. Using the congressionally man-dated definition, the National Advisory Mental Health Council found that "2.8% of Americans experience severe mental disorders in a one-year time period." The council found that without accounting for overlaps, schizo-phrenia affected 1.5 percent of adults; bipolar disorder, 1percent; major depression, 1.1 percent; panic disorder, 0.4 percent; and obsessive-compul-sive disorder, 0.6 percent. Individuals with mental illness other than those listed above were considered to have a serious mental illness only if they had a qualifying functional impairment.

There have been other attempts to define and calculate the preva-lence of serious mental illness. The Department of Health and Human Services (HHS) conducted the National Comorbidity Survey Replication (NCS-R) by interviewing nine thousand adults between 2001 and 2002. It defined "severe" mental illness more broadly as,

> [C]ases that had any of the following: suicide attempt within the pre-ceding 12 months with serious lethality intent; work disability or substan-tial limitation due to a mental or substance disorder; psychosis; bipolar I or II disorder; substance dependence with serious role impairment (as defined by disorder-specific impairment questions); an impulse-control disorder with repeated serious violence; or any disorder that resulted in an inability to function in a particular social role for 30 or more days in the year.[8]

That study found the twelve-month prevalence of serious mental illness to be 5.8 percent. The American Psychiatric Association requires the presence of a "functional impairment" to receive a *DSM* diagnosis of schizophrenia, severe major depressive disorder, and severe bipolar disorder and therefore includes all three as serious.[9]

Colorado's civil commitment code contains a concise definition of serious mental illness that is based on diagnosis. "Serious mental illness" defines those suffering from schizophrenia, a major affective disorder, a delusional disorder, or another mental disorder with psychotic features.[10] NIMH concurs.

CONCLUSION

The best independent efforts to define serious mental illnesses in adults have concluded that schizophrenia spectrum disorders, major bipolar disorder, and severe major depression are serious and make up the bulk of people with serious mental illnesses. While other illnesses may also be serious if they substantially affect the ability to function, including them does not raise the percentage by much. The line between "any" mental illness and "serious" mental illness is debatable, but the extremities are clear. The policies promoted in this book hold validity whether or not that line moves a little to the left or right. It is only the mental health industry that insists "all" mental illness is serious.

STUDIES ON VIOLENCE
AND MENTAL ILLNESS

*"The data that have recently become available, fairly read,
suggest the one conclusion I did not want to reach: whether
the sample is people who are selected for treatment as inmates
or patients in institutions or people randomly chosen from
the open community, and no matter how many social or
demographic factors are statistically taken into account, there
appears to be a relationship between mental disorder and
violent behavior."*

—Dr. John Monahan[1]

*"I'd like to say something which I think is unpopular for many
people in the mental health community. But the data are, I
believe, fairly unambiguous. . . . An active untreated psychotic
illness is associated with irrational behavior, and violence can be
part of that. And the numbers are rather stunning. . . . There is
an association between untreated psychosis and violence, especially . . . towards family and friends. People with treated mental
illness, by contrast, are at no higher risk. . . . [There is] a fifteen
fold reduction in the risk of homicide . . . with treatment."*

—Dr. Thomas Insel[2]

Summary: People with poor mental health, mental illness, or serious mental illness are not more violent than others. People with serious mental illness that is allowed to go untreated, as a group, are more violent than the general population.

247

When the public asks, "Are the mentally ill more violent?" we believe they are asking about the homeless psychotic mentally ill on the streets and people "acting crazy," not their coworkers and family members who have anxiety, mild depression, or sadness and are easily treated. Those who argue that the mentally ill are *not* more violent generally quote studies of the treated. The studies show treatment works. No more. No less. And they rarely quote studies limited to the seriously ill. The following brings together research on mental illness and violence to others included throughout the book as well as other information. It does not include studies on violence to self or suicide. Many were culled from collections maintained by the Treatment Advocacy Center and Mental Illness Policy Org.

COMMUNITY VIOLENCE

- A recent meta-analysis of five studies of 4,480 individuals showed that 16 percent of those with schizophrenia, 27 percent of those with bipolar disorder, and 37 percent of those with major depression attempted an act of community violence. This is significantly higher than controls.[3]
- A meta-analysis of 204 studies of psychosis as a risk factor for violence reported that "compared with individuals with no mental disorders, psychosis was significantly associated with a 49–68% increase in the odds of violence."[4]
- A large study of 34,653 people published in 2012 found that "those with serious mental illness irrespective of substance abuse status, were significantly more likely to be violent than those with no mental or substance use disorders."[5]
- Eight studies of homicide and schizophrenia combined found that 6.5 percent of homicide offenders had a diagnosis of schizophrenia.[6]
- In a Swedish study of 8,003 people discharged from the hospital with a diagnosis of schizophrenia, 13.2 percent committed at least one violent crime compared with 5.3 percent of the general population. Concurrent abuse of alcohol or drugs accounted for much of the increased rate.[7]
- A study in Wales and England found the mentally ill are more likely to be murderers than murdered and that high rates of victimiza-

tion were partly due to being murdered by other people with mental illness.[8]

- A review of twenty-two studies published between 1990 and 2004 "concluded that major mental disorders per se, especially schizophrenia, even without alcohol or drug abuse, are indeed associated with higher risks for interpersonal violence."[9]
- A study of 961 young adults in New Zealand reported that individuals with schizophrenia and associated disorders were two and one-half times more likely than controls to have been violent in the past year. If the person was also a substance abuser, the incidence of violent behavior was even higher.[10]
- In Sweden, among 3,743 individuals discharged from the hospital with a diagnosis of bipolar disorder, 8.4 percent committed a violent crime compared to 3.5 percent of the general population.[11]
- An examination of studies published from 1970 to 2007 found that "sound epidemiologic research has left no doubt about a significant relation between psychosis and violence."[12]
- A 1998 study of 331 people with severe mental illness reported that 17.8 percent "had engaged in serious violent acts that involved weapons or caused injury." It also found that "substance abuse problems, medication noncompliance, and low insight into illness operate together to increase violence risk."[13]
- The 1980–1983 Epidemiological Catchment Area (ECA) survey reported much higher rates of violent behavior among people with severe mental illness living in the community compared to other community residents. For example, people with schizophrenia were twenty-one times more likely to have used a weapon in a fight.[14]
- A 1992 study comparing people with severe mental illness living in the community in New York with other community residents found the former group to be three times more likely to commit violent acts such as weapons use or "hurting someone badly." The sicker the individual, the more likely the person was to have been violent.[15]
- A study of all 2,005 individuals convicted of homicide or attempted homicide in Sweden from 1988 to 2001 reported that 229, or 11 percent, had schizophrenia or bipolar disorder. Substance abuse and medication noncompliance were significant risk factors.[16]

- In Singapore, 110 individuals were charged with murder between 1997 and 2001. Among these, 7 had schizophrenia, 1 had bipolar disorder, and 2 had delusional disorders. Thus, 10 out of 110 (9 percent) had psychotic disorders.[17]
- A 2008 study found that more than 26,000 Americans with a mental illness were incarcerated for murder.[18]

WORKPLACE VIOLENCE

- "According to the federal Bureau of Labor Statistics, half of all non-fatal injuries resulting from workplace assaults occur in health care and social service settings. . . . The most dangerous settings are psychiatric units and nursing homes, where patients are often confused, disoriented or suffering from mental ailments."[19]
- Psychiatric nurses are frequent victims of workplace violence, much of it perpetrated by patients.[20]
- "Recent studies and news reports suggest that when agitation escalates into full-blown assault, nurses are often the victims. . . . Of those physically assaulted on the job, 38% talked with a colleague afterward, but only 19% filed a formal report."[21]
- Officials at Napa State Hospital in California logged about 3,000 acts of aggression against patients and staff in 2012. This may not be surprising since 90 percent of patients admitted to the five state psychiatric hospitals in California get there only after being channeled through the criminal justice system.[22]
- According to the American Psychiatric Nurses Association position paper, 75–100 percent of the nursing staff on acute psychiatric units had been assaulted during their careers. Twenty-eight percent of the clinical staff reported an assault within the last six months. The survey reported the rate of nonfatal, job-related violent crime among general medical physicians is 16.2 per 1,000, while for psychiatrists and mental health professionals, the rate jumped to 68.2 per 1,000.[23]

VIOLENCE TARGETED TO FAMILY

- A MacArthur Foundation study of 1,136 psychiatric patients followed for one year after their discharge from a psychiatric hospital found 18 percent of those with a serious mental illness without substance abuse became violent, with family members being the targets of violence in half the cases. The researchers concluded, "The people at the highest risk are family members and friends who are in their homes or in the patient's home."[24]
- Of the approximately 4,000 family homicides in the United States in 2013, individuals with serious mental illness were estimated to be responsible for 29 percent of these, or approximately 1,150 homicides. This is 7 percent of all homicides in the US.[25]
- The National Alliance on Mental Illness (NAMI) reported that 11 percent of its members had a mentally ill family member who had physically harmed another person within the previous year.[26]
- The Department of Justice found that "family murderers were more likely than nonfamily murderers to have a history of mental illness (14% vs. 3%)." Twenty-five percent of those who killed their parents were particularly likely to have such a history. The report also found that 12 percent of those who murdered their spouses and 17 percent of those who murdered their siblings had a history of mental illness.[27]

COMPLIANCE WITH MEDICATION REDUCES VIOLENCE

- A study of 82,000 patients found "violent crime fell by 45% in patients receiving antipsychotics ... and by 24% in patients prescribed mood stabilizers."[28]
- A study of 742 released prisoners found "maintaining psychiatric treatment after release can substantially reduce violent recidivism."[29]
- One meta-analysis of ten studies of homicides and psychotic illness reported that the homicide rate in individuals never treated was twenty-two times higher than the rate in individuals treated.[30]
- A study in New York assessed sixty severely mentally ill men who had been charged with violent crimes. The author reported that medica-

tion noncompliance and lack of awareness of illness both played significant roles in causing the men's violent behavior.[31]

- A study of 907 individuals with severe mental illness reported that those who were violent were "more likely to deny needing psychiatric treatment." The authors concluded "clinical interventions that address a patient's perceived need for psychiatric treatment, such as compliance therapy and motivational interviewing, appear to hold promise as risk management strategies."[32]

- A study of 1,011 outpatients with severe psychiatric disorders in five states reported that "community violence was inversely related to treatment adherence," i.e., the less medication individuals took, the more likely they were to become violent.[33]

- In an analysis of data from the ECA study, the authors noted that "mentally ill individuals with no treatment contact in the past six months had significantly higher odds of violence in the long term" and that "moderate levels of agitation and psychoticism increase the risk of violence." They then conclude, "This would seem to provide a strong argument for providing more interventions targeted specifically to persons with combined mental illness and addictive disorders who are likely not to comply voluntarily with conventional outpatient therapies."[34]

- A study of 133 outpatients with schizophrenia showed that "13 percent of the study group were characteristically violent." Having inadequately treated symptoms of delusions and hallucinations was one of the predictions of violent behavior. Specifically, "71 percent of the violent patients ... had problems with medication compliance, compared with only 17 percent of those without hostile behaviors," a difference that was statistically highly significant.[35]

- A study of severely mentally ill patients in a state forensic hospital found a highly significant correlation between failure to take medication and a history of violent acts in the community.[36]

- A study of inpatients diagnosed with schizophrenia reported an inverse correlation between their propensity to violence and their blood level of antipsychotic medication.[37]

STUDIES CORRELATING
ANOSOGNOSIA WITH VIOLENCE

L ack of awareness of being ill is present in up to 50 percent of those with untreated schizophrenia and up to 40 percent of those with untreated bipolar disorder. It may be a form of anosognosia, damage caused to a certain area of the brain. Anosognosia has been corroborated and "photographed" using structural MRI, functional MRI, single photon emission computed tomography (PET), diffusion tensor imaging (DTI), and other techniques.[1] MRIs show better brain activation in the insula and the inferior parietal lobule (top) and medial prefrontal cortex (bottom) in schizophrenia patients with high insight as compared to schizophrenia patients with low insight.[2] However, as Dr. Robert Liberman has pointed out, "in all such studies there is considerable overlap in the normal and abnormal ratings." Conclusions are sometimes drawn from these brain imaging studies that are not warranted.[3]

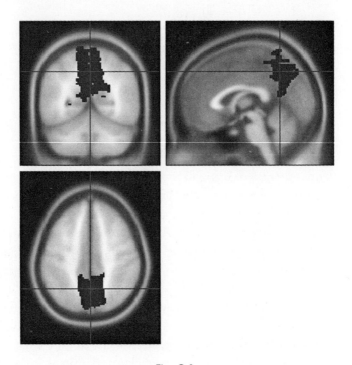

Fig. C.1.

In comparison with patients with altered insight, those with preserved insight showed significant increased perfusion in the bilateral precuneus; this perfusion was also increased in comparison to healthy controls. The figure shows the anatomical localization of hyperperfusion projected onto sections of a normal MRI.

Images courtesy of Professor Eric Guedj, Nuclear Medicine Department, Timone Hospital, Marseille, France.

Over two hundred studies document lack of insight.[4] Following are some of the studies showing the association between lack of insight (likely anosognosia) and violence as compiled by the Treatment Advocacy Center:

- In Ohio, 115 people with schizophrenia who had committed violent acts for which legal charges were incurred were compared to 111 individuals with schizophrenia who had no history of violent acts. The violent individuals had "marked deficits in insight" and were much more symptomatic. Compared to the nonviolent individuals, those who had been violent scored significantly lower on awareness of mental disorder, awareness of achieved effect of medications, and awareness of social consequences of mental disorders.[5]

- In North Carolina, 331 "severely mentally ill" individuals who had been involuntarily admitted to a psychiatric hospital were assessed for their history of assaultive and violent behavior. The findings indicated "that substance abuse problems, medication noncompliance, and low insight into illness operate together to increase violence risk."[6]

- In New York, sixty male patients with psychosis who had been charged with a violent crime were assessed. Severity of community violence was strongly associated with poor insight, medication non-adherence, and substance abuse.[7]

- In England, forty-four male inpatients in a forensic psychiatric hospital were assessed for violent behavior. It was found that "a previous diagnosis of mental illness, lack of insight, and active signs of mental illness were the most predictive of inpatient violence."[8]

- In Spain, sixty-three people with a diagnosis of schizophrenia or schizoaffective disorder were assessed for violent behavior during their brief hospitalizations. The strongest predictors of violent behavior were lack of insight into symptoms (especially delusions), being sicker, and past history of violence.[9]

- In Sweden, forty "mentally disordered" individuals with a history of "violent criminality" were discharged from two forensic hospitals and followed for between three and twelve years. Twenty-two of them committed additional violent crimes, and eighteen did not. Among the strongest predictors of those who committed additional violent crimes were lack of insight and "noncompliance with remediation attempts."[10]

- In England, 503 patients in two forensic psychiatric hospitals were assessed for aggressive and violent behavior. Lack of insight strongly correlated with higher levels of such behavior.[11]

- In Ireland, 157 individuals with first-episode psychosis were assessed for violent behavior. The strongest predictors of violent behavior in the week following admission were poor insight and a past history of violence.[12]

STUDIES ON ASSISTED OUTPATIENT TREATMENT (AOT) IN NEW YORK AND ELSEWHERE

"**A**lthough numerous AOT programs currently operate across the United States, it is clear that the intervention is vastly underutilized."

Substance Abuse and Mental Health Services Administration, "Assisted Outpatient Treatment," National Registry of Evidence-Based Programs and Practices (SAMHSA -NREPP), 2015, http://legacy.nreppadmin.net/ViewIntervention.aspx?id=401 (accessed July 12, 2016).

AOT "programs improve adherence with outpatient treatment and have been shown to lead to significantly fewer emergency commitments, hospital admissions, and hospital days as well as a reduction in arrests and violent behavior."

Agency for Healthcare Research and Quality (AHRQ), *Management Strategies to Reduce Psychiatric Readmissions* (May 2015). Summary at http://mental illnesspolicy.org/national-studies/ahrq_endorses_aot.pdf (accessed July 12, 2016).

Assisted Outpatient Treatment is an effective crime prevention program.

Department of Justice, "Program Profile: Assisted Outpatient Treatment (AOT)," 2012, www.crimesolutions.gov/ProgramDetails.aspx?ID=228 (accessed July 12, 2016).

Kendra's Law has lowered risk of violent behaviors, reduced thoughts about suicide, and enhanced capacity to function despite problems with mental illness. Patients given mandatory outpatient treatment—who were more violent to begin with—were nevertheless four times less likely than members of the control group to perpetrate serious violence after undergoing treatment. Patients who underwent mandatory treatment reported higher social functioning and *slightly less stigma*, rebutting claims that mandatory outpatient care is a threat to self-esteem.

Jo Phelan, Marilyn Sinkewicz, Dorothy Castille, et al., "Effectiveness and Outcomes of Assisted Outpatient Treatment in New York State," *Psychiatric Services* 61, no. 2 (2010): 137–43, http://ps.psychiatryonline.org/doi/pdf/10.1176/ps.2010.61.2.137 (accessed July 25, 2016).

"For those who received AOT, the odds of any arrest were 2.66 times greater (p<.01) and the odds of arrest for a violent offense 8.61 times greater (p<.05) before AOT than they were in the period during and shortly after AOT. The group never receiving AOT had nearly double the odds (1.91, p<.05) of arrest compared with the AOT group in the period during and shortly after assignment."

Bruce Link, Matthew Epperson, Brian Perron, et al., "Arrest Outcomes Associated with Outpatient Commitment in New York State," *Psychiatric Services* 62, no. 5 (2011): 504–508, http://deepblue.lib.umich.edu/bitstream/handle/2027.42/84915/Link Epperson_2010.pdf (accessed July 25, 2016).

"The odds of arrest for participants currently receiving AOT were nearly two-thirds lower (OR=.39, p<.01) than for individuals who had not yet initiated AOT or signed a voluntary service agreement."

Allison Gilbert, Lorna Mower, Richard Van Dorn, et al., "Reductions in Arrest Under Assisted Outpatient Treatment in New York," *Psychiatric Services* 61, no. 10 (2010): 996–99, http://dhs.iowa.gov/sites/default/files/GilbertReductions InArrestUnderAOT_083012.pdf (accessed July 25, 2016).

"The likelihood of psychiatric hospital admission was significantly reduced by approximately 25% during the initial six-month court order ... and by over one-third during a subsequent six-month renewal of the order. ... Similar significant reductions in days of hospitalization were evident during initial court orders and subsequent renewals. ... Improvements were also evident in receipt of psychotropic medications and intensive case management services. Analysis of data from case manager reports showed similar reductions in hospital admissions and improved engagement in services."

Marvin Swartz, Christine Wilder, Jeffrey Swanson, et al., "Assessing Outcomes for Consumers in New York's Assisted Outpatient Treatment Program," *Psychiatric Services* 61, no. 10 (2010): 976–81. http://ps.psychiatryonline.org/doi/pdf/10.1176/ps.2010.61.10.976 (accessed July 25, 2016).

A major study of Assisted Outpatient Treatment (Kendra's Law) in New York found:

Danger and violence reduced: 55% fewer recipients engaged in suicide attempts or physical harm to self; 47% fewer physically harmed others; 46% fewer damaged or destroyed property; 43% fewer threatened physical harm to others; Overall, the average decrease in harmful behaviors was 44%

Consumer outcomes improved: 74% fewer participants experienced homelessness; 77% fewer experienced psychiatric hospitalization; 56% reduction in length of hospitalization; 83% fewer experienced arrest; 87% fewer experienced incarceration; 49% fewer abused alcohol; 48% fewer abused drugs

Consumer participation and medication compliance improved: The number of individuals exhibiting good adherence to meds increased 51%; The number of individuals exhibiting good service engagement increased 103%

Consumer perceptions were positive: 75% reported that AOT helped them gain control over their lives; 81% said AOT helped them get and stay well; 90% said AOT made them more likely to keep appointments and take meds; 87% of participants said they were confident in their case manager's ability; 88% said they and their case manager agreed on what was important to work on

Effect on mental illness system

"**Improved access to services.** AOT has been instrumental in increasing accountability at all system levels regarding delivery of services to high need individuals. Community awareness of AOT has resulted in increased outreach to individuals who had previously presented engagement challenges to mental health service providers."

"**Improved treatment plan development, discharge planning, and coordination of service planning.** Processes and structures developed for AOT have resulted in improvements to treatment plans that more appropriately match the needs of individuals who have had difficulties using mental health services in the past."

"**Improved collaboration between mental health and court systems.** As AOT processes have matured, professionals from the two systems have improved their working relationships, resulting in greater efficiencies, and ultimately, the conservation of judicial, clinical, and administrative resources."

- "There is now an organized process to prioritize and monitor individuals with the greatest need. . . .; AOT ensures greater access to services for individuals whom providers have previously been reluctant to serve. . . .; There is now increased collaboration between inpatient and community-based providers."

New York State Office of Mental Health, *Kendra's Law: Final Report on the Status of Assisted Outpatient Treatment* (Albany: New York State, 2005), p. 60, http://mentalillnesspolicy.org/kendras-law/research/kendras-law-study-2005.pdf (accessed July 25, 2016).

In New York City net costs declined 50 percent in the first year after Assisted Outpatient Treatment began and an additional 13 percent in the second year. In non-NYC counties, costs declined 62 percent in the first year and an additional 27 percent in the second year. This was in spite of the fact that psychotropic drug costs increased during the first year after initiation of Assisted Outpatient Treatment, by 40 percent and 44 percent in the city and five-county samples, respectively. The increased community-based mental health costs were more than offset by the reduction in inpatient and incarceration costs. Cost declines associated with Assisted Outpatient Treatment were about twice as large as those seen for voluntary services.

Jeffrey Swanson, Richard Van Dorn, Marvin Swartz, et al., "The Cost of Assisted Outpatient Treatment: Can it Save States Money?" *American Journal of Psychiatry* 170 (2013): 1423–32, http://ajp.psychiatryonline.org/doi/pdf/10.1176/appi.ajp .2013.12091152 (accessed July 25, 2016).

"In all three regions, for all three groups, the predicted probability of a M(edication) P(ossession) R(atio) ≥80% improved over time (AOT improved by 31–40 percentage points, followed by enhanced services, which improved by 15–22 points, and 'neither treatment,' improving 8–19 points)."

Alisa Busch, Christine Wilder, Richard Van Dorn, et al., "Changes in Guideline-Recommended Medication Possession after Implementing Kendra's Law in New York," *Psychiatric Services* 61, no. 10 (2010): 1000–1005, http://ps.psychiatryonline .org/doi/full/10.1176/ps.2010.61.10.1000 (accessed July 25, 2016).

"In tandem with New York's AOT program, enhanced services increased among involuntary recipients, whereas no corresponding increase was initially seen for voluntary recipients. In the long run, however, overall service capacity was increased, and the focus on enhanced services for AOT participants appears to have led to greater access to enhanced services for both voluntary and involuntary recipients."

Jeffrey Swanson, Richard Van Dorn, Marvin Swartz, et al., "Robbing Peter to Pay Paul: Did New York State's Outpatient Commitment Program Crowd Out Voluntary Service Recipients?" *Psychiatric Services* 61, no. 10 (2010): 988–95, http:// ps.psychiatryonline.org/doi/full/10.1176/ps.2010.61.10.988 (accessed July 25, 2016).

"We find that New York State's AOT Program improves a range of important outcomes for its recipients, apparently without feared negative consequences to recipients."

- **Racial neutrality:** "We find no evidence that the AOT Program is disproportionately selecting African Americans for court orders, nor is there evidence of a disproportionate effect on other minority populations. Our interviews with key stakeholders across the state corroborate these findings."

- **Court orders add value:** "The increased services available under AOT clearly improve recipient outcomes, however, the AOT court order, itself, and its monitoring do appear to offer additional benefits in improving outcomes."
- **AOT improves the likelihood that providers will serve seriously mentally ill:** "It is also important to recognize that the AOT order exerts a critical effect on service providers stimulating their efforts to prioritize care for AOT recipients."
- **AOT improves service engagement:** "After 12 months or more on AOT, service engagement increased such that AOT recipients were judged to be more engaged than voluntary patients. This suggests that after 12 months or more, when combined with intensive services, AOT increases service engagement compared to voluntary treatment alone."
- **Consumers Approve**: "Despite being under a court order to participate in treatment, current AOT recipients feel neither more positive nor more negative about their treatment experiences than comparable individuals who are not under AOT."

Marvin Swartz, Christine Wilder, Jeffrey Swanson, et al., "Assessing Outcomes for Consumers in New York's Assisted Outpatient Treatment Program," *Psychiatric Services* 61, no. 10 (2010): 976–81, http://ps.psychiatryonline.org/doi/pdf/10.1176/ps.2010.61.10.976 (February 8, 2015); Marvin Swartz, Jeffrey Swanson, Henry Steadman, et al., "New York State Assisted Outpatient Treatment Program Evaluation," *Office of Mental Health*, June 30, 2009, https://www.omh.ny.gov/omhweb/resources/publications/aot_program_evaluation/ (accessed July 25, 2016).

Individuals in AOT stay in treatment after AOT ends. "When the court order was for seven months or more, improved medication possession rates and reduced hospitalization outcomes were sustained even when the former AOT recipients were no longer receiving intensive case coordination services."

Richard Van Dorn, Jeffrey Swanson, Marvin Swartz, et al., "Continuing Medication and Hospitalization Outcomes after Assisted Outpatient Treatment in New York," *Psychiatric Services* 61, no. 10 (2010): 982–87, http://ps.psychiatryonline.org/doi/full/10.1176/ps.2010.61.10.982 (accessed July 25, 2016).

In Nevada County, California, AOT ("Laura's Law") decreased the number of Psychiatric Hospital Days 46.7 percent, the number of Incarceration Days 65.1 percent, the number of Homeless Days 61.9 percent, and the number of Emergency Interventions 44.1 percent. Laura's Law implementation saved $1.81–$2.52 for every dollar spent, and receiving services under Laura's Law caused a "reduction in *actual* hospital costs of $213,300" and a "reduction in *actual* incarceration costs of $75,600."

Michael Heggarty, "The Nevada County Laura's Law Experience," *Behavioral Health Department*, November 15, 2011, http://lauras-law.org/states/california/nevada-aot-heggarty-8.pptx.pdf (accessed July 25, 2016).

In Los Angeles, California, the AOT pilot program reduced incarceration 78 percent, hospitalization 86 percent, hospitalization after discharge from the program 77 percent, and cut taxpayer costs 40 percent.

Marvin Southard, "Assisted Outpatient Treatment Program Outcomes Report," Department of Mental Health, February 24, 2011, http://lauras-law.org/states/california/lalauraslawstudy.pdf (accessed July 25, 2016).

In North Carolina, AOT reduced the percentage of people refusing medications to 30 percent, compared to 66 percent of patients not under AOT.

Virginia Hiday and Teresa Scheid-Cook, "The North Carolina Experience with Outpatient Commitment: a Critical Appraisal," *International Journal of Law and Psychiatry* 10, no. 3 (1987): 215–32, http://www.sciencedirect.com/science/article/pii/0160252787900264 (accessed July 25, 2016).

In Ohio, AOT increased attendance at outpatient psychiatric appointments from 5.7 to 13.0 per year. It increased attendance at day treatment sessions from 23 to 60 per year. "During the first 12 months of outpatient commitment, patients experienced significant reductions in visits to the psychiatric emergency service, hospital admissions, and lengths of stay compared with the 12 months before commitment."

Mark Munetz, Thomas Grande, Jeffrey Kleist, et al., "The Effectiveness of Outpatient Civil Commitment," *Psychiatric Services* 47, no. 11 (1996): 1251–53. Abstract at http://ps.psychiatryonline.org/article.aspx?articleID=79783 (accessed July 25, 2016).

In Arizona, "71% [of AOT patients] . . . voluntarily maintained treatment contacts six months after their orders expired" compared with "almost no patients" who were not court-ordered to outpatient treatment.

Robert Van Putten, Jose Santiago, Michael Berren, "Involuntary Outpatient Commitment in Arizona: A Retrospective Study," *Hospital and Community Psychiatry* 39, no. 9 (1988): 953–58. Abstract at http://www.ncbi.nlm.nih.gov/pubmed/3215643 (accessed July 25, 2016).

In Iowa, "it appears as though outpatient commitment promotes treatment compliance in about 80% of patients. . . . After commitment is terminated, about 3/4 of that group remain in treatment on a voluntary basis."

Barbara Rohland, "The Role of Outpatient Commitment in the Management of persons with Schizophrenia," *Iowa Consortium for Mental Health Services*, 1998, http://www.healthcare.uiowa.edu/icmh/archives/reports/finalrpt.pdf   (accessed July 25, 2016).

In New Jersey, Kim Veith, director of clinical services at Ocean Mental Health Services, noted the AOT pilot program performed "beyond wildest dreams." AOT reduced hospitalizations, shortened inpatient stays, reduced crime and incarceration, stabilized housing, and reduced homelessness. Of clients who were homeless, 20 percent are now in supportive housing, 40 percent are in boarding homes, and 20 percent are living successfully with family members.

Treatment Advocacy Center, "Success of AOT in New Jersey 'Beyond Wildest Dreams,'" September 2, 2014, http://www.treatmentadvocacycenter.org/about-us/our-blog/110-nj/2625-success-of-aot-in-new-jersey-beyond-wildest-dreams (accessed July 25, 2016).

"Subjects who were ordered to outpatient commitment were less likely to be criminally victimized than those who were released without outpatient commitment."

Virginia Hiday, Marvin Swartz, Jeffrey Swanson, et al., "Impact of Outpatient Commitment on Victimization of People with Severe Mental Illness," *American Journal of Psychiatry* 159, no. 8 (2002): 1403–11, http://ajp.psychiatryonline.org/article.aspx?articleID=175700 (accessed July 25, 2016).

"We found no evidence of racial bias. Defining the target population as public-system clients with multiple hospitalizations, the rate of application to white and black clients approaches parity."

Jeffrey Swanson, Marvin Swartz, Richard Van Dorn, et al., "Racial Disparities in Involuntary Outpatient Commitment: Are They Real?" *Health Affairs* 28, no. 3 (2009): 816–26, http://content.healthaffairs.org/content/28/3/816.full.pdf (accessed July 25, 2016).

HIPAA REFORMS

F ollowing are suggestions, many from Peter Mill, a former state leg-
islator in Maine, on how to reform HIPAA.

- Allow families to be part of the existing "financial exemption" that
  allows protected information to be disclosed to those who pay for
  treatment services, for example, insurance companies. A family
  member who is providing substantial support (housing, food,
  clothing, care, case management) for someone with mental illness
  out of love should be allowed access to the same information already
  disclosed to those who provide support for money.
- Allow families to be part of the existing "treatment and care exemption" that allows disclosure of information to those providing treatment and care.
- Exclude both historically and currently dangerous patients from
  HIPAA. For patients who are being, or have ever been, admitted
  involuntarily to a hospital because they were dangerous, doctors
  should be allowed to disclose information for a certain period after
  the admission to prevent future dangerousness.
- Implement a lack of capacity exemption. For patients who have
  ever been found to lack capacity because of a mental illness, doctors
  should be permitted or required to disclose information if it might
  help facilitate treatment or prevent the patients from deteriorating
  to the point where they lack capacity in the future.
- Implement a prisoner-based exemption. If a patient has been incarcerated because of mental illness, doctors should be allowed to disclose information during and following that period to prevent future
  incarceration.

- Implement presumptive disclosure. HIPAA requires covered entities to actively solicit patient approval before disclosing information to families, although not to others who are exempted. Regulations should allow doctors to presume that certain seriously mentally ill patients do not object unless the patient raises an objection. Alternatively, regulations that say covered entities "may" obtain consent of the individual to release information should be changed to read "shall make good faith effort to" obtain consent.
- Put those with co-occurring substance use disorders under HIPAA regulations. The limitations on disclosing information about those abusing substances are even more stringent because of criminal justice implications. Patients who are both seriously mentally ill and abuse substances should be under the HIPAA standard, not the substance abuse standard.
- Codify Reverse HIPAA/FERPA. HIPAA and FERPA prohibit covered entities from providing information to families but do not prohibit them from receiving information from families. This should be codified. Regulations should require healthcare providers to actively solicit relevant information from family members in order to deliver better care.
- Include Safe Harbor provisions. HIPAA should insulate doctors, hospitals, and treatment programs from liability or loss of funding for making a disclosure if there was a good faith belief that the disclosure was necessary to enhance the health, safety, or welfare of the person involved or members of the general public. This would help combat the intense bias toward nondisclosure.

ACKNOWLEDGMENTS

"The only kinds of fights worth fighting are those you are going to lose, because somebody has to fight them and lose and lose and lose until someday, somebody who believes as you do wins. In order for somebody to win an important, major fight 100 years hence, a lot of other people have got to be willing— for the sheer fun and joy of it—to go right ahead and fight, knowing you're going to lose. You mustn't feel like a martyr. You've got to enjoy it."

—I. F. Stone

This book describes what I've learned from over thirty years of volunteer work, study, and advocacy dedicated to improving the lives of people with serious mental illness. Many fighters educated me. Most important were my wife, Rose, my sister-in-law, Lynn, Barbara and E. Fuller Torrey, and the hundreds I've met who struggle with serious mental illness on a daily basis. They supported this book by sharing their stories in person, by letter, e-mail, and in our Facebook Mental Illness Policy Org. page and National Alliance on Serious Mental Illness group.

More immediately, I am grateful to Jacqueline Haberfield, who helped get Mental Illness Policy Org. off the ground, and Judy Miller-Templeton who provided encouragement and helped me get over the insecurity of inadequate writing skills, and Laural Fawcett for her design help with charts and tables. Rosanna Esposito and Pippa Abston are two high-powered advocates who read early versions of the manuscript, and pointed out numerous errors of omission and commission and helped me make it a more informed book. Deborah Coady, MD, author of *Healing Painful Sex: A Woman's Guide to Confronting, Diagnosing, and Treating Sexual Pain*, read a near-final version of the manuscript and suggested beautiful improvements in both content and style and provided me with additional studies.

269

Susan Adams and Tony Gibbs read parts of the manuscript and improved it. Susan Levin provided much-needed help securing images. Thank you to my agent, Tom Miller; Editor in Chief Steven L. Mitchell; Assistant Editor Jeffrey Curry (the e. e. cummings of editors); Editorial Assistant Hanna Etu; Production and Traffic Coordinator Catherine Roberts-Abel; Director of Typesetting Bruce Carle; Senior Publicist Lisa Michalski; and the others at Prometheus who brought the book to life.

I've learned much about the legal barriers to care from those at the Treatment Advocacy Center, which I helped cofound with Dr. Torrey and which Mary Zdanowicz, Ted, Vada, and Jon Stanley birthed. Their important work is brilliantly carried on by Executive Director John Snook, current and former advocates Amy Adams, Brian Stettin, Doris Fuller, Frankie Berger, Heather Carroll, Jamie Modics, Kristina Ragosta, Lisa Dailey, Carol Meyers, Betsy Johnson, Elizabeth Sinclair, Renee Smith, Talita Mrkich, and its longest-tenured advocate who was there from the beginning making it work, Sharon Day. I also appreciate the leadership of board president Stephen Segal, and the others who serve with him. I learned about the criminal justice implications of untreated serious mental illness from Chief (ret.) Michael Biasotti and his wife, Barbara, the most "can do" mental illness advocates I have ever met who are also dear friends.

Like everyone with a seriously mentally ill family member, I express my gratitude to Representative Tim Murphy (R-PA) and his current and former staff, Susan Mocyschuk, Scott Dziengelski, and Brad Grantz; Representative Eddie Bernice Johnson (D-TX); and Senator John Cornyn and his staff Stephen Tausend and Carter Burwell who are working to improve care for the seriously ill. In New York State, Senator Catharine Young, Jessica Jeune, and Assemblymember Aileen Gunther are doing the same.

Opinion leaders including Rich Lowry, of *National Review*; Dan Morain, of the *Sacramento Bee*; Josh Greenman of the *New York Daily News*; Brian Anderson of *City Journal*; Michael Judge of the *Wall Street Journal*; and Pete Earley inspired me with their calls for better care as did Rael Jean Isaac, coauthor of *Madness in the Streets*.

The research that went into this book was made possible by those who gave generously to support Mental Illness Policy Org., including our first supporter, Carla Jacobs of the Roy Smith Foundation; John Krieger and John Irwin III of the Achelis and Bodman Foundation; Liz Browning of the Browning Foundation; Larry Mone and Vanessa Mendoza of the Manhattan Institute; Joe Masciandaro of the CarePlus Foundation NJ; Stephen Segal, Mary Ann Bernard, Evelyn Burton, Rosemary DeJoy, Deborah Fabos, Jennifer Hoff, Amy O'Donell, Marty Fox, Karen Cohen, Amanda Woodward, Diane Rabinowitz, Sherry Grenz, Lynn Nanos, G. G. Burns, Karen Easter, Teresa Pasquini, Doug Reuter, and many other moms, dads, sisters, and brothers of the seriously mentally ill who gave what they could.

Thank you all. This is a battle we will win.

NOTES

INTRODUCTION: OVERVIEW OF EVERYTHING

1. Mary Louise Kerwin, Kimberly C. Kirby, Dominic Speziali, et al., "What Can Parents Do? A Review of State Laws Regarding Decision Making for Adolescent Drug Abuse and Mental Health Treatment," *Journal of Child & Adolescent Substance Abuse* 24, no. 3 (March 2016): 166–76, http://www.ncbi.nlm.nih.gov/pmc/articles/PMC4393016/ (accessed July 4, 2016).

2. Center for Behavioral Health Statistics and Quality, "*Behavioral Health Trends in the United States: Results from the 2014 National Survey on Drug Use and Health*," HHS Publication No. SMA 15-4927, NSDUH Series H-50 (September 2015), http://www.samhsa.gov/data/sites/default/files/NSDUH-FRR1-2014/NSDUH-FRR1-2014.pdf (accessed July 26, 2016).

3. About 250,000 with "any" mental illness are homeless. See chapter 1.

4. About 1,153,050 with "any" mental illness are incarcerated. See chapter 2.

5. Approximately 2,360,500 with "any" mental illness are on probation or parole. See chapter 2.

6. Treatment Advocacy Center (TAC), *The Shortage of Public Hospital Beds for Mentally Ill Persons*, a report of the Treatment Advocacy Center by E. Fuller Torrey, Kurt Entsminger, Jeffrey Geller, et al. (Arlington, VA: Treatment Advocacy Center, 2006), http://www.treatmentadvocacycenter.org/storage/documents/the_shortage_of_public hospital_beds.pdf (accessed July 12, 2016).

7. About 38,000 people with "any" mental illness kill themselves every year, and 380,000 attempt it. See chapter 1.

8. Virginia Hiday, Marvin S. Swartz, Jeffrey W. Swanson, et al., "Criminal Victimization of Persons with Severe Mental Illness," *Psychiatric Services* 50, no. 1 (January 1999): 62–68, http://www.ncbi.nlm.nih.gov/pubmed/9890581 (accessed July 8, 2016).

9. Author interview with family member, February 2016; Peter Hermann and Ann Marimow, "Navy Yard Shooter Aaron Alexis Driven by Delusions," *Washington Post*, September 25, 2013, http://www.washingtonpost.com/local/crime/fbi-police-detail-shooting -navy-yard-shooting/2013/09/25/ee321abe-2600-11e3-b3e9-d97fb087acd6_story.html (accessed July 8, 2016).

10. Paul T. Rosynsky, "One Goh, Mass Shooter from Oikos University in Oakland, Suffers from Mental Illness, Court Psychologist Finds," *San Jose* (CA) *Mercury News*, November 20, 2012, http://www.mercurynews.com/breaking-news/ci_22029838/one -goh-mass-shooter-from-oikos-university-oakland (accessed July 8, 2016).

11. Virginia Tech Review Panel, "Mass Shootings at Virginia Tech: Addendum to the Report of the Review Panel," November 2009, http://scholar.lib.vt.edu/prevail/docs/ April16ReportRev20100106.pdf (accessed July 8, 2016).

12. Office of Management and Budget (OMB), letter from OMB director Sylvia M. Burwell to Congressman Tim Murphy, Subcommittee on Oversight and Investigations of the House Energy and Commerce Committee, November 7, 2013, http://mental illnesspolicy.org/national-studies/mentalhealthexpenditurenational.pdf (accessed July 8, 2016).

13. NYS Office of Mental Health, "Fiscally Speaking: New York State Office of Mental Health's 2012–2013 Enacted Budget," November 8, 2012, https://www.omh .ny.gov/omhweb/resources/newsltr/2012/apr/budget.html (accessed July 8, 2016).

14. "California's Mental Health Service Act: A Ten Year $10 Billion Bait and Switch: An Investigation of Proposition 63 by Mental Illness Policy Org. and Individual Californians," Mental Illness Policy Org., August 14, 2013, http://mentalillnesspolicy.org/ states/california/mhsa/mhsa_prop63_bait&switchsummary.html (accessed July 8, 2016).

15. This book differentiates between "mental health" advocates and "mental illness" advocates. Mental health advocates do not advocate for the most seriously mentally ill. Mental illness advocates do.

16. Center for Behavioral Health Statistics and Quality, *Behavioral Health Trends in the United States*.

17. Ethan Watters, "The Americanization of Mental Illness," *New York Times Sunday Magazine*, January 8, 2010, http://www.nytimes.com/2010/01/10/magazine/10psyche-t .html (accessed July 8, 2016).

18. Allen Frances, *Saving Normal* (New York: HarperCollins, 2013).

19. Ron Pies, "Deborah Danner and the Suffering of Schizophrenia," *Psychiatric Times*, November 7, 2016, http://www.psychiatrictimes.com/blogs/deborah-danner-and -suffering-schizophrenia (accessed December 10, 2016).

INFAMOUS MENTALLY ILL ADULTS WHO WENT OFF TREATMENT

1. Author interview with family member, February 2016; Peter Hermann and Ann Marimow, "Navy Yard Shooter Aaron Alexis Driven by Delusions," *Washington Post*, September 25, 2013, http://www.washingtonpost.com/local/crime/fbi-police-detail -shooting-navy-yard-shooting/2013/09/25/ee321abe-2600-11e3-b3e9-d97fb087acd6 _story.html (accessed July 8, 2016).

2. Virginia Tech Review Panel, "Mass Shootings at Virginia Tech: Addendum to the Report of the Review Panel," November 2009, http://scholar.lib.vt.edu/prevail/docs/ April16ReportRev20100106.pdf (accessed July 8, 2016).

3. Bob Orr, "Newly Released Jared Lee Loughner Files Reveal Chilling Details," CBS, March 27, 2013, http://www.cbsnews.com/news/newly-released-jared-lee -loughner-files-reveal-chilling-details (accessed July 9, 2016).

4. Police found anxiety and depression medications in his home after the July 20, 2012, shootings, but no toxicology report was ordered, so it is not known if he was taking them. His psychiatrist, Dr. Lynne Fenton, testified that on June 11, Mr. Holmes cut his appointment short and refused further offers of help. Dan Elliott and Catherine Tsai, "Colorado Shooter James Holmes' Therapist Reported Threat to College," *Chicago Sun-Times*, April 4, 2013; *Denver Post* version: John Ingold, "Aurora Theater Shooting Documents: Doctor Reported James Holmes Was Threat to Public," *Denver Post*, April 4, 2013,

http://www.denverpost.com/2013/04/04/aurora-theater-shooting-documents-doctor
-reported-james-holmes-was-threat-to-public (accessed July 8, 2016); Matthew Nussbaum, Jordan Steffan, and John Ingold, "Aurora Theater Shooting Gunman Told Doctor:
'You Can't Kill Everyone,'" *Denver Post*, June 16, 2015, http://www.denverpost.com/the-
ater-shooting-trial/ci_28322297/aurora-theater-shooting-jurors-hear-from-key
-university (accessed July 8, 2016).

    5. Stuart Taylor Jr., "Hinckley's Brother and Sister Testify Father Rejected Hospi-
talization Idea," *New York Times*, May 12, 1982, http://www.nytimes.com/1982/05/12/us/
hinckley-s-brother-and-sister-testify-father-rejected-hospitalization-idea.html (accessed
July 9, 2016).

    6. Mr. Miles was incompetent to stand trial and was hospitalized to have his com-
petency restored. Elissa Rivas, "Deputy Darren Goforth's Accused Killer to Return to
Harris County," ABC Eyewitness News, September 7, 2016, http://abc13.com/news/
deputys-accused-killer-to-return-to-harris-county/1501801 (accessed December 15, 2016).

    7. Jericka Duncan, "NYPD Shooter Had Criminal Past, Struggles with Mental
Illness," CBS Evening News, December 22, 2014, http://www.cbsnews.com/news/nypd
-shooter-had-criminal-past-struggles-with-mental-illness (accessed December 15, 2016).

    8. Zawahri had been hospitalized in 2006, but author could not find media reports
showing he was in treatment in the period immediately preceding the 2013 shootings.

CHAPTER 1: HUMAN CONSEQUENCES OF IGNORING THE SERIOUSLY MENTALLY ILL

    1. National Association of State Mental Health Program Directors (NASMHPD),
*Responding to a High-Profile Tragic Incident Involving a Person with a Serious Mental
Illness: A Toolkit for State Mental Health Commissioners*, NASMHPD and the Council
of State Governments Justice Center, 2010, https://csgjusticecenter.org/wp-content/
uploads/2012/12/Responding_to_a_High-Profile_Tragic_Incident_Involving_a_Person
_with_a_Serious_Mental_Illness.pdf (accessed July 30, 2016).

    2. Dan Elliott and Catherine Tsai, "Colorado Shooter James Holmes' Therapist
Reported Threat to College," *Chicago Sun-Times*, April 4, 2013. *Denver Post* version: John
Ingold, "Aurora Theater Shooting Documents: Doctor Reported James Holmes Was
Threat to Public," *Denver Post*, April 4, 2013, http://www.denverpost.com/2013/04/04/
aurora-theater-shooting-documents-doctor-reported-james-holmes-was-threat-to-public
(accessed July 8, 2016). Matthew Nussbaum, Jordan Steffan, and John Ingold, "Aurora
Theater Shooting Gunman Told Doctor: 'You Can't Kill Everyone,'" *Denver Post*, June 16,
2015, http://www.denverpost.com/theater-shooting-trial/ci_28322297/aurora-theater
-shooting-jurors-hear-from-key-university (accessed July 8, 2016).

    3. Bob Orr, "Newly Released Jared Lee Loughner Files Reveal Chilling Details,"
CBS, March 27, 2013, http://www.cbsnews.com/news/newly-released-jared-lee-loughner
-files-reveal-chilling-details (accessed July 9, 2016).

    4. Stuart Taylor Jr., "Hinckley's Brother and Sister Testify Father Rejected Hospi-
talization Idea," *New York Times*, May 12, 1982, http://www.nytimes.com/1982/05/12/us/
hinckley-s-brother-and-sister-testify-father-rejected-hospitalization-idea.html (accessed
July 9, 2016).

5. Mark Follman, Gavin Aronsen, Deanna Pan, et al., "US Mass Shootings, 1982–2012: Data From Mother Jones' Investigation," *Mother Jones*, December 28, 2012, http://www.motherjones.com/politics/2012/12/mass-shootings-mother-jones-full-data (accessed July 9, 2016).

6. E. Fuller Torrey, "1,000 Homicides by Mentally Ill," Mental Illness Policy Org., 2011, http://mentalillnesspolicy.org/consequences/1000-homicides.html (accessed July 9, 2016).

7. Jason C. Matejkowski, Sara W. Cullen, and Phyllis L. Solomon, et al., "Characteristics of Persons with Severe Mental Illness Who Have Been Incarcerated for Murder," *Journal of the American Academy of Psychiatry and the Law* 36, no. 1 (March 2008): 74–86, http://www.jaapl.org/content/36/1/74.full (accessed July 9, 2016).

8. E. Fuller Torrey, John Snook, DJ Jaffe, et al., "Raising Cain: The Role of Serious Mental Illness in Family Homicides," Treatment Advocacy Center, 2016, http://www.treatmentadvocacycenter.org/component/content/article/218-general/3557-raising-cain (accessed December 22, 2016). See violence targeted to family in appendix B.

9. "Report: Alan Farajian Killed His Mother 'Because She Had Poisoned Him,'" WPBF (25) News, January 9, 2013, http://www.wpbf.com/article/report-alan-farajian -killed-his-mother-because-she-had-poisoned-him/1315650 (accessed December 17, 2016).

10. Arelis R. Hernández, "Daughter Accused of Stabbing Mother to Death: Meagan Jones, 21, Argued with Her Mother Prior to Stabbing Her, Deputies Said," *Orlando Sentinel*, February 19, 2013, http://articles.orlandosentinel.com/2013-02-19/news/os -daughter-stabbed-mother-death-20130219_1_steak-knife-emergency-responders -deputies (accessed July 9, 2016).

11. Christin Coyne, "Mom: 'Son Tried to Kill Me with a Hammer,'" *Weatherford (TX) Democrat*, November 29, 2012, http://www.weatherforddemocrat.com/news/local _news/mom-son-tried-to-kill-me-with-a-hammer/article_efdf1f56-97f5-529e-92c3 -f9db325f702b.html (accessed July 9, 2016).

12. Thomas Insel, "Keynote Address at the IOM Workshop," *Mental Health and Violence: Opportunities for Prevention and Early Intervention* (Washington, DC: Institute of Medicine, February 26, 2014), from the National Academy of Sciences, http://www.nationalacademies.org/hmd/Activities/Global/ViolenceForum/2014-FEB-26/Day%201/ Welcome%20and%20Morning%20Presentations/4-Insel-Video.aspx (accessed July 9, 2016).

13. John Monahan, "Mental Disorder and Violent Behavior," *American Psychologist* 47, no. 4 (April 1992): 511–21. Abstract at http://psycnet.apa.org/journals/amp/47/4/511/ (accessed July 6, 2016).

14. American Psychiatric Nurses Association, "Workplace Violence (2008 Position Statement)," *American Psychiatric Nurses Association*, 2008, http://www.apna.org/files/ public/APNA_Workplace_Violence_Position_Paper.pdf (accessed July 8, 2016).

15. See Supreme Court decisions in chapter 15.

16. The SAMHSA "National Center for Trauma Informed Care," has been renamed as the "National Center for Trauma Informed Care *and Alternatives to Seclusion and Restraint.*" SAMHSA, "About NTIC," http://www.samhsa.gov/nctic/about (accessed August 16, 2016).

17. Sixty-nine percent of them (389,000) were sheltered (living in emergency shel-

ters or transitional housing), but 31 percent (175,000) were unsheltered living on the streets or in abandoned buildings, vehicles, or parks. These estimates do not include homeless "couch-surfers" who camp out on the sofas of friends and families, move every few days, and have no permanent address. US Department of Housing and Urban Development (HUD), *The 2015 Annual Homeless Assessment Report (AHAR) to Congress*, Office of Community Planning and Development, Abt Associates, November 2015, https://www .hudexchange.info/resources/documents/2015-AHAR-Part-1.pdf (accessed July 9, 2016).

18. Jennifer Hoff, "Right to Treatment Rally" YouTube video, 6:46, posted by Joy Torres, June 19, 2014, https://www.youtube.com/watch?v=gB6kedOIyQc& (accessed July 9, 2016).

19. Lillian Gelberg and Lawrence S. Linn, "Social and Physical Health of Homeless Adults Previously Treated for Mental Health Problems," *Hospital and Community Psychiatry* 39, no. 5 (June 1988): 510–16. Abstract at http://www.researchgate.net/ publication/19777082_Social_and_physical_health_of_homeless_adults_previously _treated_for_mental_health_problems (accessed July 9, 2016); Deborah K. Padgett and E. L. Struening, "Victimization and Traumatic Injuries among the Homeless: Associations with Alcohol, Drug, and Mental Problems," *American Journal of Orthopsychiatry* 62, no. 4 (October 1992): 525–34. Abstract at http://onlinelibrary.wiley.com/doi/10.1037/ h0079369/abstract (accessed July 6, 2016).

20. Doris J. James and Lauren E. Glaze, *Mental Health Problems of Prison and Jail Inmates* (Washington, DC: special report, Bureau of Justice Statistics, DOJ, September 2006), http://bjs.gov/content/pub/pdf/mhppji.pdf (accessed July 9, 2016).

21. Substance Abuse and Mental Health Services Administration (SAMHSA), *NSDUH 2014 Report: Behavioral Health Trends in the United States: Results from the 2014 National Survey on Drug Use and Health*, HHS Publication No. SMA 15-4927, NSDUH Series H-50, http://www.samhsa.gov/data/sites/default/files/NSDUH-FRR1-2014/ NSDUH-FRR1-2014.pdf (accessed July 26, 2016).

22. American Foundation for Suicide Prevention, "Suicide Statistics," *American Foundation for Suicide Prevention*, 2014, http://afsp.org/about-suicide/suicide-statistics (accessed July 8, 2016). AFSP estimates there are twenty-five suicide attempts for every completion, but other sources put it much lower.

23. Dr. E. Fuller Torrey looked at studies of the prevalence of suicide among the seriously mentally ill and studies of the prevalence of serious mental illness among those who commit suicide, two sides of the same coin, and in both cases found about 5,000 of the then 38,000 suicides (about 13 percent) were in people with serious mental illness. E. Fuller Torrey, "5000 Suicides a Year are Likely Caused by Schizophrenia and Bipolar Disorder," Mental Illness Policy Org., http://mentalillnesspolicy.org/consequences/suicide .html (accessed July 9, 2016).

24. Kahyee Hor and Mark Taylor, "Suicide and Schizophrenia: A Systematic Review of Rates and Risk Factors," *Journal of Psychopharmacology* 24, no. 4, suppl., November 2010: 81–90, http://www.ncbi.nlm.nih.gov/pmc/articles/PMC2951591 (accessed July 9, 2016); Centers for Disease Control and Prevention (CDC), "Surveillance for Violent Deaths, National Violent Death Reporting System, 16 States, 2010," by Sharyn E. Parks, Linda L. Johnson, Dawn D. McDaniel, et al., *Morbidity and Mortality Weekly Report* 63 (January 17, 2014): 1–33, http://www.cdc.gov/mmwr/preview/mmwrhtml/ss6301a1.htm (accessed July 9, 2016).

25. Mark Olfson, Melanie Wall, Shuai Wang, et al., "Short-Term Suicide Risk after Psychiatric Hospital Discharge," *JAMA Psychiatry*, September 21, 2016, http://archpsyc .jamanetwork.com/article.aspx?articleid=2551516 (accessed September 27, 2016).

26. The study also found more than 21 percent of persons with serious mental illness had been victims of personal theft (theft of an item from one's person), more than 140 times higher than the general population. Nearly 28 percent of persons with SMI had been victims of property crimes. Linda A.Teplin, Gary M. McClelland, Karen M. Abram, et al., "Crime Victimization in Adults with Severe Mental Illness," *Archives of General Psychiatry* 62, no. 8 (August 2005): 911–21, http://archpsyc.jamanetwork.com/article .aspx?articleid=208861 (accessed July 6, 2016).

Another study found persons with mental illness are victims of violence at a rate only two and a half times greater than in the general population—8.2 percent versus 3.1 percent. Virginia A. Hiday, et al., "Criminal Victimization of Persons with Severe Mental Illness," *Psychiatric Services* 50, no. 1 (January 1999): 62–68, http://ps.psychiatryonline .org/doi/full/10.1176/ps.50.1.62 (accessed July 9, 2016). In a more recent study, 23 percent of those with schizophrenia, 38 percent of those with bipolar disorder, and 41 percent of those with major depression reported being victimized. Sarah L. Desmarais, Richard A. Van Dorn, Kiersten L. Johnson, et al., "Community Violence Perpetration and Victimization among Adults with Mental Illnesses," *American Journal of Public Health* 104, no. 12 (December 2014): 2342–49. Abstract at http://ajph.aphapublications.org/doi/ abs/10.2105/AJPH.2013.301680 (accessed July 8, 2016).

27. Tamsin Short, Stuart Thomas, and Stefan Luebbers, et al., "A Case-Linkage Study of Crime Victimisation in Schizophrenia-Spectrum Disorders over a Period of Deinstitutionalisation," *BMC Psychiatry* 13 (2013), http://www.ncbi.nlm.nih.gov/pmc/ articles/PMC3599537 (accessed July 8, 2016).

28. The practice of telling difficult patients they have a right to leave, in order to encourage them to leave, is so common that families gave it a name. They "disappeared" him.

29. Mairead C. Dolan, David Castle, and Kate McGregor, "Criminally Violent Victimisation in Schizophrenia Spectrum Disorders: The Relationship to Symptoms and Substance Abuse," *BMC Public Health* 12 (June 18, 2012): 445, http://www.ncbi.nlm.nih .gov/pmc/articles/PMC3503690 (accessed July 9, 2016).

30. Short, et al., "A Case-Linkage Study."

31. "Higher levels of manic symptoms indicate a raised risk of being a victim of violence." Federico Fortugno, Christina Katsakou, Stephen Bremner, et al., "Symptoms Associated with Victimization in Patients with Schizophrenia and Related Disorders," *PLoS One* 8, no. 3 (March 19, 2013): e58142, http://www.ncbi.nlm.nih.gov/pmc/articles/ PMC3602443 (accessed July 9, 2016).

32. Kathleen Branch, "Laws Surrounding Mental Illness Make It Harder for Victims to Get Treatment," *Baltimore Sun*, October 30, 2013, http://articles.baltimoresun .com/2013-10-30/news/bs-ed-mental-illness-guns-20131029_1_involuntary-treatment -assisted-outpatient-treatment-mental-illness-and-guns (accessed July 9, 2016).

33. Torrey, et al., "Raising Cain."

34. Rael Jean Isaac and Virginia C. Armat, *Madness in the Streets: How Psychiatry and the Law Abandoned the Mentally Ill* (New York: Free Press, 1990).

35. Monica Malowney, Sarah Keltz, Daniel Fischer, et al., "Availability of Outpatient Care from Psychiatrists: A Simulated-Patient Study in Three US Cities," *Psychiatric Ser-*

vices 66, no. 1 (January 2015): 94-96, October 2014. Abstract at http://www.ncbi.nlm
.nih.gov/pubmed/?term=%22Availability+of+Outpatient+Care+From+from+Psychiatrists
%3A+A+Simulated-Patient+Study+in+Three+U.S.+Cities.%22 (accessed July 9, 2016).

36. Chirlane McCray, "How We Will Shatter the Mental Illness Stigma," *Daily News*, February 26, 2015, http://nydn.us/1AMy98u (accessed July 9, 2016).

37. "Mother of Western Psych Shooter Gives Deposition in Lawsuit," CBS Pittsburgh, December 5, 2013, http://pittsburgh.cbslocal.com/2013/12/05/mother-of -western-psych-shooter-gives-deposition-in-lawsuit (accessed July 9, 2016).

38. Paula Reed Ward, "Deposition Shows Mom Reaching Out to Western Psych Shooter," *Pittsburgh Post-Gazette*, December 4, 2013, http://www.post-gazette.com/local/ city/2013/12/04/Judge-orders-release-of-deposition-by-mother-of-man-who-shot-six-at -Western-Psych/stories/201312040153#ixzz3CG1iqG00 (accessed July 6, 2016).

CHAPTER 2: CRIMINAL JUSTICE CONSEQUENCES OF IGNORING THE SERIOUSLY MENTALLY ILL

1. House Subcommittee on Oversight and Investigations of the Committee on Energy and Commerce, "Where Have All the Patients Gone? Examining the Psychiatric Bed Shortage," Michael Biasotti testimony, 113th Cong., March 26, 2014, http:// mentalillnesspolicy.org/imd/biasottipsychhospitaltestimony.pdf (accessed July 9, 2016).

2. Nick Welsh, "Mental Health Hearing Gets Hot: And the County ADMHS Director Loses Her Cool," *Santa Barbara Independent*, December 15, 2015, http://www .independent.com/news/2015/dec/17/mental-health-hearing-gets-hot (accessed July 9, 2016).

3. National Law Center on Homelessness and Poverty, *Criminalizing Crisis: The Criminalization of Homelessness in US Cities* (Washington, DC: report, National Law Center on Homelessness and Poverty, November 2011), http://www.nlchp.org/ Criminalizing_Crisis (accessed July 9, 2016).

4. Half of stalkers have a mental illness and 15 percent have a serious mental illness. K. Mohandie and R. Meloy, "The RECON Typology of Stalking: Reliability and Validity Based Upon a Large Sample of North American Stalkers," *Journal of Forensic Science* 51, no. 1 (2006) 147–55, http://www.victimsofcrime.org/docs/default-source/src/ mohandie-k-meloy-r-green-mcgowan-m-_-williams-j-2005.pdf?sfvrsn=2 (accessed July 9, 2016).

5. Michael Biasotti, "Management of the Severely Mentally Ill And Its Effects on Homeland Security," (master's thesis, Monterey, CA: Naval Postgraduate School, September 2011), http://mentalillnesspolicy.org/crimjust/homelandsecuritymentalillness.pdf (accessed July 9, 2016).

6. Michael Biasotti, "State's Mentally Ill Need Treatment, Not Incarceration," *Times Union* (Albany, NY), October 14, 2013, http://www.timesunion.com/opinion/ article/State-s-mentally-ill-need-treatment-not-4894707.php (accessed July 9, 2016).

7. Heather Jacobson, in e-mail correspondence with the author, December 14, 2016.

8. "115 Law Enforcement Officers Killed by Mentally Ill," Mental Illness Policy Org., 2009, http://mentalillnesspolicy.org/crimjust/120LEOSkilledbyMentallyIll.htm (accessed July 9, 2016); Treatment Advocacy Center, *Justifiable Homicides by Law Enforce-*

ment Officers: What is the Role of Mental Illness? (Arlington, VA: report, Treatment Advocacy Center and the National Sheriffs' Association, September 2013), http://www.treatmentadvocacycenter.org/storage/documents/2013-justifiable-homicides.pdf (accessed January 1, 2017).

9. Nick Breul and Mike Keith, "Deadly Calls and Fatal Encounters, Analysis of US Law Enforcement Line of Duty Deaths when Officers Responded to Dispatched Calls for Service and Conducted Enforcement (2010-2014)," Department of Justice, Community Oriented Policing Services, 2016, p. 48, http://www.nleomf.org/assets/pdfs/officer-safety/Primary-Research-Final-10-0.pdf (accessed August 11, 2016).

10. Ben Chapman, Joe Kemp, and Larry McShane, "Subway Shooter Peter Jourdan's Sister Rails at System, Wonders Why Her Brother Was Able to Buy a Gun," *New York Daily News,* January 5, 2013, http://www.nydailynews.com/new-york/subway-shooter-peter-jourdan-sister-rails-system-article-1.1233949 (accessed December 15, 2016).

11. Mr. Miles was incompetent to stand trial and was hospitalized to have his competency restored. Elissa Rivas, "Deputy Darren Goforth's Accused Killer to Return to Harris County," ABC Eyewitness News (Houston, Texas), September 7, 2016, http://abc13.com/news/deputys-accused-killer-to-return-to-harris-county/1501801 (accessed December 15, 2016).

12. Jericka Duncan, "NYPD Shooter Had Criminal Past, Struggles With Mental Illness," CBS Evening News, December 22, 2014, http://www.cbsnews.com/news/nypd-shooter-had-criminal-past-struggles-with-mental-illness (accessed December 15, 2016).

13. Tux Turkel, "When Police Pull the Trigger in Crisis, the Mentally Ill Often are the Ones Being Shot," *Portland* (ME) *Press Herald,* December 8, 2012, http://www.pressherald.com/news/projects/Shoot-Maine-misfiring-on-deadly-force.html (accessed July 9, 2016).

14. Tom Moroney and Lindsey Rupp, "Bullets Are Safety Net as 64 Mentally Ill Die at Hands of Police," *Bloomberg News,* December 27, 2012. Version available at http://www.bloomberg.com/news/articles/2012-12-27/bullets-are-safety-net-as-64-mentally-ill-die-at-hands-of-police (accessed July 9, 2016).

15. US Department of Justice, Civil Rights Division, "Investigation of the Baltimore City Police Department," August 10, 2016, https://www.justice.gov/opa/file/883366/download (accessed September 18, 2016).

16. Lori Fullbright, "Tulsa Man Frustrated over Death of Roommate Shot and Killed by Officer" News9.com (Oklahoma), February 19, 2013, http://www.news9.com/story/21242353/man-shot-and-killed-by-tulsa-police-officer-identified (accessed December 15, 2016).

17. Justifiable homicides by law enforcement "decreased overall by 5% between 1980 and 2008 but justifiable homicides resulting from an attack on a law enforcement increased by 67%, from an average of 153 to 255 such homicides per year and many appear mental illness related." Treatment Advocacy Center, *Justifiable Homicides.*

18. Ibid.

19. Todd Lewan, "Suicide at the Hands of Police," CBS News, April 26, 1998, http://www.cbsnews.com/news/suicide-at-the-hands-of-police (accessed July 9, 2016).

20. Michael Biasotti, "Pass Kendra's Law Improvement Act, Says Vice President of New York State Association of Chiefs of Police," Syracuse (blog), June 15, 2011, http://blog.syracuse.com/opinion/2011/06/wednesdays_readers_page_center_6.html (accessed July 9, 2016).

21. Matt Spina, "Today's Mental Health Squad: The Police," *Buffalo News*, May 18, 2013, http://www.buffalonews.com/city-region/todays-mental-health-squad-the -police-20130518 (accessed July 9, 2016).

22. Council of State Governments, Criminal Justice/Mental Health Consensus Project, New York, "Mental Health Courts," CSG Justice Center, 2013, http://csgjustice center.org/mental-health-court-project (accessed July 9, 2016).

23. Jails are generally run by counties for those serving short sentences or awaiting trials. Prisons are for those serving longer sentences and can be run by the state or federal government. There were 1,561,500 people in prisons and 744,600 in jail or 2,306,100 total. Lauren E. Glaze and Erika Parks, *Correctional Populations in the United States, 2011* (Washington, DC: Bureau of Justice Statistics, November 2012), p. 5, http://bjs.gov/ content/pub/pdf/cpus14.pdf (accessed December 21, 2016). More than 50 percent of those (1,153,050) have a mental health problem. Doris J. James and Lauren E. Glaze, *Mental Health Problems of Prison and Jail Inmates* (Washington, DC: Bureau of Justice Statistics, September 2006), http://bjs.gov/content/pub/pdf/mhppji.pdf (accessed July 9, 2016). However only about 16 or 17 percent of individuals in federal prisons (265,455) and 17 percent of those in jails (126,582) have "serious" mental illness. Fred Osher, David A. D'Amora, and Martha Plotkin, et al., "Adults with Behavioral Health Needs under Correctional Supervision," Council of State Governments Justice Center, 2012, https:// www.bja.gov/Publications/CSG_Behavioral_Framework.pdf (accessed July 9, 2016).

24. There are 4,721,000 individuals under probation or parole. Glaze and Parks, *Correctional Populations*. If the proportion of the mentally ill on probation and parole is the same as the proportion incarcerated, 50 percent (2,360,500) have any mental illness and 16 percent (755,360) have serious mental illness.

25. E. Fuller Torrey, Mary T. Zdanowicz, Aaron D. Kennard, et al., "The Treatment of Persons with Mental Illness in Prisons and Jails: A State Survey," Treatment Advocacy Center, April 8, 2014, http://tacreports.org/storage/documents/treatment-behind-bars/ treatment-behind-bars.pdf (accessed July 9, 2016).

26. A recent study of a Correctional Center in Oklahoma found, that of "the 10 psychiatric medications the Department of Corrections spent the most on in 2013, seven were antipsychotics and three were anti-depressants." Clifton Adcock and Shaun Hittle, "Prison Drug Data Reveals Disorders are Severe for Many Mentally Ill Inmates," *Miami News-Record*, February 15, 2014. Version at http://oklahomawatch.org/2014/02/01/ prison-meds-reveal-disorders-severe-for-mentally-ill-inmates (accessed July 9, 2016). In Muskegon, Michigan, "at least 10 to 20% of people charged or convicted of crimes can clearly be classified as having significant mental illness. Common diagnoses are schizophrenia, bipolar disorder . . . or post-traumatic stress disorder" and the cost is 50 percent higher than for other inmates. John S. Hausman, "Mental Illness and Criminal Justice: Law Enforcement Copes with Issues Hospitals Once Handled," *Muskegon* (MI) *Chronicle*, December 16, 2013, http://www.mlive.com/news/muskegon/index.ssf/2013/12/mental _health-criminal_justice.html (accessed July 9, 2016). In 2010, people with mental illness were only 29% of the New York City jail population. By 2014 they represented 38%. Approximately one third of this 38% had serious mental illness. Bill de Blasio, *Mayor's Task Force on Behavioral Health and the Criminal Justice System* (New York: 2014), http:// www1.nyc.gov/assets/criminaljustice/downloads/pdfs/annual-report-complete.pdf (accessed July 26, 2016).

27. James and Glaze, "Mental Health Problems."

28. Tom Dart, "Untreated Mental Illness an Imminent Danger?" *60 Minutes*, CBS, September 29, 2013. Video by subscription available at http://www.cbsnews.com/videos/untreated-mental-illness-an-imminent-danger-2/ (accessed July 9, 2016). The interview is approximately 11:40 into broadcast.

29. Mary Beth Pfeiffer, *Crazy in America: The Hidden Tragedy of Our Criminalized Mentally Ill* (New York: Carroll & Graf, 2007).

30. Dart, "Imminent Danger."

31. Judge Steve Leifman, "Give People with Mental Illness Treatment, Not a Jail Cell," *Miami Herald*, May 17, 2014, http://miamidda.com/pdf/5.17.14%20Miami%20Herald.%20Give%20people%20with%20mental%20illness%20treatment%20not%20a%20jail%20cell.pdf (accessed July 9, 2016).

32. E. Fuller Torrey, Aaron D. Kennard, Don Eslinger, et al., "More Mentally Ill Persons Are in Jails and Prisons than Hospitals: A Survey of the States," Treatment Advocacy Center, May 2010, http://www.treatmentadvocacycenter.org/storage/documents/final_jails_v_hospitals_study.pdf (accessed July 9, 2016).

33. Torrey, et al., "More Mentally Ill Persons."

34. Leonica Valentine, "Squeegee Man Is City's Latest Blast from the Past," *New York Post*, July 9, 2015, http://nypost.com/2015/07/19/squeegee-man-is-citys-latest-blast-from-the-past (accessed on December 15, 2016).

35. Cynthia L. Blitz, Nancy Wolff, and Jing Shi, "Physical Victimization in Prison: The Role of Mental Illness," *International Journal of Law and Psychiatry* 31, no. 5 (October/November 2008): 385–93. Abstract at http://www.ncbi.nlm.nih.gov/pmc/articles/PMC2836899 (accessed July 9, 2016).

36. James and Glaze, "Mental Health Problems."

37. Pete Earley, *Crazy: A Father's Search through America's Mental Health Madness* (New York: G. P. Putnam's Sons, 2006).

38. CBS Miami, "CBS4's Michelle Gillen Revisits 'The Forgotten Floor,'" CBS Miami, July 8, 2013, http://miami.cbslocal.com/2013/07/18/cbs4s-michelle-gillen-revisits-the-forgotten-floor (accessed July 9, 2016).

39. Stephen B. Seager, *Behind the Gates of Gomorrah: A Year with the Criminally Insane* (New York: Gallery Books, 2014). Dr. Seager gave a speech about the conditions at NAPA on CSPAN: http://www.c-span.org/video/standalone/?322243-1%2Fbook-discussion-behind-gates-gomorrah (accessed July 9, 2016).

40. Lindsay M. Hayes, *National Study of Jail Suicide: 20 Years Later* (Washington, DC: National Institute of Corrections, DOJ, April 2010) http://static.nicic.gov/Library/024308.pdf (accessed July 9, 2016).

CHAPTER 3: FINANCIAL CONSEQUENCES

1. Office of Management and Budget (OMB), letter from OMB director Sylvia M. Burwell to Congressman Tim Murphy, Subcommittee on Oversight and Investigations of the House Energy and Commerce Committee, November 7, 2013, http://mental illnesspolicy.org/national-studies/mentalhealthexpenditurenational.pdf (accessed July 19, 2016). The exact amount spent is disputed due to different methods of calculating, which

costs are included, and how to account for indirect costs. It is hard to tease out spending on serious mental illness from "mental health." Substance abuse is also included in some estimates.

2. Substance Abuse and Mental Health Services Administration (SAMHSA), "Projections of National Expenditures for Treatment of Mental and Substance Use Disorders, 2010–2020," HHS Publication No. SMA-14-4883 (Rockville, MD: SAMHSA, 2014), http://store.samhsa.gov/shin/content//SMA14-4883/SMA14-4883.pdf (accessed July 19, 2016).

3. John J. Boronow and Steven S. Sharfstein, "Close the Mental Health Revolving Door," *Baltimore Sun*, December 29, 2013, http://www.baltimoresun.com/news/opinion/oped/bs-ed-commitment-20131228%2C0%2C3608071.story (accessed July 19, 2016).

4. Bill de Blasio, *Mayor's Task Force on Behavioral Health and the Criminal Justice System* (New York: 2014), http://www1.nyc.gov/assets/criminaljustice/downloads/pdfs/annual-report-complete.pdf (accessed July 20, 2016).

5. Mandatory spending ("entitlements") are paid to individuals who meet certain qualifications, for example, those entitled to social security disability. "Discretionary funds" are programs that Congress allocates funds for. For example, Congress can elect how much, if any, to appropriate for mental health block grants.

6. Dr. Insel calculated only $24 billion of combined SSI and SSDI spending was for serious mental illness, but does not explain the calculation. It is possible his is a more accurate number if he did indeed segregate benefits to those with serious mental illness from those with all mental illness. Thomas R. Insel, "Assessing the Economic Costs of Serious Mental Illness," *American Journal of Psychiatry* 165, no. 6 (June 2008): 663–65, http://ajp.psychiatryonline.org/doi/full/10.1176/appi.ajp.2008.08030366 (accessed July 19, 2016).

7. Social Security Administration, *Annual Statistical Report on the Social Security Disability Insurance Program, 2014* (Washington, DC: Office of Research, Evaluation, and Statistics, 2015), https://www.socialsecurity.gov/policy/docs/statcomps/di_asr/2014/di_asr14.pdf (accessed July 19, 2016).

8. Rachel L. Garfield and Kaiser Foundation, *Mental Health Financing in the United States: A Primer* (Menlo Park, CA: Henry J. Kaiser Family Foundation, April 2011), http://kaiserfamilyfoundation.files.wordpress.com/2013/01/8182.pdf (accessed July 19, 2016).

9. "Research Weekly: The 'National Bill' for Severe Mental Illness," Treatment Advocacy Center, January 21, 2016, http://www.treatmentadvocacycenter.org/about-us/our-blog/69-no-state/2997-the-national-bill-for-severe-mental-illness (accessed July 20, 2016). Statistics sourced from the Healthcare Cost and Utilization Project (HCUP) administered by the Agency for Healthcare Research and Quality (AHRQ).

10. The amount in state funds is likely $27 billion calculated as follows. Forty-two percent of NASMHPD spending is identified as state funds, and 48 percent are Medicaid funds (state plus local). Assuming state contribution to Medicaid is 50 percent, then only half the Medicaid spending is state funds. Robert W. Glover, Joel E. Miller, and Stephanie R. Sadowski, "Proceedings on the State Budget Crisis and the Behavioral Health Treatment Gap: The Impact on Public Substance Abuse and Mental Health Treatment Systems," National Association of State Mental Health Program Directors, March 22, 2012, http://www.nasmhpd.org/sites/default/files/Summary-Congressional%20Briefing

_March%2022_Website(1).pdf (accessed July 19, 2016); Ted Lutterman, ed., "Shifting Challenges: Mental Health in the ACA Era," July 2, 2013, http://www.allhealth.org/briefingmaterials/UPDATEDTEDLUTTERMANPRESENTATION2JUL2013_SB.PDF (accessed July 19, 2016).

11. Between 2011 and 2012, "New York cut $95.2 million, Illinois $62.2 million and North Carolina $48.2 million." "State Mental Health Cuts: The Continuing Crisis," National Alliance on Mental Illness, November 2011, http://www.nami.org/get attachment/About-NAMI/Publications/Reports/StateMentalHealthCuts2.pdf (accessed July 19, 2016).

12. "Approximately 1 million detentions in county jails involve persons with serious mental illnesses." Haya Ascher-Svanum, Allen W. Nyhuis, Douglas E. Faries, et al., "Involvement in the US Criminal Justice System and Cost Implications for Persons Treated for Schizophrenia," *BMC Psychiatry* 10 (January 2010), http://www.ncbi.nlm.nih.gov/pmc/articles/PMC2848217 (accessed July 19, 2016). This study was funded by Eli Lilly and therefore may be suspect.

13. E. Q. Wu, H. G. Birnbaum, L. Shi, et al., "The Economic Burden of Schizophrenia in the United States in 2002," *Journal of Clinical Psychiatry* 66, no. 9 (September 2005): 1122–29. Abstract at http://www.ncbi.nlm.nih.gov/pubmed/16187769 (accessed July 19, 2016).

14. Steve Leifman, "Give People with Mental Illness Treatment, Not a Jail Cell," *Miami Herald*, May 17, 2014, http://miamidda.com/pdf/5.17.14%20Miami%20Herald.%20Give%20people%20with%20mental%20illness%20treatment%20not%20a%20jail%20cell.pdf (accessed July 19, 2016).

15. Kurt Erickson, "Cost of Mental Illness on the Rise in Illinois Prison System," *Quad-City Times* (IL, IA), August 5, 2014, http://qctimes.com/news/local/government-and-politics/cost-of-mental-illness-on-the-rise-in-illinois-prison/article_ae86e85d-4b77-50e1-855f-0bd4cf6c303d.html (accessed July 19, 2016).

16. Jeffrey Swanson, L. K. Frisman, A. G. Robertson, et al., "Costs of Criminal Justice Involvement among Persons with Serious Mental Illness in Connecticut," *Psychiatric Services* 64, no. 7 (July 2013): 630–37. Abstract at http://www.ncbi.nlm.nih.gov/pubmed/23494058 (accessed July 19, 2016).

17. Ronald C. Kessler, Steven Heeringa, Matthew D. Lakoma et.al, "Individual and Societal Effects of Mental Disorders on Earnings in the United States: Results from the National Comorbidity Survey Replication," *American Journal of Psychiatry* 165, no. 6 (June 2008): 703–11, https://www.ncbi.nlm.nih.gov/pmc/articles/PMC2410028/ (accessed July 19, 2016). Martin Cloutier, Myrlene Sanon Aigbogun, Annie Guerin, et al., "The Economic Burden of Schizophrenia in the United States in 2013," *Journal of Clinical Psychiatry* 77, no. 6 (June 2016): 764–71. Note that the study is funded by a pharmaceutical company that sells a medicine for schizophrenia.

18. Bazelon Center for Mental Health Law, "How Will Health Care Reform Help People with Mental Illnesses," Bazelon Center for Mental Health Law, 2010, http://www.bazelon.org/News-Publications/Publications/CategoryID/8/List/1/catpageindex/2/Level/a/ProductID/54.aspx (accessed July 19, 2016).

19. The *New York Times* (October 23, 2011) ran a front-page story on Keris Myrick, a woman with schizoaffective disorder who became "a CEO." The article failed to state that she was the CEO of a peer group that had a government contract that likely required

it to be peer-led. The 10 percent employment rate of seriously mentally ill quoted by Bazelon includes individuals in these supported and subsidized positions. After roughly thirty years of advocacy, this author knows less than ten people with schizophrenia in nonsubsidized employment outside the arts and mental health fields.

20. Christina Hoff Sommers and Sally Satel, *One Nation Under Therapy: How the Helping Culture is Eroding Self-Reliance* (New York: St. Martin's Press, 2005).

CHAPTER 4: WHAT SERIOUS MENTAL ILLNESS IS NOT

1. The National Survey on Drug Use and Health (NSDUH) is a large methodologically sound survey authorized by Section 505 of Public Health Act and conducted by SAMHSA's Center for Behavioral Health Statistics and Quality (CBHSQ), http://www.gpo.gov/fdsys/pkg/USCODE-2010-title42/pdf/USCODE-2010-title42-chap6A-subchapIII-A-partA-sec290aa-4.pdf. Since 2011, estimates varied from 3.9 percent of population over eighteen to 4.9 percent, largely due to different calculation methodologies. The most recent estimate is 4 percent. Center for Behavioral Health Statistics and Quality, "Behavioral Health Trends in the United States: Results from the 2014 National Survey on Drug Use and Health," HHS Publication No. SMA 15-4927, NSDUH Series H-50 (2015), http://www.samhsa.gov/data/sites/default/files/NSDUH-FRR1-2014/NSDUH-FRR1-2014.pdf (accessed July 26, 2016). Other sources report results that are generally consistent with these. See chapter 5 and appendix A.

2. The World Health Organization defines "mental health" as "a state of well-being in which every individual realizes his or her own potential, can cope with the normal stresses of life, can work productively and fruitfully, and is able to make a contribution to her or his community. . . . Mental health is more than the absence of mental disorders." "Fact Sheet: Mental Health: Strengthening Our Response," World Health Organization, August 2014, http://www.who.int/mediacentre/factsheets/fs220/en/ (accessed July 10, 2016).

3. The surgeon general defines mental health as "a state of successful performance of mental function, resulting in productive activities, fulfilling relationships with other people, and the ability to adapt to change and to cope with adversity." US Surgeon General, *Mental Health: A Report of the US Surgeon General* (Rockville, MD: report, Department of Health and Human Services, 1999), http://profiles.nlm.nih.gov/ps/access/NNBBHS.ocr (accessed July 10, 2016).

4. American Psychiatric Association (APA) "Mental Health Checkup: Lack of Illness vs Health." No longer available at psychiatry.org. Copy in possession of author.

5. Ethan Watters, "The Americanization of Mental Illness," *New York Times Sunday Magazine*, January 8, 2010, http://www.nytimes.com/2010/01/10/magazine/10psyche-t.html (accessed July 10, 2016).

6. Andrew Cuomo, "Governor Cuomo Announces More than 700 'Project Hope' Counselors Deployed to Provide Crisis Counseling in Areas Hit Hardest by Hurricane Sandy," Governor.ny.gov, December 18, 2012, http://www.governor.ny.gov/press/12182012-project-hope-counselors (accessed July 10, 2016).

7. SAMHSA sent out several tweets offering counseling for those affected by a blizzard, "24/7 crisis counseling is available for those affected by the #Blizzardof2015. . . ." It then gave out the phone number. SAMHSA, Twitter post, January 26, 2015.

8. APA, *Diagnostic and Statistical Manual of Mental Disorders: DSM-5* (Washington, DC: American Psychiatric Association, 2013).

9. Ronald C. Kessler, Patricia Berglund, Olga Demler, et al., "Prevalence, Severity, and Comorbidity of 12-Month DSM-IV Disorders in the National Comorbidity Survey Replication," *Archives of General Psychiatry* 6, no. 2 (June 2005): 617–27, http://archpsyc .jamanetwork.com/article.aspx?articleid=208671 (accessed July 10, 2016).

10. Allen Frances, *Saving Normal* (New York: HarperCollins, 2013).

11. Allen Frances, "DSM-5 Is a Guide, Not a Bible: Simply Ignore Its 10 Worst Changes," *Huffington Post*, December 3, 2012, http://www.huffingtonpost.com/allen -frances/dsm-5_b_2227626.html (accessed July 10, 2016).

12. Centers for Disease Control and Prevention (CDC), "Mental Illness Surveillance among Adults in the United States," *Morbidity and Mortality Weekly Report (MMWR) Supplement* 60 (September 2, 2011), http://www.cdc.gov/mmwr/pdf/other/ su6003.pdf (accessed July 10, 2016).

13. Allen Frances, "Psychiatric Diagnosis Gone Wild: The 'Epidemic' of Childhood Bipolar Disorder," *Psychiatric Times*, April 8, 2010, http://www.psychiatrictimes.com/ articles/psychiatric-diagnosis-gone-wild-epidemic-childhood-bipolar-disorder (accessed July 10, 2016).

14. Alan Schwarz and Sarah Cohen, "More Diagnoses of Hyperactivity in New Centers for Disease Control Data," *New York Times*, April 1, 2013, http://www.nytimes .com/2013/04/01/health/more-diagnoses-of-hyperactivity-causing-concern.html (accessed July 10, 2016).

15. "More US Children Being Diagnosed with Youthful Tendency Disorder," *Onion*, September 27, 2000, http://www.theonion.com/article/more-us-children-being -diagnosed-with-youthful-ten-248 (accessed December 17, 2016).

16. Frances, *Saving Normal*.

17. Andres Barkil-Oteo, "Collaborative Care for Depression in Primary Care: How Psychiatry Could 'Troubleshoot' Current Treatments and Practices," *Yale Journal of Biology and Medicine*, 86-(2):139-146 (2013), https://www.ncbi.nlm.nih.gov/pmc/articles/ PMC3670434/ (accessed December 17, 2016).

18. National Institute of Mental Health (NIMH), "Post-Traumatic Stress Disorder (PTSD)," http://www.nimh.nih.gov/health/topics/post-traumatic-stress-disorder-ptsd/ index.shtml (accessed July 10, 2016).

19. National Advisory Mental Health Council, Basic Behavioral Science Task Force, *Basic Behavioral Science Research for Mental Health: A National Investment* (Rockville, MD: National Institute of Mental Health, 1995).

20. John M. Grohol, "The Lie of Focusing on Those with Serious Mental Illness," *PsychCentral*, April 17, 2014, http://psychcentral.com/blog/archives/14/04/17/the-lie-of -focusing-on-those-with-serious-mental-illness (accessed July 10, 2016).

CHAPTER 5: WHAT SERIOUS MENTAL ILLNESS IS
AND HOW THAT SHOULD DRIVE POLICY

1. Substance Abuse and Mental Health Services Administration (SAMHSA), "NSDUH 2014 Report: Behavioral Health Trends in the United States: Results from the 2014 National Survey on Drug Use and Health," HHS Publication No. SMA

15-4927, NSDUH Series H-50, http://www.samhsa.gov/data/sites/default/files/ NSDUH-FRR1-2014/NSDUH-FRR1-2014.pdf (accessed July 26, 2016).

2. Jonathan Silver, "Panetti Case Argued Again Before 5th Circuit," *Texas Tribune*, September 23, 2015, http://www.texastribune.org/2015/09/23/panetti-case-argued-5th -circuit (accessed July 10, 2016).

3. Center for Mental Health Services (CMHS), "Estimation Methodology for Adults with Serious Mental Illness (SMI)," *Federal Register* 64, no. 121 (June 24, 1999): 33890–97, http://www.gpo.gov/fdsys/pkg/FR-1999-06-24/html/99-15377.htm (accessed July 10, 2016).

4. Schizophrenia-spectrum disorders include schizoaffective disorder, catatonic schizophrenia, paranoid schizophrenia, and disorganized schizophrenia. In this book, we group them as schizophrenia. In *DSM* "severe bipolar" requires more symptoms than bipolar disorder. In this book, we shorten both to bipolar because there are not enough statistics that separate out the two. In *DSM* "severe major depression" requires more symptoms than either "depression" or "major depression." American Psychiatric Association, *Diagnostic and Statistical Manual of Mental Disorders: DSM-5* (Washington, DC: American Psychiatric Association, 2013).

5. For example, severe OCD affects just .5 percent of adults. National Institute of Mental Health, "Obsessive-Compulsive Disorder (OCD) Statistics," 2005, http://www .nimh.nih.gov/statistics/1ocd_adult.shtml (accessed July 10, 2016).

6. Thomas R. Insel, "Director's Update, Mental Disorders as Brain Disorders: Thomas Insel at TEDxCaltech," YouTube video, 1:19, posted by "TEDx Talks," February 8, 2013, https://www.youtube.com/watch?v=u4m65sbqbhY (accessed July 10, 2016).

7. Depression: NIMH, "What is Depression?" NIMH, http://www.nimh.nih.gov/ health/topics/depression/index.shtml (accessed July 10, 2016). Bipolar: NIMH, "Bipolar Disorder in Adults," NIMH, http://www.nimh.nih.gov/health/publications/bipolar -disorder/index.shtml (accessed July 10, 2016). Schizophrenia: E. Fuller Torrey, "Schizo- phrenia and Bipolar Disorder are Diseases of the Brain," Mental Illness Policy Org., 2010, http://mentalillnesspolicy.org/medical/schizophrenia-brain-studies.html (accessed July 10, 2016).

8. Torrey, "Schizophrenia and Bipolar Disorder."

9. Caleb M. Adler, John Adams, Melissa P. DelBello, et al., "Evidence of White Matter Pathology in Bipolar Disorder Adolescents Experiencing Their First Episode of Mania: A Diffusion Tensor Imaging Study," *American Journal of Psychiatry* 163, no. 2 (February 2006): 322–24, http://psychiatryonline.org/doi/full/10.1176/appi.ajp.163.2.322 (accessed July 10, 2016).

10. Michael Craig Miller, *Understanding Depression* (Cambridge, MA: Harvard Health Publications, Harvard Medical School, 2013), http://www.health.harvard.edu/ special_health_reports/Understanding_Depression (accessed July 10, 2016).

11. E. Fuller Torrey, "Brain Structure in People with Mental Illness Who Have Never Been Treated," Mental Illness Policy Org., 2013, http://mentalillnesspolicy.org/ myths/medications.html (accessed July 10, 2016).

12. Schizophrenia Working Group of the Psychiatric Genomics Consortium, "Biological Insights from 108 Schizophrenia-Associated Genetic Loci," *Nature* 511, no. 7510 (July 2014): 421–27, http://www.nature.com/nature/journal/v511/n7510/full/ nature13595.html (accessed July 10, 2016).

13. NIMH, "What is Schizophrenia?" NIMH, http://www.nimh.nih.gov/health/topics/schizophrenia/index.shtml (accessed July 12, 2016). Severe bipolar: NIMH, "Bipolar Disorder in Adults," NIMH. Psychotic depression: NIMH, "What is Depression?" NIMH, http://www.nimh.nih.gov/health/topics/depression/index.shtml (accessed July 10, 2016).

14. Robert Keers, Simone Ullrich, Bianca L. DeStavola, et al., "Association of Violence with Emergence of Persecutory Delusions in Untreated Schizophrenia," *American Journal of Psychiatry* 171, no. 3 (March 2014): 332–39, http://ajp.psychiatryonline.org/doi/pdf/10.1176/appi.ajp.2013.13010134 (accessed July 10, 2016).

15. Harvard Medical School, "The Negative Symptoms of Schizophrenia, 2006 Update," *Harvard Health*, October 1, 2006, http://www.health.harvard.edu/fhg/updates/update0706c.shtml (accessed July 10, 2016).

16. Terry E. Goldberg and Michael F. Green, "Neurocognitive Functioning in Patients with Schizophrenia: An Overview," in Kenneth L. Davis, Dennis Charney, Joseph T. Coyle, et al. (eds.), *Neuropsychopharmacology: The Fifth Generation of Progress* (Philadelphia, PA: Lippincott/Williams & Wilkins, 2002), pp. 657–69, http://www.acnp.org/Docs/G5/CH48_657-670.pdf (accessed July 10, 2016).

17. For an example of a word salad, watch video: "Disorganized Speech Schizophrenia," YouTube video, 1:18, posted by "Nouuuuranlovesadam," July 16, 2011, https://www.youtube.com/watch?v=avbfd_OkLoU (accessed July 26, 2016).

18. T. E. Goldberg, J. D. Ragland, E. F. Torrey, et al., "Neuropsychological Assessment of Monozygotic Twins Discordant for Schizophrenia," *Archives of General Psychiatry* 47, no. 11 (November 1990): 1066–72. Abstract at http://www.ncbi.nlm.nih.gov/pubmed/2241508 (accessed July 10, 2016).

19. V. Stergiopoulos, A. Cusi, T. Bekele, et al., "Neurocognitive Impairment in a Large Sample of Homeless Adults with Mental Illness," *Acta Psychiatrica Scandinavica* [Epub ahead of print] 131, no. 4 (January 21, 2015). Abstract at http://www.ncbi.nlm.nih.gov/pubmed/25604122 (accessed July 10, 2016).

20. Laurent Boyer, Michel Cermolacce, Daniel Dassa, et al., "Neurocognition, Insight and Medication Nonadherence in Schizophrenia: A Structural Equation Modeling Approach," *PLOS One* 7, no. 10 (October 2012): e47655, http://www.ncbi.nlm.nih.gov/pmc/articles/PMC3483287 (accessed July 10, 2016).

21. Clayton E. Cramer, *My Brother Ron: A Personal and Social History of the Deinstitutionalization of the Mentally Ill* (Middletown, DE: Create Space, 2012).

22. See scans of anosognosia: Treatment Advocacy Center, "Serious Mental Illness and Anosognosia," June 2016, http://www.treatmentadvocacycenter.org/key-issues/anosognosia/3628-serious-mental-illness-and-anosognosia (accessed December 11, 2016) and appendix C.

23. Xavier Amador, *I Am Not Sick, I Don't Need Help: How to Help Someone with Mental Illness Accept Treatment* (Peconic, NY: Vida Press, 2007).

24. Frank Bruni, "Behind the Jokes, a Life of Pain and Delusion; For Letterman Stalker, Mental Illness Was Family Curse and Scarring Legacy," *New York Times*, Nov. 22, 1998, http://www.nytimes.com/1998/11/22/nyregion/behind-jokes-life-pain-delusion-for-letterman-stalker-mental-illness-was-family.html (accessed July 12, 2016).

25. Lee N. Robins and Darrel A. Regier, *Psychiatric Disorders in America: The Epidemiologic Catchment Area Study* (New York: Free Press, 1991).

26. Ronald C. Kessler, Patricia Berglund, Olga Demler, et al., "Lifetime Prevalence

and Age-of-Onset Distributions of DSM-IV Disorders in the National Comorbidity Survey Replication," *Archives of General Psychiatry* 62, no. 6 (June 2005): 593–602, http://archpsyc.jamanetwork.com/article.aspx?articleid=208678 (accessed July 10, 2016).

27. The study used to support the age fourteen claim, included all mental illness with only 23 percent of those in it having a serious disorder. The results also skewed young because the study folded substance abuse in. Kessler, et al., "Lifetime Prevalence and Age-of-Onset." Recently, there have been suggestions that major depression begins earlier, but this may be due to diagnosing less severe forms as "major."

28. Thomas R. Insel, NIMH Director's Blog: "AIDS: A Cautionary Tale," NIMH. nih.gov, June 20, 2014, http://www.nimh.nih.gov/about/director/2014/aids-a-cautionary -tale.shtml (accessed July 10, 2016).

29. There are many theories of causality, and there are likely multiple causes. Genetics and epigenetics have been receiving more attention as gene sequencing becomes cheaper. Neurodevelopmental and neurodegenerative theories are receiving attention as imaging technology advances. Some believe infections, like toxoplasmosis, incurred during the third trimester of pregnancy may heighten schizophrenia in those genetically predisposed. E. Fuller Torrey and Robert H. Yolken, "*Toxoplasma gondii* and Schizophrenia," *Emerging Infectious Diseases* (Center for Disease Control and Prevention) 9, no. 11 (November 2003), http://wwwnc.cdc.gov/eid/article/9/11/03-0143_article (accessed July 10, 2016). Others postulate that serious mental illness is caused by trauma to the brain or chemical abnormalities. The jury is out in spite of breathless media reports to the contrary.

30. Thomas R. Insel, Research Plenary: "The Quest for the Cure: The Science of Mental Illness (+ Four Inconvenient Truths)," NAMI Annual Meeting, September 5, 2014.

31. Institute of Medicine (IOM), *Reducing Risk for Mental Disorders: Frontiers for Preventative Intervention Research*, Patricia Beezley Mrazek and Robert J. Haggerty (eds.) (Washington, DC: National Academy of Sciences, 1994), http://www.nap.edu/catalog.php?record_id=2139 (accessed July 10, 2016). IOM is located within the National Academy of Sciences and is a premier arbiter of research.

32. The President's New Freedom Commission on Mental Health, *Achieving the Promise: Transforming Mental Health Care in America* (Rockville, MD: Department of Health and Human Services, 2003). Executive summary at http://store.samhsa.gov/product/Achieving-the-Promise-Transforming-Mental-Health-Care-in-America -Executive-Summary/SMA03-3831 (accessed July 10, 2016).

33. IOM, *Preventing Psychological Disorders in Service Members and Their Families: An Assessment of Programs*, Laura Aiuppa Denning, Marc Meisnere, and Kenneth E. Warner (eds.) (Washington, DC: National Academies Press, 2014), http://www.national academies.org/hmd/Reports/2014/Preventing-Psychological-Disorders-in-Service -Members-and-Their-Families.aspx (accessed July 10, 2016).

34. Shirley S. Wang, "Military's Mental-Health Efforts are Ineffective, Report Finds: Study Fails to Find Evidence That Programs for Soldiers and Families Prevent Psychological Disorders," *Wall Street Journal*, February 10, 2014, http://www.wsj.com/articles/SB100 0142405270230491420457939494103966972 (accessed July 10, 2016).

35. There are many illnesses and side effects of medications that can mimic the symptoms of mental illness. Whenever mental illness is suspected, there should be a comprehensive medical exam to rule out those other causes. Ron Diamond, "How to Tell If Someone Diagnosed with a Mental Illness Has Another Medical Disorder That May

Have Led to a Misdiagnosis," Mental Illness Policy Org., 1998, http://mentalillnesspolicy .org/coping/misdiagnosis.html (accessed July 10, 2016).

36. Serious mental illnesses are believed to be "neurodevelopmental," in that there is a risk phase and a prodromal phase before an active phase. Insel, "Quest for the Cure." "Prodromal" refers to precursor symptoms. The North American Prodrome Longitudinal Study (NAPLS) is trying to determine how to predict who will develop serious mental illness. The best current thinking is that *all* of the following, if found in a single individual, might be one way to predict psychosis, without generating the false positives if any single factor were used: (1) genetic vulnerability to schizophrenia with recent deterioration in functioning, (2) higher levels of unusual thought content, (3) higher levels of suspicion-paranoia, (4) greater social impairment. One day, we might be able to predict psychosis by measuring the neuroanatomical, neurophysiological, neurohormonal, and neurocognitive abnormalities that precede it. J. Addington, Kristin Cadenhead, Barbara A. Cornblatt, et al., "North American Prodrome Longitudinal Study (Napls 2): Overview and Recruitment," *Schizophrenia Research* 142, no. 1–3 (2012), http://www.ncbi.nlm.nih .gov/pmc/articles/PMC3502644/pdf/nihms411004.pdf (accessed July 10, 2016). The Recovery after Initial Schizophrenia Episode (RAISE) study is trying to determine if we can prevent people with first episode psychosis (FEP) from having it become chronic.

37. Bipolar: Stanley Center for Psychiatric Research, "Genetics of Bipolar and Schizophrenia," *Broad Institute*, http://www.broadinstitute.org/science/programs/ psychiatric-disease/stanley-center-psychiatric-research/genetics-bipolar-and-schizo (accessed July 10, 2016). Schizophrenia: NIMH, *Recovery After an Initial Schizophrenia Episode (RAISE)*, 2015, http://www.nimh.nih.gov/health/topics/schizophrenia/raise/ index.shtml (accessed July 10, 2016)

38. Irv Gottesman, T. M. Laursen, A. Bertelsen, et al., "Severe Mental Disorders in Offspring with 2 Psychiatrically Ill Parents," *Archives of General Psychiatry* 67, no. 3 (March 2010): 252–57. Abstract at http://www.ncbi.nlm.nih.gov/pubmed/20194825 (accessed July 10, 2016).

39. Ibid. We could not find genetics statistics that tease out severe bipolar from bipolar or severe major depression from depression. Gottesman's figures are likely the closest, because they are based on data from children of those hospitalized for bipolar disorder. It is reasonable to suspect that those hospitalized for bipolar disorder are seriously ill. Another study shows children of a parent or sibling who has bipolar disorder are four to six times more likely to develop the illness, compared with children who do not have a family history of bipolar disorder. J. I. Nurnberger and T. Foroud, "Genetics of Bipolar Affective Disorder," *Current Psychiatry Reports* 2, no. 2 (April 2000): 147–57. Abstract at http://www.ncbi.nlm.nih.gov/pubmed/11122948 (accessed July 10, 2016).

40. N. Antypa and A. Serretti, "Family History of a Mood Disorder Indicates a More Severe Bipolar Disorder," *Journal of Affective Disorders* 156 (March 2014): 178–86. Abstract at http://www.ncbi.nlm.nih.gov/pubmed/24439249 (accessed July 10, 2016).

41. Douglas F. Levinson and Walter E. Nichols, "Major Depression and Genetics,"

Stanford University, 2016, http://depressiongenetics.stanford.edu/mddandgenes.html (accessed July 10, 2016).

42. E. Fuller Torrey, *Surviving Schizophrenia: A Family Manual*, 6th ed. (New York: HarperCollins, 2014).

CHAPTER 6: WHAT SCIENCE TELLS US ABOUT TREATMENT THAT SHOULD BE REFLECTED IN POLICY

1. Medicine for schizophrenia: Anthony F. Lehman, Jeffrey A. Lieberman, Lisa B. Dixon, et al. (work group on schizophrenia), *Practice Guideline for the Treatment of Patients with Schizophrenia*, 2nd ed. (Washington, DC: American Psychiatric Association, February 2004), http://psychiatryonline.org/pb/assets/raw/sitewide/practice_guidelines/guidelines/schizophrenia.pdf (accessed March 20, 2015). Medicine for bipolar disorder: Robert M. A. Hirschfeld, Charles L. Bowden, Michael J. Gitlin, et al. (work group on Bipolar Disorder), *Practice Guideline for the Treatment of Patients with Bipolar Disorder*, 2nd ed. (Washington, DC: American Psychiatric Association, 2002), http://psychiatryonline .org/pb/assets/raw/sitewide/practice_guidelines/guidelines/bipolar.pdf (accessed July 12, 2016). Also see 2005 update at http://www.valueoptions.com/providers/Handbook/treatment/Bi-Polar_Disorder_Guideline_Watch.pdf (accessed July 12, 2016).

The utility of medicines was known as far back as 1959, when researchers noted that the hospital discharge rate for patients treated with medications was twice that for those not treated. Henry Brill and Robert E. Patton, "Analysis of Population Reduction in New York State Mental Hospitals during the First Four Years of Large-Scale Therapy with Psychotropic Drugs," *American Journal of Psychiatry* 116, no. 6 (December 1959): 495–509, http://psychiatryonline.org/doi/abs/10.1176/ajp.116.6.495 (accessed July 12, 2016).

In 2013, recognizing the importance of antipsychotics, the National Committee for Quality Assurance (NCQA) added "Adherence to Antipsychotic Medications for Individuals with Schizophrenia" as a metric to be tracked by healthcare organizations seeking its seal of approval. NCQA, "Adherence to Antipsychotic Medications for People with Schizophrenia," NCQA, 2014, http://www.ncqa.org/report-cards/health-plans/state-of -health-care-quality/2015-table-of-contents/antipsychotic-medications (accessed July 12, 2016).

2. S. K. Erickson, R. Ciccone, S. B. Schwarzkopf, et al., "Legal Fallacies of Antipsychotic Drugs," *Journal of the American Academy of Psychiatry and the Law* 35, no. 2 (2007): 235–46, http://mentalillnesspolicy.org/medical/antipsychotics.pdf (accessed July 12, 2016).

3. There is no way to predict what medication will work best. However, if a first-degree relative has been treated successfully with a certain medication, that medication might be effective for a family member.

4. E. Fuller Torrey, *Surviving Schizophrenia: A Family Manual*, 6th ed. (New York: HarperCollins, 2013).

5. E. Fuller Torrey, Kurt Entsminger, Jeffrey Geller, et al., "The Shortage of Public Hospital Beds for Mentally Ill Persons," Treatment Advocacy Center, 2006, http://www .treatmentadvocacycenter.org/storage/documents/the_shortage_of_publichospital_beds .pdf (accessed July 12, 2016).

6. Torrey, Entsminger, Geller, et al., *Shortage of Public Hospital Beds.*

7. In California, over 90 percent of state psychiatric hospital occupants got there through the criminal justice system. Jerry Brown, *Governor Budget Summary 2014–2015,* January 10, 2014.

Seventy-three percent of those in Oregon State Hospital are court ordered to be there. These include mentally ill prisoners, people unfit to stand trial, those found not guilty by reason of insanity, and those having psychiatric examinations as part of court proceedings. Joseph D. Bloom, "CRIPA, *Olmstead,* and the Transformation of the Oregon Psychiatric Security Review Board," *Journal of the American Academy of Psychiatry and the Law* 40 (November 2012): 383–89, http://www.jaapl.org/content/40/3/383.full.pdf (accessed July 12, 2016).

8. Doris A. Fuller, Elizabeth Sinclair, Jeffrey Geller, et al., *Going, Going, Gone: Trends and Consequences of Eliminating State Psychiatric Beds, 2016* (Arlington, VA: Treatment Advocacy Center, 2016), http://www.tacreports.org/storage/documents/going-going -gone.pdf (accessed July 12, 2016).

9. House Committee on Energy and Commerce Subcommittee on Oversight and Investigations, "Where Have All the Patients Gone? Examining the Psychiatric Bed Shortage, Hearings Before the House Subcommittee on Oversight and Investigations of the Committee on Energy and Commerce," Jon Mark Hirshon statement on behalf of the American College of Emergency Physicians, 113th Cong., March 26, 2014, http://mental illnesspolicy.org/imd/emergencydocpsychhospitaltestimony.pdf (accessed July 12, 2016).

10. Stephanie McCrummen, "A Father's Scars: For Va.'s Creigh Deeds, Tragedy Brings Unending Questions," *Washington Post,* November 1, 2014, https://www .washingtonpost.com/national/a-fathers-scars-for-deeds-every-day-brings-questions/ 2014/11/01/2217a604-593c-11e4-8264-deed989ae9a2_story.html (accessed December 17, 2016).

11. Julian E. Barnes, "Insanity Defense Fails for Man Who Threw Woman onto Track," *New York Times,* March 23, 2001, http://www.nytimes.com/2000/03/23/nyregion/ insanity-defense-fails-for-man-who-threw-woman-onto-track.html (accessed December 17, 2016).

12. CDC, "Number and Rate of Discharges from Short-Stay Hospitals," CDC, 2010, http://www.cdc.gov/nchs/data/nhds/2average/2010ave2_firstlist.pdf (accessed July 12, 2016).

13. American College of Emergency Physicians (ACEP), "ACEP Psychiatric and Substance Abuse Survey 2008," *American College of Emergency Physicians,* http://www.acep .org/uploadedFiles/ACEP/Advocacy/federal_issues/PsychiatricBoardingSummary.pdf (accessed July 12, 2016).

14. "Waits for Care and Hospital Beds Growing Dramatically for Psychiatric Emergency Patients," American College of Emergency Physicians, October 17, 2016, http:// newsroom.acep.org/2016-10-17-Waits-for-Care-and-Hospital-Beds-Growing -Dramatically-for-Psychiatric-Emergency-Patients (accessed December 10, 2016).

15. Cynthia Hubert, Phillip Reese, and Jim Sanders, "Nevada Buses Hundreds of Mentally Ill Patients to Cities around Country," *Sacramento Bee,* April 14, 2013, http:// www.sacbee.com/2013/04/14/5340078/nevada-buses-hundreds-of-mentally.html (accessed July 12, 2016).

16. Following are some studies on the relationship between lack of inpatient capacity and increased homelessness, arrest, crime, and violence.

- A study of 132 patients discharged from Columbus State Hospital in Ohio reported that 36 percent became homeless within six months. J. R. Belcher, "Rights versus Needs of Homeless Mentally Ill Persons," *Social Work* 33, no. 5 (September–October 1988): 398–402.
- In reviewing early studies on discharged psychiatric patients, Dr. Judith Rabkin concluded, "Arrest and conviction rates for the subcategory of violent crimes were found to exceed general population rates in every study in which they were measured." J. G. Rabkin, "Criminal Behavior of Discharged Mental Patients: A Critical Appraisal of the Research," *Psychological Bulletin* 86, no. 1 (1979): 1–27. Abstract at https://www.ncjrs.gov/App/publications/Abstract.aspx?id=75899 (accessed July 12, 2016).
- In a follow-up of patients released from a psychiatric hospital, Dr. Henry Steadman, et al. reported, "27% of released male and female patients report at least one violent act within a means of four months after discharge." John Monahan, "Mental Disorder and Violent Behavior," *American Psychologist* 47, no. 4 (April 1992): 511–21. Abstract at http://psycnet.apa.org/journals/amp/47/4/511 (accessed July 12, 2016).
- In 2006, Markowitz published data on eighty-one US cities, and found a direct correlation between the decreasing availability of psychiatric hospital beds and the increase in crime, arrest rates, and homelessness. Fred E. Markowitz, "Psychiatric Hospital Capacity, Homelessness, and Crime and Arrest Rates," *Criminology* 44, no. 1 (February 2006): 45–72. Abstract at http://onlinelibrary.wiley.com/doi/10.1111/j.1745-9125.2006.00042.x/abstract (accessed July 12, 2016).

17. Bernard E. Harcourt, "An Institutionalization Effect: The Impact of Mental Hospitalization and Imprisonment on Homicide in the United States, 1934–2001," *Journal of Legal Studies* 40, no. 1 (January 2011), http://www.jstor.org/stable/10.1086/658404 (accessed July 12, 2016).

18. Drew Alexander, "Jail Not the Place for Mentally Ill, Says Summit County Sheriff," (letter to the editor), *South Side Leader* (Akron, OH), April 12, 2012, http://www.akron.com/akron-ohio-opinions.asp?aID=15743 (accessed July 12, 2016).

19. Patty B. Wight, "Mental Blocks, Part 1: Needing a Psychiatric Bed, Ending up in Jail," *Maine Public Broadcasting Network*, December 23, 2013.

20. Steve Johnson, "Erlanger Gets Go-Ahead for $25 Million Mental Health Hospital," *Times Free Press*, August 25, 2016, http://www.timesfreepress.com/news/local/story/2016/aug/24/regulators-new-25-million-88-bed-mental-hospital-chattanooga/382841 (accessed August 25, 2016).

21. "No Room at the Inn: Trends and Consequences of Closing Public Psychiatric Hospitals 2005–2010" (Arlington, VA: Treatment Advocacy Center, July 19, 2012), http://tacreports.org/storage/documents/no_room_at_the_inn-2012.pdf (accessed July 12, 2016).

22. House Committee on Energy, "Where Have all the Patients Gone?" Hirshon, statement.

23. "Psychotherapies," *National Institute of Mental Health*, http://www.nimh.nih.gov/health/topics/psychotherapies/index.shtml (accessed July 14, 2016).

24. National Institute for Health and Care Excellence (NICE), "Psychosis and Schizophrenia in Adults: Prevention and Management," NICE, February 12, 2014, https://www.nice.org.uk/guidance/cg178/resources/psychosis-and-schizophrenia-in-adults-prevention-and-management-35109758952133 (accessed July 14, 2016).

25. Keith Laws, "Assessing the Potential Benefits and Harm of Cognitive Behavioural Therapy for Psychosis," *Mental Health Today*, March/April 2015, https://www.mentalhealthtoday.co.uk/assessing-the-potential-benefits-and-harm-of-cognitive-behavioural-therapy-for-psychosis.aspx (accessed July 14, 2016).

26. US Department of Health and Human Services, *Federal Register* 80, no. 249 (December 29, 2015): 81223, https://www.gpo.gov/fdsys/pkg/FR-2015-12-29/pdf/2015-32592.pdf (accessed August 31, 2016). As the *Washington Post* reported, "After years of consideration, the Food and Drug Administration has determined that for carefully selected patients with profound depression, the benefits of electroconvulsive therapy, long demonized, outweigh the risks of possible memory loss caused by its use." Dan Hurley, "FDA: Electroshock Has Risks But Is Useful to Combat Severe Depression," *Washington Post*, July 18, 2016, https://www.washingtonpost.com/national/health-science/fda-electroshock-has-risks-but-is-useful-to-combat-severe-depression/2016/07/18/4a109cbc-2f4e-11e6-9de3-6e6e7a14000c_story.html (accessed August 31, 2016). ECT for depression: Alan J. Gelenberg, Marlene P. Freeman, John C. Markowitz, et al. (work group on Major Depressive Disorder), *Practice Guideline for the Treatment of Patients with Major Depressive Disorder*, 3rd ed. (Washington, DC: American Psychiatric Association, October 2010), http://psychiatryonline.org/pb/assets/raw/sitewide/practice_guidelines/guidelines/mdd.pdf (accessed July 12, 2016).

27. Cochrane Schizophrenia Group, "Electroconvulsive Therapy for Schizophrenia," *Cochrane Database of Systematic Reviews*, April 20, 2005. Abstract at http://onlinelibrary.wiley.com/wol1/doi/10.1002/14651858.CD000076.pub2/abstract (accessed August 30, 2016).

28. NIMH, "Brain Stimulation Therapies," NIMH, June 2016, http://www.nimh.nih.gov/health/topics/brain-stimulation-therapies/brain-stimulation-therapies.shtml (accessed August 30, 2016).

29. DJ Jaffe, "Save the Hospitals," *National Review*, September 18, 2013, http://www.nationalreview.com/article/358796/save-hospitals-d-j-jaffe (accessed December 15, 2016).

30. Cochrane Collaborative, "Consumer-Providers of Care for Adult Clients of Statutory Mental Health Services," by Veronica Pitt, Dianne Lowe, Sophie Hill, et al., *Cochrane Database of Systematic Reviews* no. 3 (2012), http://onlinelibrary.wiley.com/doi/10.1002/14651858.CD004807.pub2/full (accessed July 12, 2016).

31. Lisa Dixon, Diana Perkins and Christine Calmes, "Guideline Watch: Practice Guideline for the Treatment of Patients with Schizophrenia" (Washington, DC: American Psychiatric Association, September 2009), http://psychiatryonline.org/pb/assets/raw/sitewide/practice_guidelines/guidelines/schizophrenia-watch.pdf (accessed July 12, 2016).

32. Brynmor Lloyd-Evans, Evan Mayo-Wilson, Bronwyn Harrison, et al., "A Systematic Review and Meta-Analysis of Randomised Controlled Trials of Peer Support for People with Severe Mental Illness," *BMC Psychiatry* 14 (2014), http://www.ncbi.nlm.nih.gov/pmc/articles/PMC3933205 (accessed July 12, 2016).

33. Researchers said, "Peer support was associated with $5,991 higher total Medicaid cost. Peer support was also associated with higher crisis stabilization cost and lower psychiatric hospitalization cost, but the relationships were not statistically significant. Peer support was associated with $2,100 higher prescription drug cost, $5,116 higher professional services cost, and $1,225 lower facility cost." Researchers chose the politi-

cally correct path. While finding no benefit to peer support, they concluded, "While the implementation of Medicaid financed peer support programs may not result in savings from reductions of costly crisis stabilizations and psychiatric hospitalizations, it does support the principles of self-direction and recovery from severe mental illness. State policy makers must weigh the potential higher cost associated with peer support programs with efforts to redesign the delivery of mental health services." Glenn Landers and Mei Zhou, "The Impact of Medicaid Peer Support Utilization on Cost," *Medicaid & Medicare Research Review* 4, no. 1 (2014): E1–E14, http://www.cms.gov/mmrr/Downloads/ MMRR2014_004_01_a04.pdf (accessed July 12, 2016).

34. "The Evidence," Peer Support Resources, http://www .psresources.info/the-evidence (accessed August 15, 2016).

35. Even adding together "might cause neighbors/community to have negative opinion," "did not want others to find out," and "might have negative effect on job," stigma still comes behind "could not afford cost" and "could handle problem without treatment." Substance Abuse and Mental Health Services Administration (SAMHSA), *Results from the 2011 National Survey on Drug Use and Health: Mental Health Findings*, NSDU Series H-45, HHS Publication No. (SMA) 12-4725 (Rockville, MD: SAMHSA, 2012); Fig. 2.1, p. 26, http://www.samhsa.gov/data/NSDUH/2k11MH_FindingsandDetTables/ 2K11MHFR/NSDUHmhfr2011.pdf (accessed July 12, 2016).

36. The military's stigma study found, "Despite popular opinion and a strong theoretical base that stigma deters treatment-seeking, we were unable to identify empirical literature to support this link. . . . The regression analyses revealed that stigma did not predict initiation of treatment-seeking. . . . However, a variety of other factors (e.g., availability of providers, time off of work to seek care) may affect whether intentions to seek treatment translate into actual behavior." Joie Acosta, Amariah Becker, Jennifer L. Cerully, et al., *Mental Health Stigma in the Military* (Santa Monica, CA: Rand Corporation, 2014), http://www.rand.org/pubs/research_reports/RR426.html (accessed July 12, 2016).

Another paper found that "[T]he majority of studies found no association between anticipated stigma and mental health service use or intentions to seek help." Marie-Louise Sharp, Nicola T. Fear, and Roberto J. Rona, "Stigma as a Barrier to Seeking Health Care Among Military Personnel with Mental Health Problems," *Epidemiologic Reviews* 37 (Oxford University Press, October 2014), http://www.kcl.ac.uk/kcmhr/publications/ assetfiles/2015/Sharp2015.pdf (accessed July 12, 2016).

37. The Field Poll, "Tabulations from a Survey of California Adults about Behavioral Health Issues," Prepared for the California HealthCare Foundation (San Francisco, CA: Field Research Corporation, June 2014), http://media.sacbee.com/ smedia/2014/09/16/16/27/16xg5H.So.4.pdf (accessed July 12, 2016).

38. S. Clement, O. Schauman, T. Graham, et al., "What Is the Impact of Mental Health-Related Stigma on Help-Seeking? A Systematic Review of Quantitative and Qualitative Studies," *Psychological Medicine* 45, no. 1 (January 2015): 11–27. Abstract at http://www.ncbi.nlm.nih.gov/pubmed/24569086 (accessed July 12, 2016).

39. Ramin Mojtabai, Mark Olfson, Nancy A. Sampson, et al., "Barriers to Mental Health Treatment: Results from the National Comorbidity Survey Replication (NCS-R)," *Psychological Medicine* 41, no. 8 (August 2011): 1751–61, http://www.ncbi.nlm.nih.gov/ pmc/articles/PMC3128692 (accessed July 12, 2016).

40. Centers for Disease Control and Prevention (CDC), National Center for Health

Statistics, "Antidepressant Use in Persons Aged 12 and Over: United States, 2005–2008," by Laura A. Pratt, Debra J. Brody, and Qiuping Gu (NCHS Data Brief, Hyattsville, MD: National Center for Health Statistics, CDC, 2011), http://www.cdc.gov/nchs/data/databriefs/db76.pdf (accessed July 12, 2016).

41. One study found that the duration of first-episode psychosis going untreated was fifty-five weeks in jurisdictions with broad commitment criteria but went up to seventy-nine weeks in jurisdictions with narrow dangerousness criteria. Matthew Large and Olav Nielssen, "Evidence for a Relationship between the Duration of Untreated Psychosis and the Proportion of Psychotic Homicides Prior to Treatment," *Social Psychiatry and Psychiatric Epidemiology* 43, no. 1 (January 2008): 37–44. Abstract at http://www.ncbi.nlm.nih.gov/pubmed/17960314 (accessed July 12, 2016).

One-third of the current state-to-state variation in murder rates can be explained by differences in the strictness of involuntary commitment laws, with easier commitment correlating with lower murder rates. Steven P. Segal, "Civil Commitment Law, Mental Health Services, and US Homicide Rates," *Social Psychiatry and Psychiatric Epidemology* 47, no. 9 (September 2012): 1449–58. Abstract at http://www.ncbi.nlm.nih.gov/pubmed/22072224 (accessed July 12, 2016).

42. Kendra's Law is named after Kendra Webdale who was pushed to her death in front of a subway car by Andrew Goldstein, who had a long history of doing well in treatment, going off treatment, deteriorating, being put back on medications in a hospital, going off, and repeating again.

43. The criteria for admission are appropriately narrow: The person must be

(1) eighteen years of age or older; and
(2) suffering from a mental illness; and
(3) unlikely to survive safely in the community without supervision, based on a clinical determination; and
(4) have a history of lack of compliance with treatment for mental illness that has:
    (i)   prior to the filing of the petition, at least twice within the last thirty-six months been a significant factor in necessitating hospitalization in a hospital, or receipt of services in a forensic or other mental health unit of a correctional facility or a local correctional facility, not including any current period, or period ending within the last six months, during which the person was or is hospitalized or incarcerated; or
    (ii) prior to the filing of the petition, resulted in one or more acts of serious violent behavior toward self or others or threats of, or attempts at, serious physical harm to self or others within the last forty-eight months, not including any current period, or period ending within the last six months, in which the person was or is hospitalized or incarcerated; and
(5) as a result of his or her mental illness, unlikely to voluntarily participate in outpatient treatment that would enable him or her to live safely in the community; and
(6) in view of his or her treatment history and current behavior, in need of assisted outpatient treatment in order to prevent a relapse or deterioration which would be likely to result in serious harm to the person or others . . . and
(7) likely to benefit from assisted outpatient treatment. New York State Legislature,

NY MHY. LAW § 9.60: NY Code—Section 9.60: Assisted Outpatient Treatment, 2010, http://codes.lp.findlaw.com/nycode/MHY/B/9/9.60 (accessed July 12, 2016).

44. Lynn Gibbs, "Notes from Presentation by Judge Anderson to Ventura County Laura's Law Workgroup," Mental Illness Policy Org., January 2015, http://mental illnesspolicy.org/states/california/judgeandersonpresentation.html (accessed September 11, 2016); Mad in America, "Disability Rights Will Challenge California's Outpatient Commitment Laws in Court," Mental Illness Policy Org., December 14, 2014, http://mentalillnesspolicy.org/states/california/p&aopposition.pdf (accessed September 11, 2016).

45. National Sheriffs' Association, "National Sheriffs' Association Supports Mission of Treatment Advocacy Center," Sheriffs.org, March 2013, http://www.sheriffs.org/sites/default/files/uploads/documents/GovAffairs/2013-03%20Treatment%20Advocacy%20Center.pdf (accessed July 13, 2016); IACP endorsement: International Association of Chiefs of Police (IACP), Resolution: "Assisted Outpatient Treatment," Mental Illness Policy Org., October 21, 2014, http://mentalillnesspolicy.org/crimjust/iacpadoptsaot.pdf (accessed July 12, 2016); DOJ endorsement: US Department of Justice, National Institute of Justice, "Program Profile: Assisted Outpatient Treatment (AOT)," Crime Solutions, March 26, 2012, www.crimesolutions.gov/ProgramDetails.aspx?ID=228 (accessed July 12, 2016).

46. NAMI (National Alliance on Mental Illness), "Involuntary Commitment and Court-Ordered Treatment," NAMI, 1995, http://www.nami.org/About-NAMI/Policy-Platform/9-Legal-Issues (accessed July 12, 2016). NAMI National's staff has refused to support the grassroots by encouraging the adoption of AOT. This is largely due to NAMI's move away from focusing on serious mental illness.

47. SAMHSA endorsement: SAMHSA, National Registry of Evidence-Based Programs and Practices (SAMHSA-NREPP), "Assisted Outpatient Treatment," 2015, http://legacy.nreppadmin.net/ViewIntervention.aspx?id=401 (accessed July 12, 2016). AHRQ endorsement: Agency for Healthcare Research and Quality (AHRQ), "Management Strategies to Reduce Psychiatric Readmissions," Mental Illness Policy Org., May 2015. Summary at http://mentalillnesspolicy.org/national-studies/ahrq_endorses_aot.pdf (accessed July 12, 2016).

48. Reverend Thomas G. Wenski, Committee on Domestic Justice and Human Development, United States Conference of Catholic Bishops, Letter to US House of Representatives, July 6, 2016.

49. K. J. Brennan, *Kendra's Law: Final Report on the Status of Assisted Outpatient Treatment* (Appendix 2), New York State Office of Mental Health (Albany, NY: 2005), http://mentalillnesspolicy.org/kendras-law/research/kendras-law-study-2005.pdf (accessed July 12, 2016). Unpublished revision at http://mentalillnesspolicy.org/kendras-law/kendras-law-constitutional.html (accessed July 12, 2016). *Parens patriae* are the powers the state has to protect those who can't protect themselves, and is often invoked to help children, the elderly and those with mental impairments.

50. Tom Barnidge, "Contra Costa Supervisors to Hear the Case for Laura's Law," *Contra Costa (CA) Times*, April 4, 2014, http://www.contracostatimes.com/barnidge/ci_25501045/barnidge-contra-costa-supervisors-hear-case-lauras-law (accessed July 12, 2016).

51. Pat and Bruce Goodale, "Our Failing the Mentally Ill Has High Societal Costs,"

(letter), *Wall Street Journal*, February 12, 2013, http://www.wsj.com/articles/SB100014241 2788732419620457829816157478742 (accessed July 12, 2016).

52. Dan Roberts, "Secret Service Allowed Armed Man with Assault Charge into Elevator with Obama," *Guardian*, September 30, 2014, http://www.theguardian.com/world/2014/sep/30/secret-service-white-house-intruder-omar-gonzalez (accessed July 14, 2016).

CHAPTER 7: SUBSTANCE ABUSE AND MENTAL HEALTH SERVICES ADMINISTRATION (SAMHSA)

1. Conference Committee, "Conference Report on ADAMHA Reorganization Act (S. 1306)," US Congress, *Congressional Record* (Washington, DC: US Government Printing Office, May 19, 1992); *Alcohol, Drug Abuse, Mental Health Administration (ADAMHA) Reorganization Act*, Pub. L. 102–321, July 10, 1992, http://history.nih.gov/research/downloads/PL102-321.pdf (accessed July 12, 2016).

2. US Congress, *Public Health Service Act*, Section 1912 of Title XIX, Part B, Subpart I of the PHS Act (42 USC §300x-2) http://www.gpo.gov/fdsys/pkg/USCODE -2010-title42/pdf/USCODE-2010-title42-chap6A-subchapXVII-partB.pdf (accessed July 12, 2016).

3. As a result of lobbying by non-SAMHSA-funded groups, some congressional appropriations are required to be used for the seriously ill and SAMHSA disingenuously claims credit for them. For example, Congress allocated funds to be used for First Episode Psychosis (FEP), and SAMHSA now claims its FEP activities as "proof" it does focus on the seriously ill. Another example. SAMHSA conducted an online survey asking how SAMHSA could improve care. The third-highest vote-getter was expanding the use of AOT. SAMHSA ignored the results. But, Congress forced SAMHSA to fund AOT (2015 "Doc Fix" bill), and SAMHSA now uses its AOT activities as proof it focuses on serious mental illness. US Department of Health and Human Services (HHS), "Fiscal Year 2017, SAMHSA, Justification of Estimates for Appropriations Committees," SAMHSA, p. vii, http://www.samhsa.gov/sites/default/files/samhsa-fy-2017 -congressional-justification.pdf (accessed September 25, 2016). SAMHSA, "Stakeholder Feedback: Strategic Initiatives." First page archived at http://web.archive.org/web/20140803130542/http://feedback.samhsa.gov/forums/77283--closed-samhsa-s -strategic-initiatives/filters/top (accessed December 20, 2016).

4. Substance Abuse and Mental Health Services Administration (SAMHSA), *Leading Change: A Plan for SAMHSA's Roles and Actions 2011–2014*, HHS Publication No. (SMA) 11–4629 (Rockville, MD: SAMHSA, 2011), http://store.samhsa.gov/shin/content/SMA11-4629/01-FullDocument.pdf (accessed July 12, 2016).

5. Josh Sanburn, "Inside the National Suicide Hotline: Preventing the Next Tragedy," *Time*, September 13, 2013, http://healthland.time.com/2013/09/13/inside-the -national-suicide-hotline-counselors-work-to-prevent-the-next-casualty/print (accessed July 12, 2016).

6. SAMHSA, *Leading Change 2.0: Advancing the Behavioral Health of the Nation 2015–2018*, HHS Publication No. (PEP) 14-LEADCHANGE2 (Rockville, MD: SAMHSA, 2014), http://store.samhsa.gov/shin/content//PEP14-LEADCHANGE2/PEP14-LEADCHANGE2.pdf (accessed July 12, 2016).

7. Paul Summergrad, "SAMHSA Strategic Plan Falls Short on Serious Mental Illness," *Psychiatric News*, September 11, 2014, http://psychnews.psychiatryonline.org/doi/full/10.1176/appi.pn.2014.9b17 (accessed July 12, 2016).

8. Tim Murphy, "Examining SAMHSA's Role in Delivering Services to the Severely Mentally Ill," Hearings Before the House Subcommittee on Oversight and Investigations of the Committee on Energy and Commerce, 113th Cong. (May 22, 2013), http://mentalillnesspolicy.org/samhsa/tim-murphy-statement-5.22.13.pdf (accessed July 12, 2016).

9. *Wall Street Journal* editorial board, "The Definition of Insanity: How a Federal Agency (SAMHSA) Undermines Treatment for the Mentally Ill," *Wall Street Journal*, March 31, 2014, http://mentalillnesspolicy.org/samhsa/wsj_samhsa_hurts_3.23.14.html (accessed July 12, 2016).

10. HHS, "Fiscal Year 2017, SAMHSA," p. vii.

11. Elinore F. Mccance-Katz, "The Federal Government Ignores the Treatment Needs of Americans With Serious Mental Illness," *Psychiatric Times*, April 21, 2016, http://www.psychiatrictimes.com/depression/federal-government-ignores-treatment-needs-americans-serious-mental-illness/page/0/1 (accessed July 12, 2016).

12. Partnership for Public Service, "Agency Report: Substance Abuse and Mental Health Services Administration (HHS)," Best Places to Work in the Federal Government, 2016, http://bestplacestowork.org/BPTW/rankings/detail/HE32 (accessed July 12, 2016).

13. US Government Accountability Office (GAO), *Mental Health: HHS Leadership Needed to Coordinate Federal Efforts Related to Serious Mental Illness*, Report to the Subcommittee on Oversight and Investigations, Committee on Energy and Commerce, US House of Representatives (Washington, DC: February 5, 2015), http://www.gao.gov/assets/670/667644.pdf (accessed July 12, 2016).

14. The Recovery Model was previously promoted in chapter 14 of the 2003 *New Freedom Commission Report on Mental Health*, which described recovery as "the process by which people are able to live, work, learn, and participate fully in their communities." But it never gained traction. SAMHSA started their quest to invent their own definition of recovery in August 2010, with a "Dialogue Meeting," followed by a year-long "Public Engagement Process," followed by four months of internal reviews and then followed by a vote by 8,500 interested parties they had marshaled. SAMHSA, "Stakeholder Feedback: Recovery," SAMHSA, 2011, http://blog.samhsa.gov/2011/08/12/recovery-defined-give-us-your-feedback/ (accessed July 12, 2016).

After sorting through 259 online comments, 500 ideas from 1,000 participants, and over 1,200 comments, SAMHSA finally issued its definition. "SAMHSA's Definition and Guiding Principles of Recovery: Answering the Call for Feedback," SAMHSA (blog), December 11, 2011, http://blog.samhsa.gov/2011/12/22/samhsas-definition-and-guiding-principles-of-recovery-answering-the-call-for-feedback (accessed July 12, 2016).

SAMHSA then took four months to revise it. This became the "Recovery Model" and the Ten "Guiding Principles of Recovery" designed to foster "physical and emotional well-being." Paolo del Vecchio, "SAMHSA's Working Definition of Recovery Updated," SAMHSA (blog), March 23, 2012, http://blog.samhsa.gov/2012/03/23/defintion-of-recovery-updated/#.U3YZFShJ-6k (accessed July 12, 2016).

15. del Vecchio, "SAMHSA's Working Definition of Recovery Updated."

16. Erika Jääskeläinen, Pauliina Juola, Noora Hirvonen, et al., "A Systematic Review

and Meta-Analysis of Recovery in Schizophrenia," *Schizophrenia Bulletin* 39, no. 6 (2013): 1296–1306, http://schizophreniabulletin.oxfordjournals.org/content/39/6/1296.full (accessed July 30, 2013).

17. E. Fuller Torrey and DJ Jaffe, "After Newtown," *National Review*, August 14, 2013, http://www.nationalreview.com/article/355826/after-newtown-e-fuller-torrey-d-j-jaffe (accessed December 19, 2016).

18. Sally Satel and Mary Zdanowicz, "Commission's Omission: The President's Mental-Health Commission in Denial," *National Review*, July 29, 2003, http://mental illnesspolicy.org/mentalhealth/new-freedom-commission.html (accessed July 12, 2016).

19. Sally Satel, "A Statement of Madness: The New Guidelines for Treating Mental Illness Need Help," *National Review*, April 5, 2006, http://www.nationalreview.com/article/217240/statement-madness-sally-satel?target=author&tid=901248 (accessed July 12, 2016).

20. SAMHSA supports recovery newsletters, a "Recovery to Practice" initiative, a "Partners for Recovery" initiative, recovery webinars, conferences and brochures. In its three-year plan, the word "recovery" is mentioned 206 times. "Recovery Model" programs dominate the SAMHSA National Registry of Evidence-Based Programs and Practices (NREPP).

21. Mental Health America (MHA) "is committed to the notion that every individual with a mental health or substance use condition can recover." Mental Health America, "Position Statement 72: Violence: Community Mental Health Response," *Mental Health America*, September 17, 2011, http://www.mentalhealthamerica.net/positions/violence#.UxuhvShJ-5c (accessed July 12, 2016).

California's Mental Health Services Act has raised over $1 billion annually to help "people with severe mental illness," but by specifically referencing the Recovery Model, the Oversight Commission is able to justify withholding help from people with serious mental illness who can't self-direct their own care. California State Treasurer, "Investment in Mental Health Wellness Grant Program: Frequently Asked Questions (FAQ)," (Sacramento, CA: California State Treasurer), January 14, 2014, http://www.treasurer.ca.gov/chffa/imhwa/faq.pdf (accessed July 12, 2016).

22. SAMHSA, *Leading Change 2.0: 2015–2018*.

23. del Vecchio, "SAMHSA's Working Definition of Recovery Updated."

24. Charlotte Walker, "Jagged Little Pill: Has the Recovery Narrative Gone Too Far?" *purplepersuasion*, June 11, 2014, https://purplepersuasion.wordpress.com/2014/06/11/jagged-little-pill-has-the-recovery-narrative-gone-too-far (accessed July 12, 2016).

25. SAMHSA, "National Registry of Evidence-Based Programs and Practices (SAMHSA-NREPP)," SAMHSA-NREPP, 2016, http://www.nrepp.samhsa.gov (accessed July 12, 2016).

26. SAMHSA does not use the term "certifies," but that is the essence of what NREPP does.

27. SAMHSA-NREPP, "Mental Health First Aid," NREPP, May 2012, http://legacy.nreppadmin.net/ViewIntervention.aspx?id=321 (accessed July 12, 2016).

28. Mental Illness Policy Org., "Mental Health First Aid is Unproven Yet SAMHSA Subsidized," Mental Illness Policy Org., 2013, http://mentalillnesspolicy.org/samhsa/mental-health-first-aid-fails.html (accessed July 12, 2016).

29. Barack Obama, *Now is the Time: The President's Plan to Protect Our Children and*

Our Communities by Reducing Gun Violence (Washington, DC: White House, January 16, 2013), http://www.whitehouse.gov/sites/default/files/docs/wh_now_is_the_time_full.pdf (accessed July 12, 2016); Lynn Jenkins (R–KS), *Mental Health First Aid Act of 2015*, HR 1877, 114th Cong. (September 13, 2016), https://www.congress.gov/bill/114th-congress/house-bill/1877/all-actions (accessed September 19, 2016). Also see Gene Green (R–TX), *Comprehensive Behavioral Health Reform and Recovery Act of 2016*, HR 4435, 114th Cong. (February 2, 2016), https://www.congress.gov/bill/114th-congress/house-bill/4435 (accessed July 12, 2016).

30. Bill de Blasio, *ThriveNYC: A Mental Health Roadmap for All* (New York City: 2015), https://thrivenyc.cityofnewyork.us/wp-content/uploads/2015/11/Mental HealthRoadmap.pdf (accessed July 12, 2016).

31. SAMHSA-NREPP, "Triple P-Positive Parenting Program," May 15, 2014. Link expired.

32. Philip Wilson, Robert Rush, Susan Hussey, et al., "How Evidence-Based is an 'Evidence-Based Parenting Program'? A PRISMA Systematic Review and Meta-Analysis of Triple P," *BMC Medicine* 10 (November 2012), http://www.biomedcentral.com/content/pdf/1741-7015-10-130.pdf (accessed July 12, 2016); James C. Coyne and Linda Kwakkenbos, "Triple P-Positive Parenting Programs: The Folly of Basing Social Policy on Underpowered Flawed Studies," *BMC Medicine* 11 (January 2013), http://bmcmedicine .biomedcentral.com/articles/10.1186/1741-7015-11-11 (accessed July 12, 2016).

33. SAMHSA-NREPP, "Wellness Recovery Action Plan," NREPP, September 2010, http://legacy.nreppadmin.net/ViewIntervention.aspx?id=208 (accessed September 19, 2016).

34. Mental Illness Policy Org., "WRAP is Certified as 'Evidence Based' by SAMHSA, But Is It?" Mental Illness Policy Org., 2013, http://mentalillnesspolicy.org/samhsa/wrapunproven.html (accessed July 12, 2016). SAMHSA recently awarded a program run by Ms. Copeland $330,000 for each of three years.

35. Mental Illness Policy Org., "Teen Screen Certified by SAMHSA in Spite of Zero Research," Mental Illness Policy Org., 2013, http://mentalillnesspolicy.org/samhsa/teenscreenunproven.html (accessed July 12, 2016).

36. Mental Illness Policy Org., "Kognito At-Risk for College Students Certified by SAMHSA as Effective Way to Identify Mentally Ill Students in Spite of Lack of Evidence," Mental Illness Policy Org., 2013, http://mentalillnesspolicy.org/samhsa/kognitounproven.html (accessed July 12, 2016).

37. US House of Representatives Committee on Energy and Commerce Subcommittee on Oversight and Investigations, "Examining SAMHSA's Role in Delivering Services to the Severely Mentally Ill: Hearings Before the House Subcommittee on Oversight and Investigations of the Committee on Energy and Commerce," Sally Satel testimony, 113th Cong., May 22, 2013, http://mentalillnesspolicy.org/samhsa/satel.5.22.13 .samhsa.testimony.pdf (accessed July 12, 2016). The American Psychiatric Association also criticized SAMHSA for failing to "develop explicit goals for evidence-based medical care for serious psychiatric illnesses." Summergrad, "SAMHSA Strategic Plan Falls Short."

38. One reason SAMHSA hasn't certified these is that SAMHSA requires programs to be submitted to them for review. When programs help persons with mental illness, but no one profits from them, there is no submitter.

39. HHS, "Fiscal Year 2017, SAMHSA," p. 55 (accessed September 25, 2016). Block

grants are federal funds that are supposed to be distributed to states ("block granted") with little federal direction. Before Congress established the block grants, the funds were appropriated for specific legislatively mandated programs, including Community Mental Health Centers. Block granting was supposed to give states more flexibility.

40. Mental Illness Policy Org., "How SAMHSA Mental Health Block Grant Guidance and Application Form Encourages States to Not Use Block Grants for the Most Seriously Ill," Mental Illness Policy Org., February 3, 2013, http://mentalillnesspolicy.org/samhsa/samhsa-block-grant-problems.pdf (accessed July 12, 2016).

41. SAMHSA, "FY 2014–2015 Block Grant Application," SAMHSA, 2014, http://www.samhsa.gov/sites/default/files/fy2014-2015-bg-application.pdf (accessed July 12, 2016). Substance Abuse and Mental Health Services Administration (SAMHSA), "FY 2012–2013 Block Grant Application," SAMHSA, 2012, http://beta.samhsa.gov/sites/default/files/bg_planning_section.pdf (accessed July 12, 2016).

42. SAMHSA, "Block Grant Public Comment Log," 2012. Archived at http://web.archive.org/web/20130213155030/http://www.samhsa.gov/grants/blockgrant/docs/BGComment-Question-Log-Continuous.pdf (accessed July 12, 2016).

43. In 1986, states were required to conduct mental health planning as a condition for receiving the block grant, but the statute put providers in the planning groups. Family members of the seriously ill on the planning councils are simply outvoted by the industry representatives. Joseph N. de Raismes, III, "The Evolution of Federal Mental Health Planning Legislation" (paper, National Association of Mental Health Planning & Advisory Councils, 2005). Link to article available under Frequently Asked Questions, http://www.namhpac.org/about.html (accessed July 12, 2016).

44. US Congress, *Consolidated Appropriations Act of 2014*, HR 3547, 113th Congress (2013–2014) enacted as Public Law 113-76, January 17, 2014, https://www.gpo.gov/fdsys/pkg/PLAW-113publ76/pdf/PLAW-113publ76.pdf (accessed July 12, 2016). The legislative history is at https://beta.congress.gov/bill/113th-congress/house-bill/3547/text. The accompanying Senate Report 113-71 (2014) is at http://www.gpo.gov/fdsys/pkg/CRPT-113srpt71/pdf/CRPT-113srpt71.pdf (accessed July 12, 2016). When the 21st Century Cures Act (H.R. 34) was passed in December 2016, the set-aside was raised to ten percent. US Congress, "21st Century Cures Act," https://www.congress.gov/bill/114th-congress/house-bill/34/text (accessed December 10, 2016).

45. SAMHSA, "Guidance for Revision of the FY 2014–2015 MHBG Behavioral Health Assessment and Plan," SAMHSA, 2014, http://www.samhsa.gov/sites/default/files/mhbg-5-percent-set-aside-guidance.pdf (accessed July 12, 2016). See chapter 12 for a discussion of peer support and SAMHSA support for it.

46. SAMHSA, "Stakeholder Feedback: Trauma," SAMHSA, December 31, 2010. First page archived at http://web.archive.org/web/20140728143636/http://feedback.samhsa.gov/forums/186681--closed-definition-of-trauma (accessed July 12, 2016). The idea of focusing on trauma started at a 1994 SAMHSA-sponsored conference that was supposed to address victimized women. Instead, it promoted SAMHSA's anti-treatment narrative by highlighting alleged "re-victimization experienced in residential or inpatient settings through such practices as seclusion and restraint." SAMHSA, "About the National Center for Trauma Informed Care," SAMHSA, 2005. Archived at http://web.archive.org/web/20140406182517/http://samhsa.gov/nctic/about.asp (accessed July 12, 2016).

47. SAMHSA, "Trauma Definition," SAMHSA, December 10, 2012. First page archived at http://web.archive.org/web/20140701164137/http://samhsa.gov/trauma justice/traumadefinition/definition.aspx (accessed July 12, 2016).

48. Boris Vatel, "Unmasking Trauma-Informed Care," *Clinical Psychiatry News*, October 9, 2015, http://www.clinicalpsychiatrynews.com/views/single-view/unmasking -trauma-informed-care/dfa0935dfbb07b1c60fc7c3bc3ed5fac.html (accessed July 12, 2016).

49. HHS, "Fiscal Year 2017, SAMHSA," p. 56.

50. Christina Hoff Sommers and Sally Satel, *One Nation Under Therapy: How the Helping Culture is Eroding Self-Reliance* (New York: St. Martin's Press, 2005).

51. The National Center for Trauma-Informed Care seems to have morphed into anti-treatment territory. Its original purpose was "to offer technical assistance to stimulate and support interest in and implementation of trauma-informed care in publicly funded systems and programs." SAMHSA, "About the National Center for Trauma-Informed Care," SAMHSA, 2005. But the active website says it was renamed the National Center for Trauma-Informed Care *and Alternatives to Seclusion and Restraint* (emphasis added): http://www.samhsa.gov/nctic/about (accessed July 12, 2016). We don't know what alternatives they are proposing. Most likely it is not medication or treatment.

52. Mental Illness Policy Org., "SAMHSA Supports Groups That Lobby Against Improved Treatment," Mental Illness Policy Org., 2012, http://mentalillnesspolicy.org/ samhsa/samhsa-support-antipsychiatry.pdf (accessed July 12, 2016).

53. SAMHSA's Resource Center to Promote Acceptance, Dignity, and Social Inclusion Associated with Mental Health (ADS Center), "Mental Illness Awareness Week Guide," SAMHSA, October 2010, http://mentalillnesspolicy.org/samhsa/samhsa_miaw _guide.pdf (accessed July 12, 2016).

54. Mindfreedom, "The Truth Behind the MFI Truth Brochure," Mindfreedom, September 6, 2008, http://www.mindfreedom.org/kb/mental-health-system/truth (accessed July 12, 2016).

55. Icarus Project, "Welcome to the Icarus Project," Icarus Project, 2014, http://www .theicarusproject.net (accessed February 28, 2015).

56. National Coalition for Mental Health Recovery (NCMHR), "Coalition of Individuals with Psychiatric Labels Supports Protestors' Efforts to 'Occupy' the American Psychiatric Association Convention," press release, May 3, 2012, http://www.ncmhr.org/ press-releases/5.3.12.htm (accessed July 12, 2016).

57. Mental Illness Policy Org., "SAMHSA Supports Groups."

58. Joseph Rogers, interview by Joanne Silberner, "The Closing of Haverford State: A Special Report," *NPR: The Infinite Mind*, June 21, 2000.

59. SAMHSA, "Listing of Active Contracts," May 2011. Archived at https://web .archive.org/web/20140530185530/http://www.hhs.gov/about/smallbusiness/small business/pdf/samhsa.pdf (accessed July 12, 2016).

60. Pat Risser, "Pat Risser Highlights," http://www.patrisser.com/personalinfo/res .html (accessed July 12, 2016).

61. Pat Risser, "Personal Stories," MindFreedom, http://www.mindfreedom.org/ personal-stories/risserpat (accessed December 19, 2016).

62. Dr. Sally Satel told a House subcommittee, "Despite the fact that we were called an 'advisory council,' it was clear that CMHS did not want our advice." House Committee on Energy and Commerce, "Examining SAMHSA's Role," Satel testimony.

63. SAMHSA, "Building Blocks: Sing-Along Songs," SAMHSA, 2011, formerly at https://bblocks2015-stage.icfwebservices.com/activities/songs/healthy-snacks.aspx (accessed July 12, 2014).

64. US Government Accountability Office (GAO), "Federal Efforts on Mental Health: Why Greater HHS Leadership is Needed," Transcript of Hearings on the GAO Report on SAMHSA, Before the Subcommittee on Oversight and Investigations of the Committee on Energy and Commerce, 114th Cong., February 11, 2015, http://docs .house.gov/meetings/IF/IF02/20150211/102944/HHRG-114-IF02-Transcript -20150211.pdf (accessed July 12, 2016).

65. E. Fuller Torrey, "The Ridiculous 'National Wellness Week,'" *National Review*, September 17, 2014, http://www.nationalreview.com/article/388140/ridiculous-national -wellness-week-e-fuller-torrey (accessed July 12, 2016).

66. Treatment Advocacy Center, "SAMHSA Receives Worst Government Agency Award," *National Review*, November 10, 2011, http://www.nationalreview.com/ article/388140/ridiculous-national-wellness-week-e-fuller-torrey (accessed December 21, 2016). Until recently, SAMHSA also put on an annual in-house musical to celebrate World AIDS Day.

67. Tom Coburn (then US Senator, R–OK), *2013 Wastebook*, Analysis, United States Congress, Washington, DC, 2013, p. 175.

68. US Congress, "21st Century Cures Act (H.R. 34) 114th Cong. 2015," Congress .gov, https://www.congress.gov/bill/114th-congress/house-bill/34/text (accessed December 10, 2016).

CHAPTER 8: THE MENTAL HEALTH NONPROFIT COMPLEX AND ITS CRITICS

1. National Coalition for Mental Health Recovery (NCMHR), "Member Organizations and Friends of the National Coalition," NCMHR, http://www.ncmhr .org/members.htm (accessed July 13, 2016). NCMHR is partially funded by dues from members, many of whom receive SAMHSA funds.

2. NCMHR, "Coalition of Individuals with Psychiatric Labels Supports Protestors' Efforts to 'Occupy' the American Psychiatric Association Convention," press release, May 3, 2012, http://www.ncmhr.org/press-releases/5.3.12.htm (accessed July 13, 2016).

3. Lauren Spiro, "From the Director," *National Coalition News*, June 2013, http:// www.ncmhr.org/newsletters.htm (accessed July 13, 2016).

4. Virginia Organization of Consumers Asserting Leadership, "About VOCAL," VOCAL, 2002, http://www.vocalvirginia.org/#/about-vocal/4534688342 (accessed July 13, 2016).

5. NCMHR claims "studies have shown that psychiatric diagnosis and labeling can result in increased stigma and discrimination in employment, housing, and community relationships." So, presumably letting and encouraging people to go undiagnosed is the goal. National Coalition for Mental Health Recovery, "Coalition of Individuals with Psychiatric Labels."

6. Substance Abuse and Mental Health Services Administration (SAMHSA), "FY 2010 SAMHSA Grant Awards," SAMHSA, October 13, 2010, http://media.samhsa.gov/ Grants/2010/awards/SM-10-008.aspx (accessed July 13, 2016).

7. E. Fuller Torrey and DJ Jaffe, "After Newtown: The Existing Federal Mental-Health Agency Actually Opposes Efforts to Treat Mental Illness," *National Review*, August 13, 2013, http://www.nationalreview.com/article/355826/after-newtown-e-fuller-torrey-d-j-jaffe (accessed July 13, 2016).

8. National Empowerment Center (NEC), "Home page," NEC, http://www.power2u.org/ (accessed July 13, 2016).

9. Oryx Cohen, "Welcome Page," Freedom Center, http://freedom-center.org/welcome (accessed July 13, 2016).

10. NEC, "Emotional CPR: Saving Lives, Healing Communities (webinar and slides)," NEC, http://emotional-cpr.org. Also see "Emotional CPR: Saving Lives, Healing Communities," YouTube video, 1:30:17, posted by "Emotional CPR," April 19, 2013, https://www.youtube.com/watch?v=cfriXNOq40w&feature=youtu.be (accessed July 13, 2016).

11. SAMHSA, "FY 2010 SAMHSA Grant Awards"; Substance Abuse and Mental Health Services Administration (SAMHSA), "FY 2001 Grant Funding Awards as of October 2001," October 19, 2001. Archived at http://web.archive.org/web/20140714054112/http://www.samhsa.gov/grants/content/2001/awardees/sm01-003.awardees.htm (accessed July 13, 2016).

12. Joseph Rogers, interview by Joanne Silberner, "The Closing of Haverford State: A Special Report," *NPR: The Infinite Mind*, June 21, 2000.

13. National Mental Health Consumers' Self-Help Clearinghouse, "Who We Are!" Mental Health Association of Southeastern Pennsylvania, 2015, http://www.mhselfhelp.org/about-us/ (accessed July 13, 2016). In 2016, SAMHSA gave the Clearinghouse a grant to another organization without explaining why, leading to rumors.

14. National Alliance on Mental Illness (NAMI), "About NAMI: Who We Are, What We Do," NAMI, 2014, http://www.nami.org/template.cfm?section=About_NAMI (accessed July 13, 2016). The author was a former board member of the New York City, New York State, and national organizations.

Examples of NAMI national's historic focus on serious mental illness: In 1993, when President Clinton was formulating a national health plan, the industry argued it should cover all mental health problems. Recognizing that that would drive up costs and likely result in the plan excluding all mental health benefits, NAMI national broke with the industry and proposed a compromise that "would concentrate mental health coverage on treatment of the most severe illnesses." Daniel Goleman, "Mental Health Professionals Worry over Coming Change in Health Care," *New York Times*, May 10, 1993, http://www.nytimes.com/1993/05/10/us/mental-health-professionals-worry-over-coming-change-in-health-care.html (accessed July 13, 2016). In 1995, NAMI again broke with the industry by endorsing various forms of involuntary treatment when needed. NAMI, "Involuntary Commitment and Court-Ordered Treatment," NAMI, 1995, http://www.nami.org/About-NAMI/Policy-Platform/9-Legal-Issues (accessed July 21, 2016). As late as 1999, NAMI and its executive director were criticizing the National Institute of Mental Health (NIMH) for conducting useless research like that on the mating habits of birds. E. Fuller Torrey, Michael B. Knable, John M. Davis, et al., *A Mission Forgotten: The Failure of the National Institute of Mental Health to Do Sufficient Research on Severe Mental Illnesses* (Arlington, VA: NAMI and the NAMI Research Institute/Stanley Research Programs, December 1999), http://www.treatmentadvocacycenter.org/storage/documents/amission forgotten_-_nimh.pdf (accessed July 13, 2016).

But by 2002, everything changed. NAMI was defending the research they previously criticized. NAMI, "NAMI Condemns CBS's *60 Minutes* for 'Sound Bite Journalism,'" press release, April 24, 2002, http://www.nami.org/Press-Media/Press-Releases/2002/NAMI-Condemns-CBS-s-60-Minutes-for-Sound-Bite-Jou (accessed July 13, 2016). They committed to ignoring the policy on involuntary treatment they used to support and embraced many politically correct, wasteful programs described in this book.

15. Mental Illness Policy Org., "WRAP Certified as 'Evidence-Based,' by SAMHSA, But is It?" Mental Illness Policy Org., 2012, http://mentalillnesspolicy.org/samhsa/wrapunproven.html (accessed July 13, 2016).

16. Rael Jean Isaac and Virginia C. Armat, *Madness in the Streets: How Psychiatry and the Law Abandoned the Mentally Ill* (New York: Free Press, 1990); E. Fuller Torrey, *Nowhere to Go: The Tragic Odyssey of the Homeless Mentally Ill* (New York: Harper & Row, 1988).

17. Amanda Peters, "Lawyers Who Break the Law: What Congress Can Do to Prevent Mental Health Patient Advocates from Violating Federal Legislation," *Oregon Law Review* 89, no. 1 (2010): 133–74, http://mentalillnesspolicy.org/myths/mental-health-bar.pdf (accessed July 13, 2016).

18. Morton Birnbaum, "The Right to Treatment," *American Bar Association Journal* 46 (1960): 499–504.

19. See *Wyatt v. Stickney*, chapter 15.

20. For example, Disability Rights California continually raises the specter of suits to prevent treatment of the mentally ill who have a history of incarceration. Dan Morain, "Mentally Ill Deserve More of Our Attention," *Sacramento Bee*, October 5, 2014, http://www.sacbee.com/opinion/opn-columns-blogs/dan-morain/article2620121.html (accessed July 13, 2016).

21. Darold Treffert, "Dying with Their Rights On," *Prism* 2, no. 2 (February 1974): 49–52. Originally published in *American Journal of Psychiatry* 130, no. 9 (September 1973): 1041, http://www.dorotheadixthinktank.org/Portals/0/Literature/Dying%20with%20Their%20Rights%20On_Darold%20Treffert_MD_AMA_1974.pdf (accessed July 13, 2013).

22. Bazelon Center for Mental Health Law, "Who We Are," *Bazelon*, 2013, http://www.bazelon.org/Who-We-Are.aspx (accessed July 13, 2016).

23. Bazelon CEO Robert Bernstein told the Institute of Medicine, "We are writing into [Olmstead] settlement agreements . . . peer support. Peer support is being incorporated as part of the remedy." Robert Bernstein, "Mental Health and Violence: Opportunities for Prevention and Early Intervention—A Workshop," 13:54, National Academy of Sciences, February 26, 2014, http://www.nationalacademies.org/hmd/Activities/Global/ViolenceForum/2014-FEB-26/Day%201/Panel%201/19-Bernstein-Video.aspx (accessed July 13, 2016).

24. US Congress, *Protection and Advocacy for Mentally Ill Individuals Act of 1986*, Pub. L. 99-319, 1986, http://www.gpo.gov/fdsys/pkg/STATUTE-100/pdf/STATUTE-100-Pg478.pdf (accessed July 13, 2016). See chapter 14.

25. Elizabeth Bernstein and Nathan Koppel, "A Death in the Family: Aided by Advocates for the Mentally Ill, William Bruce Left the Hospital—Only to Kill His Mother," *Wall Street Journal*, August 16, 2008, http://online.wsj.com/news/articles/SB121883750650245525 (accessed July 13, 2016).

26. PsychRights, "Involuntary Commitment/Treatment," *PsychRights*, http://psychrights.org/Research/nypainvol.htm (accessed July 13, 2016).

27. State and county mental health officials do support beds when the federal government will pay. NASMHPD sagely identified how certain provisions of the Affordable Care Act will hurt the ability to provide hospital beds. National Association of State Mental Health Program Directors, *The Vital Role of State Hospitals*, Joe Parks and Alan Q. Radke (eds.) (Alexandria, VA: NASMHPD, July 2014), http://nasmhpd.org/content/vital-role-state-psychiatric-hospitals-0 (accessed July 13, 2016). Robert W. Glover and Joel E. Miller, "The Interplay between Medicaid DSH Payment Cuts, the IMD Exclusion, and the ACA Medicaid Expansion Program: Impacts on State Mental Health Services (policy statement)," April 13, 2013, http://nasmhpd.org/sites/default/files/TheDSH Interplay04_26_13WebsiteFINAL.pdf (accessed July 13, 2016). National Association of State Mental Health Program Directors, "Position Statement on Repeal of the Medicaid IMD Exclusion," NASMHPD, June 6, 2000, http://nasmhpd.org/content/position -statement-repeal-medicaid-imd-Exclusion (accessed July 26, 2016).

28. In 2013, the Mental Health Liaison Group lobbied for more money for prevention, in spite of the fact that serious mental illness can't be prevented. Mental Health Liaison Group, letter to Senators Tom Harkin and Lamar Alexander, Senate Committee on Health, Education, Labor, and Pensions, April 8, 2013, http://mhlg.org/issue -statements/mental-health (accessed July 13, 2016).

29. Mental Health America (MHA), "Who We Are," MHA, http://www.mental healthamerica.net/who-we-are (accessed July 13, 2016).

30. DJ Jaffe, "Just Say No, Governor Cuomo: New York State Should Not Close Its Psychiatric Hospitals," *City Journal*, February 13, 2014, http://www.city-journal.org/2014/eon0213dj.html (accessed July 13, 2016).

31. See chapter five for anosognosia. Eduardo Vega, "Forced Treatment and Constitutional Rights: Can They Coexist?" YouTube video, 53:59, posted by "sfpublicdefender," March 19, 2013, http://www.youtube.com/watch?v=EYJDbDEeOzg (accessed July 13, 2016).

32. Mr. Davison regularly calls for common sense policies like preventing persons with serious mental illness from owning firearms and allowing treatment before tragedy.

33. National Council for Behavioral Health, *2014 Annual Report, 2013–2014*, http://www.thenationalcouncil.org/about/annual-report/ (accessed July 13, 2016). Also see their press releases. In 2014, the National Council merged with the State Associations of Addiction Services (SAAS).

34. DJ Jaffe, "Counterproductive Craziness at Federal Agency," *Washington Times*, September 16, 2011, http://www.washingtontimes.com/news/2011/sep/16/counterproductive-craziness-at-federal-agency/ (accessed December 19, 2016).

35. National Council for Behavioral Health, "Mental Health and Addiction Policy Agenda," National Council for Behavioral Health, 2014, http://www.thenationalcouncil.org/policy-action/policy-agenda/ (accessed July 13, 2016).

36. "Mental Health First Aid Legislation," National Council for Behavioral Health, https://www.thenationalcouncil.org/about/mental-health-first-aid/mental-health-first -aid-legislative-activity/ (accessed December 19, 2016).

37. American Hospital Association, "Trend Watch: Bringing Behavioral Health into the Care Continuum: Opportunities to Improve Quality, Costs and Outcomes," January 2012, aha.org/research/reports/tw/12jan-tw-behavhealth.pdf (accessed July 13, 2016).

American Hospital Association (AHA), Letter to Senators Max Baucus and Orrin Hatch, Senate Finance Committee, September 30, 2013, http://www.aha.org/advocacy-issues/letter/2013/130930-let-aha-senate-behave-health.pdf (accessed July 13, 2016). See IMD Exclusion in Chapter 14.

38. National Association of Psychiatric Health Systems (NAPHS), "NAPHS History, 2008," https://www.naphs.org/about/history (accessed July 13, 2016).

39. Allen Frances, *Saving Normal* (New York: HarperCollins, 2013).

40. *Psychiatry Under the Influence* documented both real and imagined problems with pharmaceutical research, and his suggested "fixes" will likely make the problem worse. Robert Whitaker and Lisa Cosgrove, *Psychiatry Under the Influence: Institutional Corruption, Social Injury, and Prescriptions for Reform* [prepub version] (New York: Palgrave Macmillan, 2015).

41. Mike Debonis, "Congress passes 21st Century Cures Act, Boosting Research and Easing Drug Approvals," *Washington Post*, December 7, 2016, https://www.washingtonpost.com/news/powerpost/wp/2016/12/07/congress-passes-21st-century-cures-act-boosting-research-and-easing-drug-approvals/ (accessed December 20, 2017).

42. Inae Oh, "John Oliver: Big Pharma Is Like Your High School Boyfriend, Only Concerned With 'Getting Inside You,'" *Mother Jones*, February 9, 2015, http://www.motherjones.com/mixed-media/2015/02/john-oliver-big-pharma (accessed December 20, 2016).

43. The NYAPRS board of directors is comprised of those who run mental health programs. Some are not peers. Membership in the National Coalition for Mental Health Recovery (NCMHR) is limited to genuine peer organizations. NYAPRS is not a member.

44. DJ Jaffe, "Just Say No, Governor Cuomo"; Mental Illness Policy Org., "Analysis of NYAPRS Opposition to Kendra's Law," Mental Illness Policy Org., June 2012, http://mentalillnesspolicy.org/kendras-law/nyaprs-opposition-kendras-law.html (accessed July 13, 2016).

45. House Committee on Energy and Commerce Subcommittee on Oversight and Investigations, "Where Have All the Patients Gone? Examining the Psychiatric Bed Shortage, Hearings Before the House Subcommittee on Oversight and Investigations of the Committee on Energy and Commerce," Jon Mark Hirshon statement on behalf of the American College of Emergency Physicians, 113th Cong., March 26, 2014, http://mentalillnesspolicy.org/imd/emergencydocpsychhospitaltestimony.pdf (accessed July 12, 2016).

46. American Psychiatric Nurses Association, *Workplace Violence* (position statement) (Falls Church, VA: American Psychiatric Nurses Association, 2008), http://www.apna.org/files/public/APNA_Workplace_Violence_Position_Paper.pdf (accessed July 13, 2016).

47. Jeffrey Lieberman, *Shrinks: The Untold Story of Psychiatry* (New York: Little, Brown, 2015).

48. Paul Summergrad, "SAMHSA Strategic Plan Falls Short on Serious Mental Illness," *Psychiatric News*, September 11, 2014, http://psychnews.psychiatryonline.org/doi/full/10.1176/appi.pn.2014.9b17 (accessed July 13, 2016).

49. Some psychiatrists see relatively easy-to-treat, insured patients with depression or other issues during the day in their private practice. These patients are often grateful for their services. Public-sector psychiatrists see difficult-to-treat, seriously mentally ill, uninsured patients in hospitals, jails or clinics. They are often overworked, underpaid, and under intense pressure to check the right boxes on forms or to deny services to the ill. They are called on at nights and weekends to handle emergencies. Many burn out and get out.

50. American Psychological Association, "Most Popular Topics," APA, 2014, http://apa.org (accessed July 13, 2015).

51. 1199SEIU United Healthcare Workers East, "About 1199SEIU United Healthcare Workers East," SEIU, 2013, http://www.1199seiu.org/about#sthash.KNxM9xch.dpbs (accessed July 13, 2016).

52. Roger Glass, "PEF Cautiously Optimistic about New Mental Health Plan," Public Employees Federation, January 8, 2014, http://www.aft.org/news/pef-cautiously -optimistic-about-new-mental-health-plan (accessed December 20, 2016).

53. One Mind for Research, "Gemini, Apollo, the Stigma," One Mind for Research, 2014.

54. Patrick Kennedy, "Patrick Kennedy Speaks at Mental Health Liaison Group's Annual Meeting," Patrick J. Kennedy, January 27, 2014, http://patrickjkennedy.net/patrick -kennedy-speaks-at-mental-health-liaison-groups-annual-meeting/ (accessed August 17, 2016).

55. Patrick Kennedy, "Speech 2014 NAMI," C-Span video, 20:47, September 7, 2014, http://www.c-span.org/video/?c4507851/patrick-kennedy-speech-2014-nami (accessed July 13, 2016).

56. Carter Center, "The 30th Annual Rosalynn Carter Symposium on Mental Health Policy," Carter Center, 2013, https://www.cartercenter.org/health/mental_health/ symposium/2014/index.html (accessed July 13, 2016).

57. Katharine Mieszkowski, "Scientology's War on Psychiatry," *Salon*, July 1, 2005, http://www.salon.com/2005/07/01/sci_psy (accessed March 4, 2015).

58. Mental Illness Policy Org., "Mindfreedom and Scientology," Mental Illness Policy Org., 2011, http://mentalillnesspolicy.org/myths/mindfreedom-scientology-oaks -cchr.html (accessed March 4, 2015).

59. National Sheriffs' Association, "National Sheriffs' Association Supports Mission of Treatment Advocacy Center," Sherrifs.org, March 2013, http://www.sheriffs.org/sites/ default/files/uploads/documents/GovAffairs/2013-03%20Treatment%20Advocacy%20 Center.pdf (accessed July 13, 2016).

60. Kevin Fritz, "Thank You, Sheriff," *Lake Mary News*, October 31, 2016, https:// www.lakemarylife.com/lake-mary-news/article/thank-you-sheriff (accessed December 22, 2016).

61. International Association of Chiefs of Police (IACP), Resolution: "Assisted Out-patient Treatment," Mental Illness Policy Org., October 21, 2014, http://mentalillness-policy .org/crimjust/iacpadoptsaot.pdf (accessed July 13, 2016).

62. Michael Biasotti, "State's Mentally Ill Need Treatment, Not Incarceration," *Times Union* (Albany, NY), October 14, 2013, http://www.timesunion.com/opinion/ article/State-s-mentally-ill-need-treatment-not-4894707.php (accessed July 13, 2016)

63. "CIT Center," University of Memphis, http://www.cit.memphis.edu (accessed July 19, 2016); "Welcome to CIT International," http://citinternational.org (accessed July 19, 2016).

CHAPTER 9: THE INDUSTRY FIGHTS EFFORTS TO REDUCE VIOLENCE

1. Thomas R. Insel, "Mental Health and Violence: Opportunities for Prevention and Early Intervention," 30:19, keynote address, Washington, DC, National Academy of Sciences, Institute of Medicine, February 26, 2014, http://www.national-academies.org/hmd/Activities/Global/ViolenceForum/2014-FEB-26/Day%201/Welcome%20and%20Morning%20Presentations/4-Insel-Video.aspx (accessed July 13, 2016).

2. SAMHSA's Resource Center to Promote Acceptance, Dignity and Social Inclusion Associated with Mental Health (ADS Center), "Violence and Mental Illness: The Facts," SAMHSA. Original link expired. First page available at https://web.archive.org/web/20150125014241/http://www.promoteacceptance.samhsa.gov/publications/facts.aspx.

3. Various mental health lobbyists, "Mental Health Advocates Blast Rep. Tim Murphy's Bill as a Costly Step Backward, to the Days When a Mental Illness Diagnosis Was a Life Sentence," PR Newswire, December 12, 2013, http://www.prnewswire.com/news-releases/mental-health-advocates-blast-rep-tim-murphys-bill-as-a-costly-step-backward-to-the-days-when-a-mental-illness-diagnosis-was-a-life-sentence-235602341.html (accessed July 13, 2016).

4. After mentally ill Jared Loughner shot Representative Giffords, NCMHR wrote, "Contrary to popular belief, research has shown we [people with lived experience] are no more violent than the general population" and repeated the claim when Congress tried to reform the mental health treatment system. NCMHR, "National Coalition of Individuals with Mental Health Conditions Calls for Reasonable Response to Arizona Tragedy," press release, January 10, 2011, http://www.ncmhr.org/press-releases/1.10.11.htm (accessed July 13, 2016). NCMHR, "Mental Health Advocates Decry Forced Treatment Provision in 'Doc Fix' Bill," press release, March 28, 2014, http://ncmhr.org/press-releases/3.28.14.htm (accessed July 13, 2016).

"No connection between mental illness and violence" was also trumpeted in press releases from the National Federation of Families for Children's Mental Health. Admin, "The National Federation Responds to Rep. Tim Murphy's Mental Health Bill," National Federation of Families for Children's Mental Health, December 18, 2013, https://www.ffcmh.org/blog/national-federation-responds-rep-tim-murphys-mental-health-bill (accessed July 13, 2016).

After the Sandy Hook shootings, Bazelon proclaimed, "[P]eople with mental illnesses are no more violent than people without mental illnesses." "The Relationship between the Availability of Psychiatric Hospital Beds, Murders Involving Firearms, and Incarceration Rates," Bazelon, January 15, 2013, http://www.bazelon.org/portals/0/Archives/Statements%20&%20Releases/Relationship%20Between%20Psychiatric%20Hospital%20Beds%20and%20Firearm%20Murder1.15.13.pdf (accessed July 13, 2016).

The National Association of State Mental Health Program Directors created a toolkit for state mental health commissioners on how to avoid community pressure to take steps to reduce violence. NASMHPD, *Responding to a High-Profile Tragic Incident Involving a Person with a Serious Mental Illness: A Toolkit for State Mental Health Commissioners*, NASMHPD and the Council of State Governments Justice Center, 2010.

5. Mental Health America (MHA), "Position Statement 72: Violence: Community Mental Health Response," September 17, 2011, http://www.mentalhealthamerica.net/positions/violence (accessed July 13, 2016).

6. Associated Press, "FBI Prevented 148 Mass Shootings in 2013," *New York Post*, December 16, 2013, http://nypost.com/2013/12/16/fbi-stopped-148-mass-shootings-in -2013-eric-holder (accessed July 13, 2016).

7. Henry J. Steadman, Edward P. Mulvey, John Monahan, et al., "Violence by People Discharged from Acute Psychiatric Inpatient Facilities and by Others in the Same Neighborhoods," *Archives of General Psychiatry* 55, no. 5 (May 1998): 393–401. Abstract at http://www.ncbi.nlm.nih.gov/pubmed/9596041 (accessed July 13, 2016).

8. The researchers only included patients released from short-term, acute-care hospitals, i.e., patients who were receiving treatment. The authors counted as violence only acts that produced bodily harm. If you're a good ducker, your relative is not considered violent. They did not include setting fires or trashing rooms as violence. They compared their sample of mentally ill to residents of high-crime areas of Pittsburgh, thereby making the high violence rate among mentally ill seem more normal. Sally Satel and DJ Jaffe, "Violent Fantasies," *National Review*, July 28, 1998, http://mentalillnesspolicy.org/ consequences/macarthur-violence-mental-illness.html (accessed July 13, 2016).

9. Eighteen percent of the patients without a drug or alcohol problem committed at least one act of violence (e.g., throwing objects, kicking, hitting, using a weapon), and an additional 33 percent engaged in at least one act of aggression (same as above except that no harm resulted). Violence was 31 percent among mentally ill people who also abused drugs and alcohol. Those who received six or fewer mental health treatment sessions per quarter were significantly more likely to become violent than those who received seven or more. E. Fuller Torrey, Jonathan Stanley, John Monahan, et al., "The MacArthur Violence Risk Assessment Study Revisited: Two Views Ten Years after Its Original Publication," *Psychiatric Services* 59, no. 2 (February 2008): 147–52, http://mentalillnesspolicy.org/ consequences/Torrey-McArthur-Foundation.pdf (accessed July 13, 2016).

10. John Monahan, H. Steadman, and E. Silver, *Rethinking Risk Assessment: The MacArthur Study of Mental Disorder and Violence* (New York: Oxford University 2001).

11. A. Sariaslan, H. Larsson, and S. Fazel, "Genetic and Environmental Determinants of Violence Risk in Psychotic Disorders: A Multivariate Quantitative Genetic Study of 1.8 Million Swedish Twins and Siblings," *Molecular Psychiatry*, December 2015, http://www.nature.com/mp/journal/vaop/ncurrent/full/mp2015184a.html (accessed July 13, 2016).

12. Michael Luo and Mike McIntire, "When the Right to Bear Arms Includes the Mentally Ill," *New York Times*, December 21, 2013, http://www.nytimes.com/2013/12/22/ us/when-the-right-to-bear-arms-includes-the-mentally-ill.html (accessed July 13, 2016).

13. Jeffrey Swanson, Charles E. Holzer, Vijay K. Ganju et al, "Violence and Psychiatric Disorder in the Community: Evidence from the Epidemiologic Catchment Area Surveys," *Hospital and Community Psychiatry* 41, no. 7 (July 1990): 761–70. Abstract at http://www.ncbi.nlm.nih.gov/pubmed/2142118 (accessed July 13, 2016).

14. Various mental health lobbyists, "Mental Health Advocates."

15. More than one-quarter of persons with serious mental illness claim to have been victims of violent crime in the past year, a rate more than eleven times that of the general population. Linda A. Teplin, Gary M. McClelland, Karen M. Abram, et al., "Crime Victimization in Adults with Severe Mental Illness: Comparison With the National Crime Victimization Survey," *Archives of General Psychiatry* 62, no. 8 (August 2005): 911–21, http://archpsyc.jamanetwork.com/article.aspx?articleid=208861 (accessed July 13, 2016).

16. Jeffrey W. Swanson, Marvin S. Swartz, Susan M. Essock, et al., "The Social-Environmental Context of Violent Behavior in Persons Treated for Serious Mental Illness," *American Journal of Public Health* 92, no. 9 (September 2002): 1523–31, http://www.ncbi.nlm.nih.gov/pmc/articles/PMC1447272 (accessed July 13, 2016).

17. The significant finding that people with mental illness were more likely to perpetrate injury-causing violence than be victims of it was in the study but not the abstract. The authors created two descriptions of "violence." One definition ("community violence") did not require having received or given an injury. The other definition ("violence") did. The abstract focused on community violence—violence without injury—and reported that people with mental illness are more likely to be victims than perpetrators. But when injury occurred, the results were reversed. Sarah L. Desmarais, Richard A. Van Dorn, Kiersten L. Johnson, et al., "Community Violence Perpetration and Victimization among Adults with Mental Illnesses," *American Journal of Public Health* 104, no. 12 (December 2014): 2342–49. Abstract at http://ajph.aphapublications.org/doi/abs/10.2105/AJPH.2013.301680 (accessed July 25, 2016).

18. C. Rodway, S. Flynn, M. S. Rahman, et al., "Patients with Mental Illness as Victims of Homicide: A National Consecutive Case Series," *Lancet* 1, no. 2 (2014): 129–34.

19. Jay Carney, "Press Briefing by Press Secretary Jay Carney, 5/15/2013," White House Press Office, May 15, 2013, http://www.whitehouse.gov/the-press-office/2013/05/15/press-briefing-press-secretary-jay-carney-5152013 (accessed July 13, 2016).

20. The CDC calculates that 61 percent of all firearms fatalities in the United States, 19,393 of 31,672, were suicides, and one-third had *documented* mental illness. That would be 5,817 suicides. That figure is likely low because it does not include those who did not get treatment. Jeffrey Swanson, E. Elizabeth McGuinty, Seena Fazel, et al., "Mental Illness and Reduction of Gun Violence and Suicide: Bringing Epidemiologic Research to Policy," *Annals of Epidemiology* 25 (2015) 366e376: 366–76. The American Foundation for Suicide notes that roughly half of the 42,000 suicides in 2014 were by gun. American Foundation for Suicide Prevention, "Suicide Statistics," 2014, http://afsp.org/about-suicide/suicide-statistics/ (accessed July 13, 2016). The mental health industry claims 90% of suicides are mental illness related. That would be 18,900 gun-related suicides.

21. Vanessa O'Connell and Gary Fields, "Many Mentally Ill Can Buy Guns: Federal Law Prohibits Sales Only to People Declared Unfit by Judge; States Slow to Update Database," *Wall Street Journal*, January 12, 2011, http://www.wsj.com/articles/SB10001424052748704515904576076200491395200 (accessed July 13, 2016).

22. Michael Ollove, "States Tackle Mental Illness and Gun Ownership," Pew Charitable Trusts: Stateline, March 21, 2013, http://www.pewstates.org/projects/stateline/headlines/states-tackle-mental-illness-and-gun-ownership-85899461407 (accessed July 13, 2016).

23. David Sherfinski, "Mental Illness in Youth Could Prevent Gun Purchases in Adulthood," *Washington Times*, January 7, 2014, http://www.washingtontimes.com/news/2014/jan/7/mental-illness-in-youth-could-prevent-gun-purchase (accessed July 13, 2016).

24. Wayne Lindstorm, "Opposing View: Don't Link Violence with Mental Illness," *USA Today*, January 10, 2013, http://www.usatoday.com/story/opinion/2013/01/10/mental-health-america-wayne-lindstrom/1566226 (accessed July 13, 2016).

25. Pamela S. Hyde, "Informing Public Health Strategies: Challenges and Opportunities in Behavioral Health," (PowerPoint presentation), New Orleans, LA: 3rd Annual

Public Health Law Research Meeting, January 18, 2013, http://store.samhsa.gov/product/Informing-Public-Health-Strategies-Challenges-and-Opportunities-in-Behavioral-Health/SMA13-PHYDE011813 (accessed July 13, 2016).

26. The Bazelon report purported to show that gun violence was not correlated with a reduction in psychiatric hospital beds. But the report was a study of all gun violence and did not study gun violence by persons with mental illness.

27. Barack Obama, "Fact Sheet: New Executive Actions to Reduce Gun Violence and Make Our Communities Safer," White House, January 4, 2016, https://www.whitehouse.gov/the-press-office/2016/01/04/fact-sheet-new-executive-actions-reduce-gun-violence-and-make-our (accessed July 13, 2016).

When Texas passed an "open-carry" law that allowed guns in state psychiatric hospitals, *USA Today* and the *Texas Statesman* ran headlines like "Texas Allows Guns into State Hospitals." NAMI should have theoretically supported the law since it comported with its "mentally ill are no more violent than others" rhetoric, but families of those with serious mental illness and the public were outraged. NAMI Texas, one of the better NAMI organizations, distanced itself by relying on the old standby, "stigma," claiming it was stigmatizing to think guns were needed in psychiatric hospitals. "Stigma," which had previously been used as a justification for why people with mental illness should be allowed access to firearms, quickly became the argument for preventing it.

28. Lois Beckett, "Myth vs Fact: Violence and Mental Health," *ProPublica*, June 10, 2014, http://www.propublica.org/article/myth-vs-fact-violence-and-mental-health (accessed July 13, 2016).

29. New York State Legislature, *NY Secure Ammunition and Firearms Enforcement (SAFE) Act of 2013* (Albany, January 14, 2013), http://assembly.state.ny.us/leg/?default_fld=&bn=S02230&term=2013&Summary=Y&Actions=Y&Text=Y (accessed July 13, 2016).

30. Karen Dewitt, "Mental Health Advocates Critical of New Gun Law," WBFO 88.7 (Buffalo, NY), March 7, 2013, http://news.wbfo.org/post/mental-health-advocates-critical-new-gun-law (accessed July 13, 2016); Harvey Rosenthal, "It Shouldn't Take a Tragedy to Improve Treatment," *New York Times*, January 17, 2013, http://www.nytimes.com/roomfordebate/2013/01/17/can-mental-health-care-reduce-gun-violence/it-shouldnt-take-a-tragedy-to-improve-mental-health-care (accessed March 6, 2015).

31. Thomas Kaplan and Danny Hakim, "New York Has Gun Deal, with Focus on Mental Ills," *New York Times*, January 14, 2013, http://www.nytimes.com/2013/01/15/nyregion/new-york-legislators-hope-for-speedy-vote-on-gun-laws.html (accessed July 13, 2016).

32. DJ Jaffe, "Require Therapists to Warn Authorities of Danger," *New York Times*, January 17, 2013, http://www.nytimes.com/roomfordebate/2013/01/17/can-mental-health-care-reduce-gun-violence/require-therapists-to-warn-authorities-of-danger (accessed July 13, 2016).

33. New York State Conference of Local Mental Hygiene Directors, "Memo in Opposition to Provisions of the New York SAFE Act," scribd, 2013, http://www.scribd.com/doc/127579710/Safe-Act-9-46-Memo-Clmhd-lh (accessed July 13, 2016).

34. New York Coalition of Behavioral Health Agencies, *Hearing on the New York SAFE Act, Before the New York State Mental Health & Developmental Disabilities Committee*, Statement of Jason Lippman, May 31, 2013, http://coalitionny.org/policy_advocacy/testimony/documents/CBHATestimonyNYSAFEAct.pdf (accessed July 13, 2016).

35. Lisa Pickering, "Mental Health First Aid Discourages Gun Violence," *Guardian Liberty Voice*, February 13, 2014, http://guardianlv.com/14/02/mental-health-first-aid -discourages-gun-violence (accessed July 13, 2016).

36. Jeffrey Swanson, interview by Lois Beckett, "Myth vs. Fact: Violence and Mental Health: A Q&A with an Expert Who Studies the Relationship between Mental Illness and Violence," *Pro Publica*, June 10, 2014, http://www.propublica.org/article/myth-vs -fact-violence-and-mental-health (accessed July 13, 2016).

37. Robert N. Davison, "Gun Laws and the Mentally Ill" letter to the editor, *New York Times*, December 25, 2013, http://www.nytimes.com/2013/12/26/opinion/gun-laws -and-the-mentally-ill.html (accessed July 13, 2016).

CHAPTER 10: THE INDUSTRY FIGHTS LIFE-SAVING INVOLUNTARY INTERVENTIONS

1. Leah Harris, "First They Ignore You: Impressions From Today's Hearing on H.R. 3717," *Mad in America*, April 3, 2014, https://www.madinamerica.com/2014/04/ first-ignore-impressions-todays-hearing-h-r-3717/ (accessed December 20, 2016).

2. Don Edward Green, "We Are Making a Mockery of Civil Rights—Personally Speaking," Treatment Advocacy Center, June 23, 2014, http://www.treatmentadvocacy center.org/about-us/our-blog/69-no-state/2577-we-are-making-a-mockery-of-civil -rights-personally-speaking (accessed July 14, 2016).

3. Darold A. Treffert, "1995 Wisconsin Act 292: Finally, the Fifth Standard," *Wisconsin Medical Journal* 95, no. 8 (August 1996): 537–40.

4. Allen Frances, "When Is It Justified to Force Treatment on Someone," *Huffington Post*, October 3, 2013, http://www.huffingtonpost.com/allen-frances/when-is-it -justified-to-f_b_4038218.html (accessed July 14, 2016).

5. Adam G. Gerhardstein, "A First Episode Standard for Involuntary Treatment," *University of St. Thomas Law Journal* 10, no. 2 (Fall 2012): 469, http://ir.stthomas.edu/cgi/ viewcontent.cgi?article=1312&context=ustlj (accessed December 20, 2016).

6. Bellevue: New York's Bellevue Pilot Program was conducted in the 1990s and had numerous problems. For example, there was no procedure in place to bring the non-compliant in for reevaluation. Researchers learned much from the pilot program and *did not* take it statewide. Instead, they fixed the problems and introduced it as Kendra's Law, which has proven very successful. See appendix B. Rand: The 2001 Rand Study only includes data prior to 2000. Per Brian Stettin of the Treatment Advocacy Center, "the RAND authors acknowledged multiple studies finding substantial patient improvements after AOT. Their objection was that none had attempted to isolate the court order, as opposed to the enhanced quality of services, as a determinative factor in AOT's success." Subsequent research in New York ignored by those who quote Rand, shows the court order does add value.

7. Treatment Advocacy Center, "No Relevance to Assisted Outpatient Treatment (AOT) in the OCTET Study of English Compulsory Treatment," TAC, May 2013, http://www.treatmentadvocacycenter.org/storage/documents/Research/may2013-octet -study.pdf (accessed July 14, 2016).

8. Bazelon says, "Forced mental health care is never appropriate, except when there

are immediate and serious safety risks." Bazelon Center for Mental Health Law, "Self-Determination," Bazelon, http://www.bazelon.org/Where-We-Stand/Self-Determination .aspx (accessed July 14, 2016). "Force is not treatment," claimed the head of MHA of San Francisco. Eduardo Vega, "Forced Treatment and Constitutional Rights: Can They Coexist?" YouTube video, 53:59, posted by "sfpublicdefender," March 19, 2013, http://www.youtube.com/watch?v=EYJDbDEeOzg (accessed July 14, 2016).

9. Medication over objection generally requires a separate hearing to determine if the individual lacks capacity or competency. That requirement is not superseded by AOT legislation.

10. New York courts have ruled that AOT is an appropriate use of the state's police powers and *parens patriae* powers. They did so by noting it is limited to those who have previously, on multiple occasions, refused treatment and had it lead to tragedy, and by observing that AOT allows people to continue to live in the community and doesn't allow for "forced" medication. K. J. Brennan, *Kendra's Law: Final Report on the Status of Assisted Outpatient Treatment* (New York State Office of Mental Health, Albany, NY: 2005) Appendix 2. Original at http://mentalillnesspolicy.org/kendras-law/research/kendras-law-study-2005.pdf. (accessed March 15, 2015). Unpublished revision available at http://mentalillnesspolicy.org/kendras-law/kendras-law-constitutional.html (accessed July 14, 2016).

11. Elizabeth Marcellino, "County Will Seek Court-Ordered Treatment of Mentally Ill: Advocates Split on Effectiveness of 'Laura's Law,'" EGP News (Los Angeles), July 17, 2014, http://egpnews.com/2014/07/county-will-seek-court-ordered-treatment-of -mentally-ill (accessed July 14, 2016).

12. Dan Fisher, letter to the editor, "Outpatient Commitment Would Harm Patients in Need," *Boston Globe*, January 1, 2013, http://www.bostonglobe.com/opinion/letters/2013/01/01/outpatient-commitment-would-harm-patients-need/EplTlGyIBg 66QTngV9iEVJ/story.html (accessed July 14, 2016). NEC also issued a press release stating that AOT "would bring America back to the dark ages before de-institutionalization, when people with mental health conditions languished in institutions, sometimes for life." NCMHR, "Mental Health Advocates Decry Forced Treatment Provision in 'Doc Fix' Bill," press release, March 28, 2014, http://ncmhr.org/press -releases/3.28.14.htm (accessed July 14, 2016). As far back as 1998, NEC lent support to opponents of New York State's AOT law. New York City Involuntary Outpatient Commitment Pilot Program, "Testimony Regarding the Results of the Research Study of the New York City Involuntary Outpatient Commitment Pilot Program," Harvey Rosenthal testimony, National Association for Rights Protection and Advocacy, December 16, 1998, http://www.narpa.org/testimony.ioc.nyc.htm (accessed July 14, 2016).

13. Pennsylvania Committee on Health and Human Services, *Hearings Before the Pennsylvania Committee on Health and Human Services, on House Bill 2186, Assisted Outpatient Treatment*, statement of Lynn M. Keltz on behalf of the Pennsylvania Mental Health Consumers' Association, April 8, 2010, http://www.papeersupportcoalition.org/advocacy/TestimoneyHB2186.pdf (Link expired, accessed February 28, 2015).

14. National Mental Health Consumers' Self-Help Clearinghouse, "Issues of Involuntary Intervention with Core Values and Principles," NCMHR, March 18, 1999, http://www.ncmhr.org/downloads/InvoluntaryTreatment31899.pdf (accessed July 14, 2016). Other SAMHSA-funded organizations opposing reform include the California Network for Mental Health Clients, which called for "No expansion of forced treatment or invol-

untary outpatient commitment," lobbies against Laura's Law, and organized a petition drive in opposition. The SAMHSA-supported Mental Health Empowerment Project held a demonstration in Albany protesting AOT.

15. California: Disability Rights California, "Collection of DRC Memos, California PAIMI Opposition to Laura's Law," *Mad in America*, 2013, http://mentalillnesspolicy.org/states/california/p&aopposition.pdf (accessed July 14, 2016). Colorado: Electa Draper, "Debate Rages in Colorado over Involuntary Holds for Mental Illness," *Denver Post*, May 25, 2014, http://www.denverpost.com/2014/05/24/debate-rages-in-colorado-over-involuntary-holds-for-mental-illness/ (accessed July 14, 2016). Ohio: Disability Rights Ohio, Letter to Senator Dave Burke on Ohio Senate Bill 43, March 20, 2013, http://www.disabilityrightsohio.org/news/disability-rights-ohio-sends-letter-senator-burke-ohio-senate-bill-43 (accessed July 14, 2016). Kentucky: Kentucky Protection and Advocacy, "Kentucky P&A's Response to Proposed Amendments to Hospitalization of the Mentally Ill Statute (KRS 202A)," KYPA, 2013. Washington: Brian M. Rosenthal, "Some Mental-Health Officials Oppose Commitment Bill," *Seattle Times*, February 3, 2014. Wisconsin: Disability Rights Wisconsin, "The Fifth Standard for Civil Commitment," Disability Rights Wisconsin, December 13, 1988, http://www.disabilityrightswi.org/archives/85 (accessed July 14, 2016). West Virginia: Substance Abuse and Mental Health Services Administration, *Evaluation of the Protection and Advocacy for Individuals with Mental Illness (PAIMI) Program, Phase III: Evaluation Report*, HHS Publication No. PEP12-EVALPAIMI. (Rockville, MD: Center for Mental Health Services, SAMHSA, 2011), http://store.samhsa.gov/shin/content/PEP12-EVALPAIMI/PEP12-EVALPAIMI.pdf (accessed July 14, 2016).

16. AOT was used in New York City more frequently than in the rest of New York state because it had a pilot program that enabled it to ramp up faster. Since there are more people of color in New York City, especially in the public system where AOT is more likely to be used, opponents disingenuously positioned that as an example of being non-racially neutral. New York Lawyers for the Public Interest, "Implementation of 'Kendra's Law' is Severely Biased," April 7, 2005.

17. The legislature got worried about this faux evidence and commissioned an independent study. It found no evidence of racial bias. Jeffrey Swanson, Marvin Swartz, Richard Van Dorn, et al., "Racial Disparities in Involuntary Outpatient Commitment: Are They Real?" *Health Affairs* 28, no. 3 (May/June 2009): 816–26, http://content.healthaffairs.org/content/28/3/816.full.pdf+html (accessed July 14, 2016). This finding of racial neutrality was confirmed at a December 2013 SAMHSA webinar on AOT by Dr. Stephanie Le Melle, co-director of public psychiatry at NYS Psychiatric Institute. She stated unequivocally that any racial bias within the mental health system—of which there may be a lot—is not taking place within the Kendra's Law program. Dr. Le Melle is African American. New York's Kendra's Law is also endorsed by the Harlem chapter of the National Alliance on Mental Illness, with a primarily African American membership.

18. Tim Gardner, Disability Rights New Mexico, "'Kendra's Law' won't work in NM," *Albuquerque Journal*, January 2015, http://www.abqjournal.com/521236/opinion/kendras-law-wont-work-in-nm.html (accessed July 14, 2016).

19. The only *incremental* cost is the cost of the court order and proceedings. That is around $5,000 per person and is more than offset by reduced hospitalization and incarceration. Jeffrey W. Swanson, Richard A. Van Dorn, Marvin S. Swartz, et al., "The Cost of

Assisted Outpatient Treatment: Can It Save States Money?" *American Journal of Psychiatry* 170, no. 12 (December 2013): 1423–32, http://www.treatmentadvocacycenter.org/storage/documents/2013-duke-aot-cost-study.pdf (accessed July 14, 2016).

The services AOT enrollees receive, like case management, are services that they are already entitled to. Some claim that new services are needed for those in AOT because there are not enough services to go around and that those new services are part of the cost of AOT. But it is disingenuous to "run a bill" for those in AOT (i.e., assume they are not eligible for existing services) and not run the bill for those who do volunteer. Their costs are identical. If there are not enough services to go around, the community has two choices. It can increase services or cut services for the worried well, in order to fund services for the seriously ill. AOT therefore accomplishes an important imperative: it focuses new and existing resources on the most seriously ill.

20. The following quotes from the 2011 SAMHSA evaluation of PAIMI prove that SAMHSA is aware that PAIMI programs are working to block implementation of AOT. "A number of PAIMIs worked to prevent the enactment of state laws creating outpatient commitment systems." PAIMI may "collaborate with . . . a consumer advocacy organization to block passage of a proposed expansion of an outpatient commitment law," (p. 30). "PAIMIs reported joining other advocates in activities such as: Ad hoc partnerships focused on specific issues (e.g., opposing outpatient commitment)," (p. 66). "At the state level, PAIMIs have been involved in systemic issues including outpatient civil commitment," (p. 79). "A number of PAIMIs worked to prevent the enactment of state laws creating outpatient commitment systems," (p. 94). SAMHSA, *Evaluation of the PAIMI Program*, HHS Pub. No. PEP12-EVALPAIMI.

21. NYS/OMH, *Kendra's Law: Final Report on the Status of Assisted Outpatient Treatment*.

22. William M. Greenberg, Lanna Moore-Duncan, and Rachel Herron, "Patients' Attitudes toward Having Been Forcibly Medicated," *Bulletin of the American Academy of Psychiatry and the Law* 24, no. 4 (1996): 513–24, http://www.jaapl.org/content/24/4/513.full.pdf (accessed July 14, 2016).

23. Robert A. Van Putten, Jose M. Santiago, and Michael R. Berren, "Involuntary Outpatient Commitment in Arizona: A Retrospective Study," *Hospital and Community Psychiatry* 39, no. 9 (1998): 953–58. Abstract at http://www.ncbi.nlm.nih.gov/pubmed/3215643 (accessed July 14, 2016).

24. E. Fuller Torrey, "Does Involuntary Treatment Scare People with Mental Illness Away from Treatment?" Mental Illness Policy Org., http://mentalillnesspolicy.org/ivc/ivc_doesnt_drive_ptnts_from_care.pdf (accessed December 10, 2016).

25. Jennifer Bain, "Kendra Webdale's Infamous Subway-Push Killer Says Mental-Health Law Needs to be Restructured," *New York Post*, December 29, 2012, http://nypost.com/2012/12/29/kendra-webdales-infamous-subway-push-killer-says-mental-health-law-needs-to-be-restructured (accessed July 14, 2016). The *New York Times Magazine* chronicled Mr. Goldstein starting from when he was denied voluntary admission to a hospital, causing some mental health advocates to claim that it was the lack of access to voluntary care that was responsible for the tragedy. But Mr. Goldstein had gone off medications before seeking admission to the hospital. Had the *Times* started its story at the point at which Mr. Goldstein went off treatment, the ability of AOT to prevent the tragedy would have been obvious.

26. John Stuart Mill, *On Liberty*, 1859, http://www.utilitarianism.com/ol/one.html (accessed July 14, 2016).

CHAPTER 11: THE INDUSTRY FIGHTS ACCESS TO HOSPITALS, MEDICATIONS, AND ELECTROCONVULSIVE THERAPY

1. E. Fuller Torrey, Kurt Entsminger, Jeffrey Geller, et al., "The Shortage of Public Hospital Beds for Mentally Ill Persons," Treatment Advocacy Center, 2006, http://www .treatmentadvocacycenter.org/storage/documents/the_shortage_of_publichospital_beds .pdf (accessed July 12, 2016).

2. In opposition to H.R. 2646, Val Marsh, executive director of NCMHR wrote, fixing the IMD Exclusion "advances the agenda of forced treatment." Val Marsh, "The Murphy Bill, HR 2646—a Heinous Piece of Legislation—Is Coming to a Vote. Act Now," *Mad in America*, July 5, 2016, http://www.madinamerica.com/2016/07/ hr-2646-coming-to-a-vote (accessed September 19, 2016).

3. Pete Earley, "Sending the Mentally Ill from Group Homes to an Uncertain Future," (opinion), *Washington Post*, October 30, 2014, http://www.washingtonpost.com/ opinions/pete-earley-sending-the-mentally-ill-from-group-homes-to-an-uncertain -future/14/10/30/f4bd84ce-5b22-11e4-8264-deed989ae9a2_story.html (accessed July 14, 2016).

4. Joseph Rogers, interview by Joanne Silberner, "The Closing of Haverford State: A Special Report," *NPR: The Infinite Mind*, June 21, 2000.

5. Suzy Khimm, "How the Obamacare Wars Hurt the Mentally Ill," MSNBC, January 21, 2014, http://www.msnbc.com/msnbc/how-the-obamacare-wars-hurt-the -mentally-ill (accessed July 14, 2016).

6. E. Fuller Torrey, MD, Aaron D. Kennard, Don Eslinger, et al., "More Mentally Ill Persons Are in Jails and Prisons than Hospitals: A Survey of the States," Treatment Advocacy Center, May 2010, http://www.treatmentadvocacycenter.org/storage/ documents/final_jails_v_hospitals_study.pdf (accessed July 14, 2016).

7. E. Fuller Torrey, *American Psychosis: How the Federal Government Destroyed the Mental Illness Treatment System* (New York: Oxford University Press, 2014).

8. Jon Campbell, "Mental Health Advocates Say State Has to 'Reinvest,'" *Politics on the Hudson*, July 16, 2013, http://polhudson.lohudblogs.com/2013/07/16/mental-health -advocates-say-state-has-to-reinvest (accessed July 14, 2016).

9. New York State Association of Psychiatric Rehabilitation Services (NYAPRS), "Alert: Call Albany NOW to Protect PWD's Right to Live in the Community!" NYAPRS, June 18, 2014, http://www.nyaprs.org/e-news-bulletins/2014/006383.cfm (accessed July 14, 2016).

10. Bazelon claims, "Nationwide many such beds are occupied by people who simply do not need hospital care." Bazelon Center for Mental Health Law, "Bazelon Center Statement on Sandy Hook Shooting," Bazelon, December 17, 2012, http://www.bazelon.org/ News-Publications/Press-Releases/12.17.12-Sandy-Hook-PR.aspx (accessed July 14, 2016).

11. Amanda Pustilnik, "Calling Mental Illness 'Myth' Leads to State Coercion," Cato Unbound, August 13, 2012, http://www.cato-unbound.org/2012/08/13/amanda -pustilnik/calling-mental-illness-myth-leads-state-coercion (accessed July 14, 2016).

12. Bernard E. Harcourt, "An Institutionalization Effect: The Impact of Mental Hospitalization and Imprisonment on Homicide in the United States, 1934–2001," *Journal of Legal Studies* 40, no. 1 (January 2011), http://www.jstor.org/stable/10.1086/658404 (accessed July 14, 2016).

13. John S. Hausman, "Mental Illness and Criminal Justice: Law Enforcement Copes with Issues Hospitals Once Handled," *Muskegon* (MI) *Chronicle*, December 16, 2013, http://www.mlive.com/news/muskegon/index.ssf/2013/12/mental_health-criminal_justice.html (accessed July 14, 2016).

14. Sheriff Tom Dart, interview by Steve Kroft, as part of "Imminent Danger," *60 Minutes*, CBS, New York, September 29, 2013, http://www.cbsnews.com/news/untreated-mental-illness-an-imminent-danger (accessed July 14, 2016).

15. Tony Leys, "Plan Means Fewer Beds in Southern Iowa for Mentally Ill," *Des Moines Register*, January 15, 2015, http://www.desmoinesregister.com/story/news/health/2015/01/15/eliminate-beds-mentally-southern-iowa/21836511 (accessed July 14, 2016).

16. "Forensic" patients are ones that arrived via the criminal justice system. They include the mentally ill who have been convicted of a crime, people being held for psychiatric evaluation, those who are not fit to stand trial or were found not guilty by reason of insanity.

17. A study of 348 inpatients in a Virginia state psychiatric hospital found that patients who refused to take medication "were more likely to be assaultive, were more likely to require seclusion and restraint, and had longer hospitalizations." J. A. Kasper, S. K. Hoge, T. Feucht-Haviar, et al., "Prospective Study of Patients' Refusal of Antipsychotic Medication under a Physician Discretion Review Procedure," *American Journal of Psychiatry* 154, no. 4 (1997): 483–89. Abstract at http://www.ncbi.nlm.nih.gov/pubmed/9090334 (accessed July 14, 2016).

18. Stephanie Janard, "Crisis Point: Mentally Ill and Incarcerated in the Rutherford County Jail," *Daily Courier* (Forest City, NC), March 2, 2014, http://www.thedigitalcourier.com/features/x112098019/Crisis-point (accessed July 14, 2016).

19. Foundation for Excellence in Mental Health, 2012 Form 990 filed with IRS, Guidestar, 2012, http://www.mentalhealthexcellence.org/wp-content/uploads/2013/08/2012-990-on-Guidestar.pdf (accessed July 14, 2016); MindFreedom, "Does Your Mental Health Care Need a TRUTH Injection?" MindFreedom International, July 2009, http://www.mindfreedom.org/truth/mfi-truth-200907.pdf (accessed July 14, 2016);

20. National Empowerment Center, "Resources," National Empowerment Center, May 6, 2014, http://www.power2u.org/resources.html (accessed July 14, 2016).

21. Christine Y. Lu, Fang Zhang, Matthew D. Lakoma, et al., "Changes in Antidepressant Use by Young People and Suicidal Behavior after FDA Warnings and Media Coverage: Quasi-Experimental Study," *BMJ* 348 (2014): g3596, http://www.bmj.com/content/348/bmj.g3596 (accessed July 14, 2016).

22. Followers of Whitaker argue (correctly) that double-blind, active-placebo studies are the best, except when they want to show that talk therapy works, and then any study will do. They suggest there are methodological faults with almost every study that supports the benefits of medication but don't see any faults with those that highlight problems with medications or purport to solve mental illness with talk.

23. Zebulon Taintor, Book Review: "Mad in America: Bad Science, Bad Medicine, and the Enduring Mistreatment of the Mentally Ill," *Psychiatric Services* 54, no. 1 (January

2003): 112–13, http://ps.psychiatryonline.org/doi/full/10.1176/appi.ps.54.1.112-a (accessed July 14, 2016); E. Fuller Torrey, "Anatomy of a Non-Epidemic: How Robert Whitaker Got It Wrong," Treatment Advocacy Center, http://www.treatmentadvocacy center.org/component/content/article/2085-anatomy-of-a-non-epidemic-a-review -by-dr-torrey (accessed July 14, 2016); Allen Frances, "A Debate between Allen Frances and Robert Whitaker," *Mad in America*, December 4, 2014, http://www.madinamerica .com/14/12/debate-allen-frances-robert-whitaker (accessed July 14, 2016).

24. Tyrone D. Cannon, Yoonho Chung, George He, et al., "Progressive Reduction in Cortical Thickness as Psychosis Develops: A Multisite Longitudinal Neuroimaging Study of Youth at Elevated Clinical Risk," *Biological Psychiatry* 77, no. 2 (January 2015): 147–57. Abstract at http://www.biologicalpsychiatryjournal.com/article/S0006-3223(14)00414-4/ abstract (accessed July 14, 2016). Also see E. Fuller Torrey, "Schizophrenia Changes Brain Structure: A Review of Studies of Individuals with Schizophrenia Never Treated with Antipsychotic Medications," Mental Illness Policy Org., 2013, http://mentalillnesspolicy .org/medical/brain-change-schizophrenia.html (accessed July 14, 2016).

25. Minna Torniainen, Ellenor Mittendorfer-Rutz, Antti Tanskanen, et al., "Anti-psychotic Treatment and Mortality in Schizophrenia," *Schizophrenia Bulletin* [Epub ahead of print], November 24, 2014. Abstract at http://schizophreniabulletin.oxfordjournals.org/ content/early/2014/11/24/schbul.sbu164.full.pdf+html (accessed July 14, 2016).

26. Ed Knight, "Opinion: Mental Health Advocate Ed Knight Calls for Investi-gating SAMHSA," MindFreedom International, October 29, 2010, http://www.mind freedom.org/kb/mental-health-advocacy/samhsa-alternatives/ed-knight-opinion (accessed July 14, 2016).

27. MindFreedom International, "Stop FDA from Down-Classifying the Shock Device to a Class II Device. Stop Shock Treatment," Change.org, https://www.change .org/p/fda-stop-fda-from-down-classifying-the-shock-device-to-a-class-ii-device-stop -shock-treatment (accessed August 31, 2016). NCMHR encouraged people to sign the petition on their home page. Numerous other SAMHSA-funded organizations did the same.

28. Mental Health America, "Electroconvulsive Therapy (ECT)," Mental Health America, 2016, http://www.mentalhealthamerica.net/ect (accessed August 31, 2016).

29. Dick Cavett, "Goodbye, Darkness," *People*, August 3, 1992, http://people.com/ archive/goodbye-darkness-vol-38-no-5/ (accessed December 20, 2016).

30. Lisa W. Foderaro, "With Reforms in Treatment, Shock Therapy Loses Shock," *New York Times*, July 19, 1993, B2, http://www.nytimes.com/1993/07/19/nyregion/with -reforms-in-treatment-shock-therapy-loses-shock.html (accessed August 31, 2016).

CHAPTER 12: THE INDUSTRY DIVERTS FUNDS TO PROGRAMS THAT LACK EVIDENCE AND DON'T HELP

1. Children's Mental Health Network, "Friday Update, July 3, 2015," CMH Network, July 3, 2015, http://www.cmhnetwork.org/friday-update-back-issues/friday -update-7-3-15 (accessed July 27, 2016).

2. John Grohol, "The 2015 Murphy Mental Health Crisis Act: Little Better This Time Around," PsychCentral, July 25, 2015, http://psychcentral.com/blog/

archives/2015/07/25/the-2015-murphy-mental-health-crisis-act-little-better-this-time
-around (accessed August 2, 2016).

3. Hannah Dreier, "California Mental-Health Spending Often Bypasses the Mentally Ill," *Los Angeles Daily News*, July 28, 2012, http://www.dailynews.com/20120728/
california-mental-health-spending-often-bypasses-the-mentally-ill (accessed July 16,
2016).

4. Mental Illness Policy Org., "California's Mental Health Service Act: A Ten Year
$10 Billion Bait and Switch: An Investigation of Proposition 63 by Mental Illness Policy
Org. and Individual Californians," Mental Illness Policy Org., August 14, 2013, http://
mentalillnesspolicy.org/states/california/mhsa/mhsa_prop63_bait&switchsummary.html
(accessed July 16, 2016).

5. Joy Torres, Comments on Proposed Mental Health Services Act Regulations,
proposed by Mental Health Services Oversight and Accountability Commission, July 21,
2014, p. 16, http://mentalillnesspolicy.org/states/california/mhsa/JoyTorrescomments
2mhsaRegs.pdf (accessed March 7, 2015).

6. Mental Illness Policy Org., "California's Mental Health Service Act."

7. Butte County, California, did a study on the need for housing for people of
Hmong ancestry. Eight people participated. We do not know if any had serious mental
illness or if any housing was ever built. But this "study" found participants wanted "gardens"
and a "community room." The researchers aggregated the two to conclude that if they
built housing, 58 percent wanted a "community room and garden." This formed the bases
for claiming a garden was a mental health service that would prevent mental illness from
becoming severe and disabling, thereby allowing mental health funds to be allocated to it.

8. Mental Illness Policy Org., "California's Mental Health Service Act."

9. At the May 2013 Sacramento County Mental Health Board meeting, department officials told attendees they were funding "Strengthening Families Programs." When
an advocate told the official that those are social services programs, not a mental illness
program and therefore ineligible for MHSA funding, the official simply stated, "When
the public hearings were held, the community wanted them."

10. California Mental Health Services Authority, *Annual Revenue and Expenditure
Report: Adopted Budget, June 30, 2013*, http://calmhsa.org/wp-content/uploads/2012/06/
CalMHSA-Budget-Package-2012-2013-FINAL.pdf (accessed July 16, 2016).

11. Mental Illness Policy Org., "California's Mental Health Service Act: A Ten Year
$10 Billion Bait and Switch; An Investigation of Proposition 63 by Mental Illness Policy
Org. and Individual Californians," Mental Illness Policy Org., August 14, 2013, p. 21.
http://mentalillnesspolicy.org/states/california/mhsa/mhsa.prop63.baitswitch.fullreport
.pdf (accessed July 16, 2016).

12. California State Auditor, *Mental Health Services Act*, Report 2012-122 (Sacramento, CA: California State Auditor, August 2013) http://mentalillnesspolicy.org/states/
california/mhsa/state-auditor-mhsa-report.pdf (accessed July 16, 2016); Little Hoover
Commission, *Promises Still to Keep: A Decade of the Mental Health Services Act*, Report #225
(Sacramento, CA: Little Hoover Commission, January 2015), http://www.lhc.ca.gov/
studies/225/Report225.pdf (accessed July 16, 2016); *Little Hoover Commission, Promises Still to Keep: A Second Look at the Mental Health Services Act* (Sacramento, CA: Little
Hoover Commission, September 2016), http://www.lhc.ca.gov/studies/233/Report233
.pdf (accessed September 19, 2016); Kathy Day and DJ Jaffe, "Mental Health Money 'Fix'

Will Compound the Problem," *Sacramento Bee*, February 2, 2015, http://www.sacbee.com/opinion/op-ed/soapbox/article8960117.html (accessed July 16, 2016).

13. Thomas R. Insel, "Director's Blog: Can We Prevent Psychosis?" November 20, 2014, http://www.nimh.nih.gov/about/director/2014/can-we-prevent-psychosis.shtml (accessed July 16, 2016).

14. V. B. Perez, S. W. Woods, and B. J. Roach, et al., "Automatic Auditory Processing Deficits in Schizophrenia and Clinical High-Risk Patients: Forecasting Psychosis Risk with Mismatch Negativity," *Biological Psychiatry* 75, no. 6 (March 2014): 459–69. Abstract at http://www.ncbi.nlm.nih.gov/pubmed/24050720 (accessed July 16, 2016).

15. Ron Manderscheid, "Breaking the Chains of Mental Illness That Bind Those in Poverty: Poverty Causes Mental Illness; How Can We Defeat This Trap?" *Behavioral Healthcare*, June 25, 2013, http://www.behavioral.net/blogs/ron-manderscheid/breaking-chains-mental-illness-bind-those-poverty (accessed July 16, 2016).

16. Prevention is appropriate for the substance abuse part of SAMHSA's responsibilities, not the serious mental illness part.

17. National Coalition for Mental Health Recovery, "Statement of Support for 5/5: Occupy the APA," NCMHR, 2012, http://www.ncmhr.org/statement-of-support-for-occupy-APA.html (accessed July 16, 2016).

18. Mental Health America, "Prevention and Early Intervention in Mental Health," Mental Health America, http://www.mentalhealthamerica.net/issues/prevention (accessed March 4, 2015).

19. American Mental Health Counselors Association, letter to Vice President Joe Biden, January 9, 2013, URL expired. A reference to it is at http://www.amhca.org/?page=Advocate20130202&hhSearchTerms=%22Biden%22 (accessed July 16, 2016); Ron Manderscheid, "A Time to Act for the Innocents," *Behavioral Healthcare*, January 12, 2013, http://www.behavioral.net/blogs/ron-manderscheid/time-act-innocents-0 (accessed July 16, 2016).

20. Mental Illness Policy Org., "California's Mental Health Service Act."

21. Gerald N. Grob, "Public Policy and Mental Illnesses: Jimmy Carter's Presidential Commission on Mental Health," *Milbank Quarterly* 83, no. 3 (September 2005): 425–56, http://www.ncbi.nlm.nih.gov/pmc/articles/PMC2690151/ (accessed July 16, 2016).

22. Bill Clinton, "Annual Report to Congress on the State of the Union," *Congressional Record—Senate* 145, no. 8 (January 1999): S330-335, http://beta.congress.gov/crec/1999/01/19/CREC-1999-01-19-pt1-PgS330-3.pdf (accessed July 16, 2016).

23. Paul Tonko, "It's Not the Time for Bickering," *Albany Times Union*, June 19, 2014, http://www.timesunion.com/opinion/article/It-s-not-the-time-for-bickering-5565156.php (accessed July 16, 2016).

24. Institute of Medicine (IOM), *Reducing Risk for Mental Disorders: Frontiers for Preventative Intervention Research*, ed. Patricia Beezley Mrazek and Robert J. Haggerty (Washington, DC: National Academy of Sciences, 1994), http://www.nap.edu/catalog/2139/reducing-risks-for-mental-disorders-frontiers-for-preventive-intervention-research (accessed July 16, 2016).

25. Mary Ellen O'Connell, Thomas Boat, and Kenneth E. Warner, eds., *Preventing Mental, Emotional, and Behavioral Disorders among Young People: Progress and Possibilities* (Washington, DC: National Academies Press, 2009), http://www.nap.edu/catalog/12480/preventing-mental-emotional-and-behavioral-disorders-among-young-people-progress (accessed July 16, 2016).

26. The report did find that some issues the industry considers mental "health" problems (e.g., failed marriages) could be prevented (e.g., by marriage counseling).

27. O'Connell, Boat, and Warner, *Preventing*.

28. "Peer support" colloquially means being helped by someone who has been in a similar situation. Peer support promoters almost never define peer support as "being helped by someone who has a mental illness," because that entails admitting mental illness exists. That is considered "labeling," which they consider to be offensive, perhaps traumatizing.

29. National Association of State Mental Health Program Directors (NASMHPD), "Enhancing the Peer Provider Workforce: Recruitment, Supervision and Retention," NASMHPD, September 15, 2014, http://www.nasmhpd.org/sites/default/files/ Assessment%201%20-%20Enhancing%20the%20Peer%20Provider%20Workforce _9-15-14.pdf (accessed July 16, 2016).

30. Mental Illness Policy Org., "How SAMHSA Mental Health Block Grant Guidance and Application Form Encourages States to Not Use Block Grants for the Most Seriously Ill," Mental Illness Policy Org., 2013, http://mentalillnesspolicy.org/samhsa/ samhsa-block-grant-problems.pdf (accessed July 16, 2016).

31. Peer-run respite centers are billed as an alternative to hospitalization for those in crisis and may be of utility to those in a substance abuse crisis. But consumer advocate Iris Loomknitter notes that the website for Wisconsin's peer run respite center, Iris Place, shoos the seriously ill away with a message that says, "Individuals who utilize the Peer Run Respite don't need the level of services provided by the traditional mental health system—individuals must be able to manage their own medications and support their self-care. To utilize the center, individuals must self-refer. . . . Individuals may not be homeless. . . . The respite does not have a medical-psychiatric component, guests must manage their own medications and other treatments." http://irisplacewi.org/faq (accessed July 24, 2016). The website has now moved to a new location that gives less information, so the above statements are no longer included. "About Iris Place," NAMI, http://www .namifoxvalley.org/iris-place-about.html (accessed December 20, 2016).

Arizona family advocate Lois Earley found that the website for Arizona's peer respite center, Hopes Door, states that it "is NOT [a] good option for people who: are looking for a change in medication; are seeking specialized counseling; need ongoing support from others to stay safe other than someone already in their lives, are unwilling to take responsibility for what is happening to them and for getting better." "Hope's Door," REN, http:// www.renaz.org/services/hopes-door (accessed July 27, 2016).

32. Substance Abuse and Mental Health Services Administration (SAMHSA), "SAMHSA's Working Definition of Recovery Updated," SAMHSA (blog), March 23, 2012, http://blog.samhsa.gov/2012/03/23/defintion-of-recovery-updated/#.U3YZFShJ -6k (accessed July 16, 2016).

33. SAMHSA, Bringing Recovery Supports to Scale (SAMHSA-BRSS), *Equipping Behavioral Health Systems & Authorities to Promote Peer Specialist/Peer Recovery Coaching Services* (Rockville, MD: Expert Panel Meeting Report, SAMHSA, Bringing Recovery Supports to Scale), August 17, 2012, http://www.samhsa.gov/sites/default/files/expert -panel-03212012.pdf (accessed July 16, 2016).

34. Center for Mental Health Services (CMHS), *Consumer-Operated Services: The Evidence*, HHS Publication No. SMA-11-4633 (Rockville, MD: Center for Mental

Health Services, SAMHSA, 2011).

35. Jean Campbell, "Emerging Research Base of Peer-Run Support Programs," National Empowerment Center, May 2005, http://www.power2u.org/emerging_research_base.html (accessed July 16, 2016).

36. The IOM report combined mental health with substance abuse and did not allow any conclusion to be drawn about peer support for mental illness or serious mental illness. There is evidence peer support works for substance abuse. Institute of Medicine (IOM), *Improving the Quality of Health Care for Mental and Substance-Use Conditions* (Washington, DC: National Academies Press, 2006), http://www.nap.edu/catalog/11470.html (accessed July 16, 2016).

37. Susan Eisen, Mark Schultz, Lisa Mueller, et al., "Outcome of a Randomized Study of a Mental Health Peer Education and Support Group in the VA," *Psychiatric Services* 63, no. 12 (December 2012): 1243-46. Abstract at http://www.ncbi.nlm.nih.gov/pubmed/23203360 (accessed July 16, 2016).

38. Maura Dolan, "S.F. Approves Laura's Law to Ensure Mentally Ill Receive Treatment," *Los Angeles Times*, July 8, 2014, http://www.latimes.com/local/lanow/la-me-ln-lauras-law-20140708-story.html (accessed July 16, 2016).

39. Barack Obama, *Now Is the Time: The President's Plan to Protect Our Children and Our Communities by Reducing Gun Violence* (Washington, DC: The White House, January 16, 2013), http://www.whitehouse.gov/sites/default/files/docs/wh_now_is_the_time_full.pdf (accessed July 16, 2016).

40. Mary Gibson-Leek, "Personal Accounts: Client Versus Client," *Psychiatric Services* 54, no. 8 (August 2003): 1101-2, http://mentalillnesspolicy.org/firstperson/consumers-mary-gibson-leek.html (accessed July 16, 2016).

41. National Institute of Mental Health (NIMH), "Post-traumatic Stress Disorder (PTSD)," NIMH, http://www.nimh.nih.gov/health/topics/post-traumatic-stress-disorder-ptsd/index.shtml (accessed July 16, 2016). American Psychiatric Association (APA), *Diagnostic and Statistical Manual of Mental Disorders: DSM-5* (Washington, DC: American Psychiatric Association, 2013).

42. In *DSM III-R*, a PTSD diagnosis required "an event that is outside the range of usual human experience and that would be markedly distressing to anyone." In subsequent versions this language was removed. Anyone learning about "unexpected or violent death, serious harm, or threat of death or injury experienced by a family member or other close associate" can be said to have PTSD if it affects the ability to cope. As a result, there is now a whole trauma industry, and people are encouraged to believe they have it, that it is severe, unmanageable, and chronic.

43. Sally Satel, "The Battle over Battle Fatigue: Soldiers Can Now Claim Trauma from Events They Didn't Actually Experience. Is the Diagnosis Losing Meaning?" *Wall Street Journal*, July 17, 2010, http://online.wsj.com/news/articles/SB100014240527487049133045753711308762717 08 (accessed July 16, 2016).

44. Benedict Carey, "Report Calls for Tracking Data on Stress Disorder," *New York Times*, June 20, 2014, http://www.nytimes.com/2014/06/21/us/report-calls-for-tracking-data-on-stress-disorder.html (accessed July 16, 2016).

45. Ron Manderscheid, "Response to Dr. E. Fuller Torrey Regarding Progress in Recovery," Children's Mental Health Network, October 19, 2014, http://www.cmhnetwork.org/media-center/morning-zen/manderscheid-response-torrey (accessed July

16, 2016). Trauma can cause major severe depression and depression, and those can often be treated with medications or electroconvulsive therapy. Trauma does not cause schizophrenia, bipolar disorder, or all severe depression, although it can exacerbate symptoms in those who already have them.

46. National Council on Alcoholism and Drug Dependence, "Experts Say Mental Health Effects of Hurricane Sandy Could be Powerful," DrugFree.org, 2012, Version available at http://www.drugfree.org/join-together/experts-say-mental-health-effects-of-hurricane-sandy-could-be-powerful (accessed July 16, 2016). David Ferris, "Is Climate Change a Mental Health Emergency?" *Forbes*, March 31, 2012, http://www.forbes.com/sites/davidferris/2012/03/31/is-climate-change-a-mental-health-emergency (accessed July 16, 2016). No doubt hurricanes cause stress and anxiety in people who experience them, but stress and anxiety used to be normal. The APA has defined even moderate versions as illness.

47. To put the 1.5 million in perspective, 3,000 people died in the World Trade Center attack. If each had ten people close to them, 30,000 experienced trauma. Triple it and you've still got only 90,000. Of the 1.5 million who received federally funded trauma services, 750,000 people received crisis counseling (presumably they called a phone line), and 740,000 people received public education, that is to say, probably saw or heard one of the public service announcements. Lloyd I. Sederer, "Lessons from New York City's 9/11 Mental Health Response," *Huffington Post*, September 8, 2011, http://www.huffingtonpost.com/lloyd-i-sederer-md/911-mental-health-response_b_949390.html (accessed July 16, 2016).

48. Lauren Spiro, "Our Liberation Is a Catalyst for Changing Our Culture: Escaping the Trap; Women Caught in the Mental Health System" (speech, Bethesda, MD: National Organization of Women), July 18, 2008, http://ncmhr.org/downloads/escaping-the-trap.pdf (accessed July 16, 2016).

49. Leah Harris told an audience, "Our movement goes so far beyond mental health: it is a social justice movement, a multi-issue struggle. It's radical in the sense that it seeks to address the root causes of the conditions that cause people to go into crisis in the first place—overwhelming traumatic stress, exposure to violence and abuse, isolation, *lack of access to timely support*, coupled with social ignorance, prejudice, and discrimination." She then explained how trauma causes schizophrenia: "People have extreme experiences (voices, visions, non-consensus reality) that more often than not are triggered by severe trauma[s], and are often scary to them and for those who love them. That's what's usually called schizophrenia." Leah Harris, director, National Coalition for Mental Health Recovery, "The Personal Is the Political: Reflections on an Advocacy Journey," speech at NYAPRS Conference, September 17, 2014, http://leahidaharris.com/14/09/nyaprs-speech-september-17-2014 (accessed July 16, 2016).

50. NASMHPD, "The National Center for Trauma Informed Care," NASMHPD, 2010, http://www.nasmhpd.org/content/national-center-trauma-informed-care-nctic-0 (accessed July 16, 2016).

51. Center for Mental Health Services (CMHS), "About NCTIC [National Center for Trauma Informed Care]," SAMHSA, May 20, 2014, http://www.samhsa.gov/nctic/about (accessed July 16, 2016).

52. "The need for restraint and seclusion of patients decreased and all but disappeared in inverse ratio to increase in patients receiving tranquilizing drugs." Joint Commission on Mental Illness and Health, *Action for Mental Health* (New York: Basic Books, 1961).

53. Mental Health America, "Talking to Kids about School Safety," Mental Health America, http://www.mentalhealthamerica.net/conditions/talking-kids-about-school -safety (accessed July 16, 2016).

54. Tamsin B. R. Short, Stuart Thomas, Stefan Luebbers, et al., "A Case-Linkage Study of Crime Victimisation in Schizophrenia-Spectrum Disorders over a Period of Deinstitutionalisation," *BMC Psychiatry* 13 (2013), http://www.ncbi.nlm.nih.gov/pmc/ articles/PMC3599537 (accessed July 16, 2016).

55. Virginia A. Hiday, Marvin S. Swartz, Jeffrey W. Swanson, et al., "Criminal Victimization of Persons with Severe Mental Illness," *Psychiatric Services* 50, no. 1 (January 1999): 62-68, http://www.ncbi.nlm.nih.gov/pubmed/9890581 (accessed July 16, 2016).

56. Jaakko Seikkula, Birgitta Alakare, and Jukka Aaltonen, "The Comprehensive Open-Dialogue Approach in Western Lapland: II. Long-Term Stability of Acute Psychosis Outcomes in Advanced Community Care," *Psychosis*, August 2011, http://leonardo .otwartydialog.pl/wp-content/uploads/2014/09/Materials-for-the-Tromso-Conference13 .pdf (accessed July 14, 2016).

57. Marvin Ross, "Don't Be Too Quick to Praise This New Treatment," *Huffington Post*, November 11, 2013, http://www.huffingtonpost.ca/marvin-ross/schizophrenia -treatment_b_4254350.html (accessed July 14, 2016).

58. Mary Olson, "The Promise of Open Dialogue," *Mad in America*, January 1, 2014, http://www.madinamerica.com/2014/01/promise-open-dialogue-response-marvin-ross/ (accessed July 14, 2016).

59. Alex Langford, "Open Dialogue: Reflections on the Model and the Evidence," Psychiatry SHO, March 20, 2015, https://psychiatrysho.wordpress.com/2015/03/20/133698 (accessed July 14, 2016).

60. Ibid.

61. For example, in 2012, the California mental health industry created a $32 million suicide media campaign. California Mental Health Services Authority (CalMHSA), "California Mental Health Services Authority Launches Statewide Suicide Prevention Campaign," PRWEB, December 12, 2012, http://www.prweb.com/releases/ prweb2012/12/prweb10229719.htm (accessed July 16, 2016).

62. J. John Mann, Alan Apter, Jose Bertolote, et al., "Suicide Prevention Strategies: A Systematic Review," *Journal of the American Medical Association* 294, no. 16 (October 2005): 2064–74, http://jama.jamanetwork.com/article.aspx?articleid=201761 (accessed July 16, 2016).

63. Josh Sanburn, "Inside the National Suicide Hotline: Preventing the Next Tragedy," *Time*, September 13, 2013, http://healthland.time.com/2013/09/13/inside-the -national-suicide-hotline-counselors-work-to-prevent-the-next-casualty (accessed July 16, 2016).

64. Kana Enomoto, *Hearing: Substance Abuse and Mental Health Services Administration Budget*, testimony by acting director of Substance Abuse and Mental Health Services Administration to House Appropriations Subcommittee on Labor, Health and Human Services, Education, and Related Agencies delivered March 2, 2016, http://www.c-span .org/video/?405122-1/appropriations-labor-health-human-services-education-related -agencies (accessed July 16, 2016).

65. SAMHSA, *Results from the 2011 National Survey on Drug Use and Health: Mental Health Findings.* NSDU Series H-45, HHS Publication No. (SMA) 12-4725. (Rockville, MD: SAMHSA), 2012, http://www.samhsa.gov/data/NSDUH/2k11MH

_FindingsandDetTables/2K11MHFR/NSDUHmhfr2011.pdf (accessed May 5, 2013).

66. J. John Mann, et al., "Suicide Prevention Strategies."

67. Centers for Disease Control and Prevention (CDC), "10 Leading Causes of Death by Age Group, United States: 2014," https://www.cdc.gov/injury/images/lc-charts/leading_causes_of_death_age_group_2014_1050w760h.gif (accessed December 20, 2016).

68. American Foundation for Suicide Prevention (AFSP), "Facts and Figures," AFSP, 2014, http://www.afsp.org/understanding-suicide/facts-and-figures (accessed July 16, 2016). The AFSP statistics are culled from the Center for Disease Control and Prevention 2014 Fatal Injury Reports that can be queried at http://www.cdc.gov/injury/wisqars/fatal_injury_reports.html (accessed July 16, 2016). However AFSP presents the data in useful tables.

69. Mark Olfson, Melanie Wall, Shuai Wang, et al., "Short-Term Suicide Risk after Psychiatric Hospital Discharge," *JAMA Psychiatry*, September 21, 2016, http://archpsyc.jamanetwork.com/article.aspx?articleid=2551516 (accessed September 27, 2016).

70. Diego De Leo, "Why Are We Not Getting Any Closer to Preventing Suicide?" (editorial), *British Journal of Psychiatry* 181 (2002): 372–74, http://bjp.rcpsych.org/content/181/5/372.full.pdf (accessed July 16, 2016).

71. Josh Sanburn, "Inside the National Suicide Hotline."

72. M. T. Tsuang, "Risk of Suicide in the Relatives of Schizophrenics, Manics, Depressives, and Controls," *Journal of Clinical Psychiatry* 44, no. 11 (November 1983): 398-400. Abstract at http://www.ncbi.nlm.nih.gov/pubmed/6643403 (accessed July 16, 2016).

73. Lindsay M. Hayes, *National Study of Jail Suicide: 20 Years Later* (Washington, DC: National Institute of Corrections, DOJ), April 2010, http://static.nicic.gov/Library/024308.pdf (accessed July 16, 2016).

74. Kahyee Hor and Mark Taylor, "Suicide and Schizophrenia: A Systematic Review of Rates and Risk Factors," *Journal of Psychopharmacology* 24, no. 4, suppl. (November 2010): 81-90, http://www.ncbi.nlm.nih.gov/pmc/articles/PMC2951591/ (accessed July 16, 2016).

75. Following are studies compiled by the Treatment Advocacy Center suggesting suicide is more likely in individuals with schizophrenia and bipolar disorder who are not being treated:

- A Swiss study found the suicide rate was more than twice as high among patients who had not been treated compared with those who had been treated (p = 0.04), a difference the authors called "spectacular." F. Angst, H. H. Stassen, P. J. Clayton, et al., "Mortality of Patients with Mood Disorders: Follow-up over 34–38 Years," *Journal of Affective Disorders* 68 (2002): 167-81. Abstract at http://www.ncbi.nlm.nih.gov/pubmed/12063145 (accessed July 16, 2016).
- In a study of suicide among psychiatric patients, 71.1 percent of patients who were depressed in their last episode [of hospitalization] were not receiving adequate antidepressant or lithium carbonate medication at the time of suicide. A. Roy, "Risk Factors for Suicide in Psychiatric Patients," *Archive of General Psychiatry* 39 (1982): 1089-95. Abstract at http://www.ncbi.nlm.nih.gov/pubmed/7115014 (accessed July 16, 2016).
- A study in Kentucky found that only two of twenty-eight individuals with schizophrenia who committed suicide had evidence in their blood of having taken anti-

psychotic medication. Thus, 93 percent of them were not being treated. Lisa B.
E. Shields, Donna M. Hunsaker, and John C. Hunsaker III, "Schizophrenia and
Suicide: A 10-Year Review of Kentucky Medical Examiner Cases," *Journal of Forensic
Sciences* 52, no. 4 (July 2007): 930-37. Abstract at http://onlinelibrary.wiley.com/
doi/10.1111/j.1556-4029.2007.00485.x/abstract (accessed July 16, 2016).

- A case-control study of sixty-three individuals with schizophrenia who committed suicide and sixty-three individuals with schizophrenia who did not reported
that "there were seven times as many patients who did not comply with treatment in the suicide group as there were in the control group." M. De Hert, K.
McKenzie, and J. Peuskens, "Risk Factors for Suicide in Young People Suffering
from Schizophrenia: A Long-Term Follow-up Study," *Schizophrenia Research*
47, no. 2–3 (March 2001): 127–34. Abstract at http://www.ncbi.nlm.nih.gov/
pubmed/11278129 (accessed July 16, 2016).

- A study from Germany using a case-control methodology compared twenty-seven
inpatients with schizophrenia and twenty-four inpatients with affective psychoses, all of whom suicided, with their matched inpatient case controls who did
not suicide. The authors concluded that there is "a significantly increased risk" of
suicide when medications are not used. I. Gaertner, C. Gilot, P. Heidrich, et al., "A
Case Control Study on Psychopharmacotherapy before Suicide Committed by 61
Psychiatric Inpatients," *Pharmacopsychiatry* 35, no. 2 (March 2002): 37–43. Abstract
at http://www.ncbi.nlm.nih.gov/pubmed/11951144 (accessed July 16, 2016).

76. Lithium: B. Müller-Oerlinghausen, "Arguments for the Specificity of the Anti-
suicidal Effect of Lithium," *European Archives of Psychiatry and Clinical Neuroscience* 251,
suppl. 2 (February 2001): 1172–75. Abstract at http://www.researchgate.net/publication/
11535132_Arguments_for_the_specificity_of_the_antisuicidal_effect_of_lithium
(accessed July 16, 2016). U. Lewizka, E. Severus, R. Bauer et al, "The Suicide Prevention
Effect of Lithium: More than 20 Years of Evidence—A Narrative Review, *International
Journal of Bipolar Disorder* 3, no. 15 (July 2015), http://www.ncbi.nlm.nih.gov/pmc/
articles/PMC4504869/ (accessed September 2, 2016). Clozaril: HY Meltzer, L. Alphs, Al
Green, et al., "Clozapine Treatment for Suicidality in Schizophrenia: International Suicide
Prevention Trial (InterSePT)," *Archive of General Psychiatry* 60, no. 1 (January 2003):
82–91, http://archpsyc.jamanetwork.com/article.aspx?articleid=207092 (accessed August
2, 2016). ECT: Charles H. Kellner, Erin Li, Kate Farber, et al., "Electroconvulsive
Therapy (ECT) and Suicide Prevention," *Current Treatment Options in Psychiatry* 3, no.
1 (March 2016): 73–81, http://link.springer.com/article/10.1007/s40501-016-0067-8
(accessed September 2, 2016).

77. New York State Office of Mental Health, *Kendra's Law: Final Report on the
Status of Assisted Outpatient Treatment,* Report to Legislature (Albany: New York State,
2005), http://www.omh.ny.gov/omhweb/kendra_web/finalreport/ (accessed July 16, 2016).

78. Andy Wolf, "Veteran Turned Away from VA after Requesting Mental Treatment,
Kills Himself," Popular Military, July 14, 2016, http://popularmilitary.com/veteran
-turned-away-va-requesting-mental-treatment-kills (accessed August 13, 2016).

79. Paul S. F.Yip, Eric Caine, Saman Yousuf, et al., "Means Restriction for Suicide
Prevention," *Lancet* 379, no. 9834 (June 2012): 2393–99. Abstract at http://www.the
lancet.com/journals/lancet/article/PIIS0140-6736(12)60521-2/fulltext (accessed July 16,
2016).

80. California mental health funds funded a net under the Golden Gate Bridge. But that was largely a PR ploy to defuse criticism of waste in mental health spending. Darrell Steinberg, *Steinberg Statement on Vote for Suicide Barrier at Golden Gate Bridge,* June 27, 2014.

81. Christina Hoff Sommers, and Sally Satel, *One Nation Under Therapy: How the Helping Culture is Eroding Self-Reliance* (New York: St. Martin's Press, 2005).

82. When former SAMHSA administrator Pamela Hyde told a congressional sub-committee, "Half of all lifetime cases of mental *and* substance use disorders begin by age 14 and three-fourths by age 24," she correctly noted the figure is only true if one combines mental disorders and substance abuse. Pamela Hyde, statement. See chapter 5 for age of onset explanation. *Examining SAMHSA's Role in Delivering Services to the Severely Mentally Ill. Hearings Before the House Subcommittee on Oversight and Investigations of the Energy and Commerce Committee,* 113th Cong. (May 22, 2013), http://docs.house.gov/meetings/IF/IF02/20130522/100900/HHRG-113-IF02-Wstate-HydeP-20130522.pdf (accessed July 16, 2016).

83. Robert Whitaker, *Anatomy of an Epidemic: Magic Bullets, Psychiatric Drugs, and the Astonishing Rise of Mental Illness in America* (New York: Crown Publishers, 2010).

84. Centers for Disease Control and Prevention (CDC), "ADHD Estimates Rise," May 16, 2014, http://www.cdc.gov/media/dpk/2013/dpk-ADHD-estimates-rise.html (accessed July 16, 2016). In 1999, the Surgeon General claimed 21% of children ages 9–17 had a diagnosable mental or addictive disorder that caused at least minimal impairment. US Surgeon General, *Mental Health: A Report of the U.S. Surgeon General* (Rockville, MD: Department of Health and Human Services, 1999), http://profiles.nlm.nih.gov/ps/access/NNBBHS.ocr (accessed July 16, 2016).

85. Anthony James, Uy Hoang, Valerie Seagroatt, et al., "A Comparison of American and English Hospital Discharge Rates for Pediatric Bipolar Disorder, 2000 to 2010," *Journal of the American Academy of Child & Adolescent Psychiatry* 53, no. 6 (June 2014): 614–24. Abstract at http://www.jaacap.com/article/S0890-8567(14)00160-9/abstract (accessed July 16, 2016).

86. Open Minds, "New York Court Strikes Down Limits on Executive Compensation at For-Profit Human Service Organizations," Open Minds, June 8, 2014, http://www.openminds.com/market-intelligence/news/new-york-court-strikes-state-limits-executive-compensation-profit-human-service-provider-organizations.htm (accessed July 16, 2016).

CHAPTER 13: THE INDUSTRY DIVERTS FUNDS TO IRRELEVANT STIGMA PROGRAMS

1. Joint Commission on Mental Illness and Health, *Action for Mental Health* (New York: Basic Books, 1961).

2. The *Dr. Phil* episode was removed from circulation, but parts of the interview can be found at "Dr. Phil—3 Minutes of Shelley Duvall," YouTube video, 3:00, from *Dr. Phil* televised on November 18, 2016, posted by "gerbho1," November 22, 2016, https://www.youtube.com/watch?v=2ioTXdO5qt0 (accessed December 20, 2016).

3. Joint Commission on Mental Illness and Health, *Action for Mental Health.*

4. AOT: Alli Sofer, "Effectiveness of Kendra's Law Being Debated," *Legisla-*

tive Gazette (Albany, NY), April 30, 2012; Commitment reform: Lori Ashcroft, "Life, Unrestrained," Behavioral Healthcare, January 10, 2013, http://www.behavioral.net/article/life-unrestrained (accessed July 17, 2016); Gun restrictions: Michael Fitzpatrick (then executive director of NAMI), "Gun Laws and Mental Health," NAMI (blog), August 21, 2012, http://blog.nami.org/2012/08/gun-laws-and-mental-health.html (accessed July 17, 2016). Expanding hospital care, and diagnosis, by claiming "psychiatric diagnosis and labeling can result in increased stigma": National Coalition for Mental Health Recovery, "Coalition of Individuals with Psychiatric Labels Supports Protestors' Efforts to 'Occupy' the American Psychiatric Association Convention," National Coalition for Mental Health Recovery, May 3, 2012, http://www.ncmhr.org/press-releases/5.3.12.htm (accessed July 27, 2016).

5. Barack Obama, "Obama Calls for End to Mental Illness Stigma," YouTube video, 2:14, from a televised press conference on June 3, 2013, posted by "Associated Press," June 3, 2013, https://www.youtube.com/watch?v=UqnF3UicuQs (accessed July 27, 2016).

6. National Alliance on Mental Illness, "How We Talk about NAMI," NAMI, http://www.nami.org/Extranet/NAMI-State-Organization-and-NAMI-Affiliate-Leaders/NAMI-Marketing/NAMI-Identity-Guide/How-We-Talk-About-NAMI (accessed July 27, 2016). As a result of industry pressure, the Associated Press (AP) tells its writers to "avoid descriptions that connote pity, such as afflicted with, suffers from or victim of." Associated Press, "Entry on Mental Illness Is Added to AP Stylebook," March 7, 2013, http://www.ap.org/content/press-release/2013/entry-on-mental-illness-is-added-to-ap-stylebook (accessed July 27, 2016).

7. Bazelon Center for Mental Health Law, "Bazelon Center Statement on Sandy Hook Shooting," Bazelon, December 17, 2012, http://www.bazelon.org/News-Publications/Press-Releases/12.17.12-Sandy-Hook-PR.aspx (accessed July 17, 2016).

8. Susan Rogers, "Gun Laws and the Mentally Ill" (letter to the editor), *New York Times*, December 25, 2013, http://www.nytimes.com/2013/12/26/opinion/gun-laws-and-the-mentally-ill.html (accessed July 27, 2016).

9. Bazelon Center for Mental Health Law, "Help 60 Minutes Get the Story Right on People with Schizophrenia," Bazelon, October 8, 2013, http://www.bazelon.org/What-You-Can-Do/Take-Action/Alerts/Alerts-Archive/10-8-2013-60-Minutes-Alert.aspx (accessed July 17, 2016).

10. H. Richard Lamb, "Taking Issue: Combating Stigma by Providing Treatment," *Psychiatric Services* 50, no. 6 (June 1999), http://www.treatmentadvocacycenter.org/index.php?option=com_content&id=584&Itemid=221 (accessed July 17, 2016). The former executive director of NAMI inadvertently recognized violence causes stigma when he wrote for CNN, "Stigma perpetuated by the Navy Yard tragedy will be internalized by many people living with mental health problems, causing them to stay silent and withdraw from others. This will impede their recovery in many ways." Michael Fitzpatrick, "How Shootings Stigmatize People Living with Mental Illness," CNN, September 20, 2013, http://www.cnn.com/2013/09/20/opinion/mental-health-stigma-shootings/ (accessed July 27, 2016).

11. Henry J. Steadman, "Critically Reassessing the Accuracy of Public Perceptions of the Dangerousness of the Mentally Ill," *Journal of Health and Social Behavior* 22, no. 3 (September 1981): 310-16. Abstract at http://www.jstor.org/discover/10.2307/2136524 (accessed July 27, 2016).

12. Peter C. Campanelli, "Beyond the Open Door: Challenges in Housing for People with Mental Illness (editorial),"*National Council Magazine* (of the National Council for Community Behavioral Healthcare), issue 3 (2009), http://spcsb.org/pdfs/resources/independent-living-national-council-article.pdf (accessed July 17, 2016).

13. US Surgeon General, *Mental Health: A Report of the U.S. Surgeon General* (Rockville, MD: Department of Health and Human Services, 1999), http://profiles.nlm.nih.gov/ps/access/NNBBHS.ocr (accessed July 27, 2016).

14. E. Fuller Torrey, "Stigma and Violence: Isn't It Time to Connect the Dots?" *Schizophrenia Bulletin* 37, no. 5 (September 2011): 892–96, http://mentalillnesspolicy.org/consequences/stigma.html (accessed July 27, 2016).

15. "Repeated use of the term 'stigma' in conjunction with 'mental illness' . . . may establish stigma as an element of mental illness—as inevitable and intrinsic to psychiatric conditions." Otto F. Wahl, "Is 'Stigma' the Right Word?" University of Hartford, 2003, http://uhaweb.hartford.edu/owahl/inmyopinion.htm (accessed July 27, 2016).

16. Kevin Earley, "If You Are Afraid to Tell Your Story, Stigma Wins," PeteEarley, July 14, 2014, http://www.peteearley.com/14/07/14/son-says-afraid-tell-story-stigma-wins/ (accessed July 17, 2016).

CHAPTER 14: FEDERAL POLICIES THAT FAIL THE SERIOUSLY ILL

1. E. Fuller Torrey, *Nowhere to Go: The Tragic Odyssey of the Homeless Mentally Ill* (New York: Harper & Row, 1988).

2. National Mental Health Act (1946), Pub. L. 79-487, July 3, 1946.

3. Ellen Herman, *The Romance of American Psychology: Political Culture in the Age of Experts* (Berkeley, CA: University of California Press, 1995), http://publishing.cdlib.org/ucpressebooks/view?docId=ft696nb3n8;brand=ucpress (accessed July 17, 2016).

4. Gerald N. Grob, "The National Institute of Mental Health and Mental Health Policy, 1949-1965," in Caroline Hannaway (ed.), *Biomedicine in the Twentieth Century: Practices, Policies, and Politics* (Amsterdam, NY: IOS Press, 2008), pp. 59–94.

5. Jeffrey Lieberman, *Shrinks: The Untold Story of Psychiatry* (New York: Little, Brown, 2015).

6. E. Fuller Torrey, *American Psychosis: How the Federal Government Destroyed the Mental Illness Treatment System* (New York: Oxford University Press, 2014).

7. Joint Commission on Mental Illness and Health, *Action for Mental Health* (New York: Basic Books, 1961).

8. Mental Retardation Facilities and Community Mental Health Centers Construction Act of 1963 Pub. L. 88-164, Vol. 77 (October 31, 1963) http://history.nih.gov/research/downloads/PL88-164.pdf (accessed July 17, 2016). It is colloquially known as the Community Mental Health (Centers) Act.

9. H. Goldman, N. H. Adams, C. A. Taube, "Deinstitutionalization: The Date Demythologized," *Hospital and Community Psychiatry* 34, no. 2 (February 1983): 129–34. Abstract at http://www.ncbi.nlm.nih.gov/pubmed/6860396 (accessed July 17, 2016).

10. E. Fuller Torrey, *American Psychosis*.

11. Gerald N. Grob, "The National Institute of Mental Health and Mental Health Policy."

12. E. Fuller Torrey, *American Psychosis*.

13. D. G. Langsley, "The Community Mental Health Center: Does It Treat Patients?" *Hospital and Community Psychiatry* 31, no. 12 (December 1980): 815–19. Abstract at http://www.ncbi.nlm.nih.gov/pubmed/7203401 (accessed July 17, 2016).

14. E. Fuller Torrey, *Nowhere to Go*.

15. Rachel L. Garfield, *Mental Health Financing in the United States: A Primer* (Menlo Park, CA: Henry J Kaiser Foundation, April 2011), http://kaiserfamilyfoundation .files.wordpress.com/2013/01/8182.pdf (accessed July 17, 2016).

16. Office of Management and Budget (OMB), letter from OMB director Sylvia M. Burwell to Representative Tim Murphy, Subcommittee on Oversight and Investigations of the House Energy and Commerce Committee, November 7, 2013, http://mental illnesspolicy.org/national-studies/mentalhealthexpenditurenational.pdf (accessed July 17, 2016).

17. For a listing of provisions that exempted those twenty-one and under, and sixty-four and over from the IMD Exclusion see John Fergus Edwards, "The Outdated Institution for Mental Diseases Exclusion: A Call to Re-examine and Repeal the Medicaid IMD Exclusion," Mental Health Policy Org., May 1997, http://mentalillnesspolicy.org/ imd/imd-legal-analysis.pdf (accessed July 17, 2016).

18. William Gronfein, "Incentives and Intentions in Mental Health Policy: A Comparison of the Medicaid and Community Mental Health Programs," *Journal of Health and Social Behavior* 26, no. 3 (September 1985): 192–206. Abstract at http://www.jstor.org/ discover/10.2307/2136752 (accessed July 17, 2016).

19. Jeffrey L. Geller, "Excluding Institutions for Mental Diseases from Federal Reimbursement for Services: Strategy or Tragedy?" *Psychiatric Services* 51, no. 11 (November 2000): 1397–1403 http://ps.psychiatryonline.org/article.aspx?articleID=85111 (accessed July 17, 2016).

20. Morton Kramer, *Psychiatric Services and the Changing Institutional Scene, 1950–1985* (Rockville, MD: US Department of Health Education and Welfare, 1977), as quoted in Gronfein, "Incentives and Intentions in Mental Health Policy," 1985.

21. Eddie Bernice Johnson, *An Act to Amend Title XIX of the Social Security Act to Remove the Exclusion from Medical Assistance under the Medicaid Program of Items and Services for Patients in an Institution for Mental Diseases*, H.R. 2757, 113th Cong. (July 19, 2013) https://www.congress.gov/bill/113th-congress/house-bill/2757 (accessed July 17, 2016).

22. OMB, letter from Sylvia M. Burwell.

23. Pub. L. 89–97, 79 Stat. 286.

24. E. Fuller Torrey, DJ Jaffe, Jeffrey Geller, et al., *Fraud, Waste and Excess Profits: The Fate of Money Intended to Treat People with Serious Mental Illness* (New York: report, Mental Illness Policy Org., 2015), 2015, http://mentalillnesspolicy.org/national-studies/ wastereport.pdf (accessed July 17, 2016).

25. OMB, letter from Sylvia M. Burwell.

26. Edward Berkowitz, *Disability Policy & History*, testimony, Hearings before the House Subcommittee on Social Security of the Committee on Ways and Means, 106th Cong. (July 13, 2000) http://www.ssa.gov/history/edberkdib.html (accessed July 17, 2016). Section 223(d)(1) of the Social Security Act defines disability as "an inability to engage in any substantial gainful activity by reason of any medically determinable physical or mental impairment which can be expected to result in death or which has lasted or can

be expected to last for a continuous period of not less than twelve months." A medically determinable physical or mental impairment was defined as "an impairment that results from anatomical, physiological, or psychological abnormalities that can be shown by medically acceptable clinical and laboratory diagnostic techniques. An impairment must be established by medical evidence consisting of signs, symptoms, and laboratory findings." Social Security Administration, *Annual Statistical Report on the Social Security Disability Insurance Program, 2014* (Washington, DC: Office of Research, Evaluation, and Statistics, Office of Retirement and Disability Policy, 2015), p. 2, https://www.socialsecurity.gov/policy/docs/statcomps/di_asr/2014/di_asr14.pdf (accessed July 17, 2016).

27. The Social Security Amendments of 1965 deleted the requirement that the impairment be of "long-continued and indefinite duration" and substituted in its place a requirement that the impairment "be expected to last for a continuous period of not less than 12 months." Social Security Administration, "A History of Social Security Disability Programs," SSA, 1986, https://www.ssa.gov/history/1986dibhistory.html. The 1984 Social Security Disability Benefits Reform Act changed the "mental impairment" listings and allowed for the consideration of the combined effect of all impairments when determining SSDI eligibility. It also allowed applicants to rely on their own doctors to establish illness. Social Security Administration, *Annual Statistical Report, 2014.*

28. Howard H. Goldman and Antoinette A. Gatozzi, "Murder in the Cathedral Revisited: President Regan and the Mentally Disabled," *Psychiatric Services* 39, no. 5 (May 1988): 505–509. Abstract at http://ps.psychiatryonline.org/article.aspx?articleID=72585 (accessed July 17, 2016). Social Security Administration, *Annual Statistical Report, 2014,* Table 21, p. 62.

29. In 2014, 10,261,268 individuals received SSDI benefits. Of these, 3,589,006 were receiving SSDI due to mental disabilities including 50,346 with autistic disorders; 13,890 with developmental disorders; 12,852 with childhood and adolescent disorders not elsewhere classified; 855,263 with intellectual disability; 1,418,157 with mood disorders; 336,682 with organic mental disorders; 510,082 with schizophrenic and other psychotic disorders; and 391,734 with "other." Ibid. Table 10a, p. 37.

30. Children of those who paid into SSDI are eligible for survivor benefits if they are unmarried and under eighteen (nineteen, if a full-time student) or of any age if they were disabled before age twenty-two and remain disabled.

31. Garfield, *Mental Health Financing.*

32. Ibid.

33. Social Security Administration, *History of Social Security Disability Programs.*

34. James C. McKinley, Jr., "Plea Deal for Ex-Police Officer in Huge Disability Scheme," *New York Times*, September 12, 2014, http://www.nytimes.com/2014/09/13/nyregion/plea-deal-for-ex-police-officer-in-huge-disability-scheme.html (accessed July 17, 2016).

35. Disability criteria for SSI are similar to those for SSDI but do not require prior work experience. Generally, those who qualify for SSI also qualify for Medicaid.

36. Garfield, *Mental Health Financing.*

37. Parents enter into contracts with their ill children that "charge" children for the housing and food parents provide. Parents have no desire or intent to collect the charges, but contend that the existence of a contract requiring children to pay prevents the SSI checks from being reduced by one-third.

38. President [Carter] Commission on Mental Health, *Report to the President from the President's Commission on Mental Health* (Washington, DC: US Government Printing Office, 1978), http://www.jstor.org/discover/10.2307/30015739 (accessed July 17, 2016).

39. Gerald N. Grob, "Public Policy and Mental Illnesses: Jimmy Carter's Presidential Commission on Mental Health," *Milbank Quarterly* 83, no. 3 (September 2005): 425–56, http://www.ncbi.nlm.nih.gov/pmc/articles/PMC2690151/ (accessed July 16, 2016).

40. Jimmy Carter, "Mental Health Systems Legislation Message to the Congress Transmitting the Proposed Legislation," May 15, 1979. This can be found online by Gerhard Peters and John T. Woolley on The American Presidency Project: http://www.presidency.ucsb.edu/ws/?pid=32339 (accessed July 17, 2016).

41. *Mental Health Systems Act* (S. 1177), Pub. L. 96-398, US Statutes at Large, vol. 94 (October 7, 1980), 1564–1613, https://www.gpo.gov/fdsys/pkg/STATUTE-94/pdf/STATUTE-94-Pg1564.pdf (accessed July 17, 2016).

42. Robert Epstein, interview with Tipper Gore and Rosalynn Carter, *Psychology Today*, September 1, 1999, http://www.psychologytoday.com/articles/199909/tipper-gore-and-rosalynn-carter (accessed July 17, 2016).

43. *Civil Rights of Institutionalized Persons Act*, Pub. L. 96-247, U.S. Statutes at Large, vol. 94 (May 23, 1980), pp. 349–54, https://www.gpo.gov/fdsys/pkg/STATUTE-94/pdf/STATUTE-94-Pg349.pdf (accessed July 17, 2016).

44. Department of Justice, *The Attorney General's Annual Report to Congress Describing the Department's Enforcement Efforts under the Civil Rights of Institutionalized Persons Act*, Reports 2000–2013, http://www.justice.gov/crt/publications/index.php#cripa (accessed July 17, 2016).

45. National Council on Disability (NCD), *The Civil Rights of Institutionalized Persons Act: Has It Fulfilled Its Promise?* Report to the President (Washington, DC: National Council on Disability, 2005), http://www.ncd.gov/publications/2005/08082005 (accessed July 17, 2016).

46. C. Lee Ventola, "Direct-to-Consumer Pharmaceutical Advertising: Therapeutic or Toxic?" *Pharmacy and Therapeutics* 36, no. 10 (October 2011): 669–74, 681–84, http://www.ncbi.nlm.nih.gov/pmc/articles/PMC3278148 (accessed July 17, 2016); Banning: Allen Frances, *Saving Normal* (New York: HarperCollins, 2013).

47. Some take antidepressants for reasons other than depression, and some, as a result of ongoing treatment, do not currently have depressive symptoms. Laura A. Pratt, Debra J. Brody, and Qiuping Gu, "Antidepressant Use in Persons Aged 12 and Over: United States, 2005–2008," *National Center for Health Statistics*, http://www.cdc.gov/nchs/data/databriefs/db76.pdf (accessed July 17, 2016).

48. Centers for Medicare and Medicaid Services (CMS), "Emergency Medical Treatment and Labor Act," CMS, March 26, 2012, https://www.cms.gov/Regulations-and-Guidance/Legislation/EMTALA/index.html (accessed September 10, 2012).

49. *Protection and Advocacy for Individuals with Mental Illness Act*, as amended (42 U.S.C. §§ 10801-10807, 10821-10827), https://www.gpo.gov/fdsys/pkg/STATUTE-100/pdf/STATUTE-100-Pg478.pdf (accessed August 18, 2016).

50. Amanda Peters, "Lawyers Who Break the Law: What Congress Can Do to Prevent Mental Health Patient Advocates from Violating Federal Legislation," *Oregon Law Review* 89, no. 1 (2010): 133–74, http://mentalillnesspolicy.org/myths/mental-health-bar.pdf (accessed March 6, 2015).

51. Substance Abuse and Mental Health Services Administration (SAMHSA), *Evaluation of the Protection and Advocacy for Individuals with Mental Illness (PAIMI) Program, Phase III*: Evaluation Report, HHS Publication No. PEP12-EVALPAIMI (Rockville, MD: Center for Mental Health Services, SAMHSA, 2011), http://store.samhsa.gov/shin/content/PEP12-EVALPAIMI/PEP12-EVALPAIMI.pdf (accessed July 17, 2016).

52. *Americans with Disabilities Act of 1990*, as amended by the ADA Amendments Act of 2008, Pub. L. 110-325 (June 15, 2009) http://www.ada.gov/pubs/adastatute08.htm (accessed July 17, 2016). Implementing regulations are 29 CFR Parts 1630, 1602 (Title I, EEOC); 28 CFR Part 35 (Title II, Department of Justice); 49 CFR Parts 27, 37, 38 (Title II, III, Department of Transportation); 28 CFR Part 36 (Title III, Department of Justice); 47 CFR §§ 64.601 et seq. (Title IV, FCC).

53. National Advisory Mental Health Council, *Caring for People with Severe Mental Disorders: A National Plan of Research to Improve Services* (Washington, DC: Public Health Service/ADAMHA, HHS, 1991).

54. ADAMHA Reorganization Act of 1991, Pub. L. 102-321, Public Law 102-321, U.S. Statutes at Large, Vol. 106 (July 10, 1992), pp. 323–442. https://www.gpo.gov/fdsys/pkg/STATUTE-106/pdf/STATUTE-106-Pg323.pdf (accessed July 17, 2016) History at http://history.nih.gov/research/downloads/PL102-321.pdf (accessed July 17, 2016). The act created two block grants, one for substance abuse (SABG) and one for mental health (MHBG). Two-thirds of the SAMHSA budget is allocated to substance abuse. This book only concerns itself with how SAMHSA spends its mental illness funds.

55. When presenting the July 1, 1992, conference report on S. 1306, ADAMHA Reorganization Act, to the House, Representative Henry Waxman (D-CA), chairman of the Energy and Commerce Committee's Subcommittee on Health and Environment inserted in the Congressional Record that "the funding formula for allotting block grant funds between the States is revised to more accurately target funds to populations most in need."

56. *Examining SAMHSA's Role in Delivering Services to the Severely Mentally Ill: Hearings Before the House Subcommittee on Oversight and Investigations of the Energy and Commerce Committee*, 113th Cong. (2013) (statement of Pamela S. Hyde, SAMHSA administrator), http://docs.house.gov/meetings/IF/IF02/20130522/100900/HHRG-113-IF02-Wstate-HydeP-20130522.pdf (accessed July 17, 2016).

57. Robert Pear, "Hillary Clinton Sees Hurdles in Forging Health-Care Plan," *New York Times*, February 12, 1993, http://www.nytimes.com/1993/02/12/us/hillary-clinton-sees-hurdles-in-forging-health-care-plan.html (accessed July 17, 2016).

58. Ibid.

59. C. Koyanagi, and J. Manes, "What Did the Health Care Reform Debate Mean for Mental Health Policy?" *Health Affairs* 14, no. 3 (1995): 124–30, http://content.healthaffairs.org/content/14/3/124.full.pdf (accessed July 17, 2016).

60. L. J. Scallet and J. T. Havel, "Reflections on the Mental Health Community's Experience in the Health Care Reform Debate," *Hospital and Community Psychiatry* 45, no. 9 (September 1994): 888–92. Abstract at http://www.ncbi.nlm.nih.gov/pubmed/7989019 (accessed July 17, 2016).

61. "Senate Report 102-397 Attached to HR 5677, HHS Appropriations Bill, ADAMHA Reorganization Act," Federal Register, September 10, 1993: 93. See appendix A for the definition.

62. These savings included disability payments to people with serious mental illness. However, this author is dubious that SSDI payments to people with severe mental illness would decrease significantly, because treatments are not yet efficacious enough to return the seriously ill to work in nonsubsidized positions outside the mental health field.

63. Mental Health Parity Act of 1996, Pub. L. 104-204, U.S. Statutes at Large, vol. 110 (September 26, 1997), pp. 2874–2950, https://www.gpo.gov/fdsys/pkg/STATUTE-110/pdf/STATUTE-110-Pg2874.pdf (accessed July 17, 2016).

64. Ramya Sundararaman and C. Stephen Redhead, *The Mental Health Parity Act: A Legislative History, Report to US House of Representatives*, February 8, 2008, http://congressionalresearch.com/RL33820/document.php (accessed July 17, 2016); Sarah Goodell, "Mental Health Parity," *Health Affairs*, Health Policy Briefs, April 3, 2014, http://www.healthaffairs.org/healthpolicybriefs/brief.php?brief_id=112 (accessed July 17, 2016).

65. *Health Insurance Portability and Accountability Act* of 1996, Pub. L. 104-191, US Statutes at Large, August 26, 1996, Sec. 264, http://www.gpo.gov/fdsys/pkg/PLAW-104publ191/html/PLAW-104publ191.htm (accessed July 17, 2016).

66. Department of Health and Human Services (HHS), Office for Civil Rights, "HIPAA Administrative Simplification," March 26, 2013, http://www.hhs.gov/sites/default/files/ocr/privacy/hipaa/administrative/combined/hipaa-simplification-201303.pdf (accessed July 17, 2016).

67. Department of Education, "Federal Regulations: Part 99—Family Educational Rights and Privacy (FERPA)," July 31, 2014, http://www.ecfr.gov/cgi-bin/retrieveECFR?gp=&SID=0b4547396fd9a36b869a1ea376ce85b7&r=PART&n=34y1.1.1.1.33 (accessed July 17, 2016).

68. Virginia Tech Review Panel, "Mass Shootings at Virginia Tech: Addendum to the Report of the Review Panel," November 2009, http://scholar.lib.vt.edu/prevail/docs/April16ReportRev20100106.pdf (accessed July 17, 2016).

69. Rachel Pruchno, "Mental Illness Laws Block Parents," *USA Today*, April 10, 2013 http://www.usatoday.com/story/opinion/2013/04/10/mental-illness-laws-block-parents-column/2072523 (accessed July 17, 2016).

70. Surgeon General, *Mental Health: A Report of the US Surgeon General* (Rockville, MD: Department of Health and Human Services, 1999) http://profiles.nlm.nih.gov/ps/access/NNBBHS.ocr (accessed July 17, 2016).

71. "Public health" approaches aim to improve sick societies by providing education as opposed to providing medical treatment to sick individuals. For example, educating the public on the benefits of condoms and clean needles is a public health approach that can reduce rates of contagious disorders including AIDS and hepatitis. But two Institute of Medicine (IOM) reports found that a public health approach (universal prevention) does not prevent or treat serious mental illness. Mary Ellen O'Connell, Thomas Boat, and Kenneth E. Warner, eds., *Preventing, Mental, Emotional, and Behavioral Disorders among Young People: Progress and Possibilities* (Washington, DC: National Academy of Science, IOM: 2009), http://www.nap.edu/catalog.php?record_id=12480 (accessed July 17, 2016); Patricia Beezley Mrazek and Robert J. Haggerty, eds., *Reducing Risk for Mental Disorders: Frontiers for Preventative Intervention Research* (Washington, DC: National Academy of Science, IOM: 1994), http://www.nap.edu/catalog.php?record_id=2139 (accessed July 17, 2016).

72. National Council on Disability (NCD), *From Privileges to Rights: People Labeled with Psychiatric Disabilities Speak for Themselves*, Report on Hearings (Washington, DC:

National Council on Disability, 2000) http://www.ncd.gov/publications/2000/Jan202000 (accessed July 17, 2016).

73. "Survivors" is a term used by radical antipsychiatrists to equate being diagnosed with a mental illness to surviving Nazi concentration camps or cancer. "The National Association of Psychiatric Survivors (NAPS) was founded in 1985 to espouse the ideas of Thomas Szasz that mental illness doesn't exist." Judi Chamberlin, "The Ex-Patients' Movement: Where We've Been and Where We're Going," *Journal of Mind and Behavior* 11, no. 3 (Summer 1990): 323–36, http://www.power2u.org/articles/history-project/ex-patients.html (accessed July 17, 2016); Peter Breggin, *Toxic Psychiatry: Why Therapy, Empathy and Love Must Replace the Drugs, Electroshock, and Biochemical Theories of the "New Psychiatry"* (New York: St. Martin's Press, 1991).

74. National Association for Rights Protection and Advocacy (NARPA), "In Memory and Celebration of Rae Unzicker," NARPA, March 2001, http://www.narpa.org/rae.unzicker.htm (accessed July 17, 2016).

75. NCD scheduled their 1998 hearing in Albany for November 20 so they could hear from scores of antipsychiatrists who they knew would be in Albany November 19–22, attending the radical NARPA "Redoubling Our Efforts" conference.

76. National Council on Disability (NCD), "NCD Recommendations for the Helping Families in Mental Health Crisis Act," April 17, 2014, http://www.ncd.gov/publications/2014/04172014 (accessed July 17, 2016).

77. *Medicare Prescription Drug, Improvement, and Modernization Act of 2003* (H.R. 1), Pub L. 108-173, US Statutes at Large, December 8, 2003 https://www.congress.gov/bill/108th-congress/house-bill/1 (accessed July 17, 2016). Thomas R. Oliver, Philip R. Lee, and Helene L. Lipton, "A Political History of Medicare and Prescription Drug Coverage," *Milbank Quarterly* 82.2 (2004): 283–354, http://www.ncbi.nlm.nih.gov/pmc/articles/PMC2690175 (accessed July 17, 2016)

78. George W. Bush, "Executive Order No. 13263 of April 29, 2002 Establishing President's New Freedom Commission on Mental Health," *Federal Register*, Doc. 02-11166, filed May 3, 2002, pp. 22337–38, https://www.federalregister.gov/articles/2002/05/03/02-11166/presidents-new-freedom-commission-on-mental-health (accessed July 17, 2016).

79. Michael Hogan, *2009–2013 Statewide Comprehensive Plan for Mental Health Services* (Albany, NY: NYS Office of Mental Health, October 2009)

80. Sally Satel and Mary Zdanowicz, "Commission's Omission: The President's Mental-Health Commission in Denial," *National Review*, July 29, 2003 http://mentalillnesspolicy.org/mentalhealth/new-freedom-commission.html (accessed July 17, 2016).

81. New Freedom Commission on Mental Health, *Achieving the Promise: Transforming Mental Health Care in America* (Rockville, MD: Department of Health and Human Services, 2003). Executive summary available at http://store.samhsa.gov/product/Achieving-the-Promise-Transforming-Mental-Health-Care-in-America-Executive-Summary/SMA03-3831 (accessed July 17, 2016).

82. E. Fuller Torrey, "Leaving the Mentally Ill Out in the Cold," *City Journal*, September 2003, http://mentalillnesspolicy.org/mentalhealth/new-freedom-commission.html (accessed July 17, 2016).

83. Rich Lowry, "Mistreating the Mentally Ill," *Town Hall*, July 31, 2003, http://townhall.com/columnists/richlowry/2003/07/31/mistreating_the_mentally_ill/page/full

(accessed July 17, 2016).

84. *Individuals with Disabilities Education Improvement Act of 2004* (IDEA), Pub. L. 108-446 (2004), https://www.gpo.gov/fdsys/pkg/STATUTE-118/pdf/STATUTE -118-Pg2647.pdf (accessed July 16, 2016).

85. MHPAE was signed into law as part of the Emergency Economic Stabilization Act of 2008. *Mental Health Parity and Addiction Equity Act of 2008*, Pub. L. 110-343 (2008), http://www.gpo.gov/fdsys/pkg/PLAW-110publ343/html/PLAW-110publ343 .htm (accessed July 17, 2016).

86. Department of Labor, Employee Benefits Security Administration, "Fact Sheet: The Mental Health Parity and Addiction Equity Act of 2008 (MHPAEA)," Department of Labor, January 29, 2010, http://www.dol.gov/ebsa/newsroom/fsmhpaea.html (accessed July 17, 2016).

87. Robert W. Glover and Joel E. Miller, "The Interplay between Medicaid DSH Payment Cuts, the IMD Exclusion and the ACA Medicaid Expansion Program: Impacts on State Mental Health Services (policy statement)," April 13, 2013, http://www.nasmhpd .org/sites/default/files/TheDSHInterplay04_26_13WebsiteFINAL.pdf (accessed July 17, 2016).

88. National Alliance on Mental Illness, "State Mental Health Cuts: The Continuing Crisis," NAMI, November 2011, http://www.nami.org/getattachment/About -NAMI/Publications/Reports/StateMentalHealthCuts2.pdf (accessed July 17, 2016).

89. Treatment Advocacy Center, "No Room at the Inn: Trends and Consequences of Closing Public Psychiatric Hospitals 2005–2010," Treatment Advocacy Center, July 19, 2012, http://tacreports.org/storage/documents/no_room_at_the_inn-2012.pdf (accessed July 17, 2016).

90. *Patient Protection and Affordable Care Act*, Pub. L. 111-148 (2010), http://www .gpo.gov/fdsys/pkg/PLAW-111publ148/pdf/PLAW-111publ148.pdf (accessed July 23, 2016). The Medicaid Emergency Psychiatric Demonstration was established under Section 2707.

91. Centers for Medicaid and Medicare Services (CMS) Innovation Center, "Medicaid Emergency Psychiatric Demonstration," https://innovation.cms.gov/initiatives/medicaid -emergency-psychiatric-demo (accessed September 20, 2016). The letter to the eleven participating states cancelling the program went out in late August 2016. The federal government does not look at net savings to taxpayers, i.e, include savings in state correction or hospital budgets, it only calculates savings to the federal budget. So if a program has net savings to taxpayers, but not to the federal government, it is not considered to have saved money.

92. Glover and Miller, "Interplay."

93. Barack Obama, "Now Is the Time: The President's Plan to Protect Our Children and Our Communities by Reducing Gun Violence," White House, January 16, 2013, http://www.whitehouse.gov/sites/default/files/docs/wh_now_is_the_time_full.pdf (accessed July 17, 2016).

94. Barack Obama, "Presidential Memorandum: Improving Availability of Relevant Executive Branch Records to the National Instant Criminal Background Check System," White House, January 16, 2013, http://www.whitehouse.gov/the-press-office/2013/ 01/16/presidential-memorandum-improving-availability-relevant-executive-branch (accessed July 17, 2016).

95. Helping Families in Mental Health Crisis Act of 2013, H.R. 3717, 113th Cong. (2013), https://beta.congress.gov/bill/113th-congress/house-bill/3717 (accessed January

16, 2016).

96. Helping Families in Mental Health Crisis Act of 2015, H.R. 2646, 114th Cong. (2015), https://www.congress.gov/bill/114th-congress/house-bill/2646 (accessed September 20, 2016).

97. There are provisions in the bill that guide future research and development of pharmaceuticals that will affect the mentally ill and others. We are only looking at the provisions specific to mental illness. 21st Century Cures Act, H.R. 34, 114th Cong. (2015), https://www.congress.gov/bill/114th-congress/house-bill/34/text (accessed December 10, 2016).

98. DJ Jaffe, "Stop the Madness," *City Journal*, December 6, 2016, http://www.cityjournal.org/html/stop-madness-14886.html (accessed December 10, 2016).

99. Provisions in earlier versions to rein in anti-treatment advocacy by PAIMI and significantly dismantle the IMD Exclusion did not make it into the final bill. The HIPAA provisions may not have much utility. Counterproductively Democrats added provisions that raise the stature of peer support, absent evidence it works, and embeds the recovery, stigma, prevention, and education-solves-all narratives into public law. For other important positive provisions see Treatment Advocacy Center take on bill. Treatment Advocacy Center, "Monumental: What the Cures Act Means for Mentally Ill," Treatment Advocacy Center, December 7, 2016, http://www.treatmentadvocacycenter.org/fixing-the-system/features-and-news/3706-monumental-what-the-cures-act-means-for-severe-mental-illness (accessed December 10, 2016).

CHAPTER 15: COURT DECISIONS THAT FAILED THE SERIOUSLY ILL

1. Treatment Advocacy Center, "Emergency Hospitalization for Evaluation: Assisted Psychiatric Treatment Standards by State," Treatment Advocacy Center, June 2011, http://treatmentadvocacycenter.org/storage/documents/Emergency _Hospitalization_for_Evaluation.pdf (accessed July 19, 2016).

2. Treatment Advocacy Center, "Civil Commitment Laws and Standards," Treatment Advocacy Center, October 2014, http://www.treatmentadvocacycenter.org/legal -resources/civil-commitment-laws (accessed July 19, 2016).

3. The full description of the standard is in WIS. STAT. §51.20(1)(a)2.e., http://docs.legis.wisconsin.gov/statutes/statutes/51/20/1/a/2/e (accessed July 20, 2016). In 2002, the Wisconsin Supreme Court upheld the Fifth Standard. 647 N.W.2d 851 in the Commitment of Dennis H.

4. Steven K. Erickson, Michael J. Vitacco, and Gregory J. Van Rybroek, "Beyond Overt Violence: Wisconsin's Progressive Civil Commitment Statute as a Marker of a New Era in Mental Health Law," *Marquette Law Review* 89 (Winter 2005): 359–405, http://scholarship.law.marquette.edu/cgi/viewcontent.cgi?article=1102&context=mulr (accessed July 19, 2016).

5. O'Connor v. Donaldson, 422 US 563 (1975), http://supreme.justia.com/cases/federal/us/422/563/case.html (accessed July 19, 2016).

6. Kansas v. Hendricks, 521 US 346 (1997), http://www.law.cornell.edu/supct/html/95-1649.ZS.html (accessed July 19, 2016).

7. State of Kansas, "Chapter 59: Probate Code: Article 29a: Commitment of Sexually Violent Predators: Statutes," Kansas Office of Revisor Statutes, July 1, 2007, http://

www.ksrevisor.org/statutes/ksa_ch59.html (accessed July 19, 2016).

8. Some have argued that the case does not bear on civil commitment, because Kendricks was convicted criminally, but these were civil proceedings subsequent to conviction. "It does not make criminal conviction a prerequisite for commitment."

9. Youngberg v. Romeo, 457 US 307 (1982), https://supreme.justia.com/cases/federal/us/457/307/case.html (accessed July 19, 2016).

10. Washington v. Harper, 494 US 210 (1990), https://supreme.justia.com/cases/federal/us/494/210 (accessed July 19, 2016).

11. Riggins v. Nevada, 504 US 127 (1992), http://caselaw.lp.findlaw.com/scripts/getcase.pl?court=US&vol=504&invol=127 (accessed July 19, 2016).

12. Sell v. United States, 539 US 166 (2003), http://www.law.cornell.edu/supct/html/02-5664.ZO.html (accessed July 19, 2016).

13. Olmstead v. L. C., 527 US 581 (1999), http://www.law.cornell.edu/supct/html/98-536.ZO.html (accessed July 19, 2016).

14. Department of Justice, "The Attorney General's Annual Report to Congress Describing the Department's Enforcement Efforts under the Civil Rights of Institutionalized Persons Act, Reports 2000–2013," Department of Justice, http://www.justice.gov/crt/publications/index.php#cripa (accessed July 19, 2016).

15. Mary Zdanowicz, "Keeping the Mentally Ill Out of Jail: Sheriffs as Litigants," *Albany Government Law Review* 8, no. 2 (2015): 536–62.

16. Pete Earley, "Sending the Mentally Ill from Group Homes to an Uncertain Future" (opinion), *Washington Post*, October 30, 2014, http://www.washingtonpost.com/opinions/pete-earley-sending-the-mentally-ill-from-group-homes-to-an-uncertain-future/14/10/30/f4bd84ce-5b22-11e4-8264-deed989ae9a2_story.html (accessed July 19, 2016). Stephanie McCrummen, "In Transition to Independent Living, the 'Dignity of Risk' for the Mentally Ill," *Washington Post*, December 27, 2014, http://www.washingtonpost.com/national/in-transition-to-independent-living-the-dignity-of-risk-for-the-mentally-ill/2014/12/27/dececlee-8ad6-11e4-9e8d-0c687bc18da4_story.html (accessed July 19, 2016).

17. Zdanowicz argues sheriffs could bring Olmstead suits to force localities to provide services to prisoners with a history of recidivism who are being discharged. Doing so would enable these individuals to receive treatment in a less-restrictive environment than jail. Mary Zdanowicz, "Keeping the Mentally Ill Out of Jail." Others believe Olmstead requires states to implement Assisted Outpatient Treatment because it is a "less restrictive setting" than the institutional alternatives—incarceration and hospitalization—and is "within the resources available to states" because it saves 50 percent of the cost of care.

18. Addington v. Texas, 441 US 418 (1979), http://supreme.justia.com/cases/federal/us/441/418/case.html (accessed July 19, 2016).

19. Zinermon v. Burch, 494 US 113 (1990), http://supreme.justia.com/cases/federal/us/494/113/case.html (accessed July 19, 2016)

20. Justice Blackmun wrote that "the very nature of mental illness makes it foreseeable that a person needing mental health care will be unable to understand . . . the [admission and consent to treatment] forms . . . and unable to make a 'knowing and willful decision' whether to consent to admission." Ibid.

21. Kimberly Collins, Gabe Hinkebein, and Staci Schorgl, "The John Hinckley Trial & Its Effect on the Insanity Defense," University of Missouri–Kansas City School of Law,

http://law2.umkc.edu/faculty/projects/ftrials/hinckley/hinckleyinsanity.htm (accessed July 19, 2016).

22. Clark v. Arizona, 548 US 735 (2006), http://www.law.cornell.edu/supremecourt/text/05-5966 (accessed July 19, 2016).

23. Ford v. Wainwright, 477 US 399 (June 26, 1986), http://www.law.cornell.edu/supremecourt/text/477/399#writing-USSC_CR_0477_0399_ZO (accessed March 8, 2015).

24. Panetti v. Quarterman, 551 US 930 (US Supreme Court, June 28, 2007) http://www.supremecourt.gov/opinions/06pdf/06-6407.pdf (accessed March 8, 2015).

25. Michael Perlin, *Mental Disability and the Death Penalty: The Shame of the States* (Lanham, Maryland: Rowman & Littlefield, 2013).

26. District of Columbia v. Heller, 554 US 570 (June 26, 2008), https://supreme.justia.com/cases/federal/us/554/570/opinion.html (accessed September 23, 2016). In *Tyler v. Hillsdale* [Michigan] *Sheriffs' Department*, the Sixth Court of Appeals allowed Tyler to continue his case, arguing that his involuntary commitment of thirty years ago should not preclude him from gun ownership.

27. Riese v. St. Mary's Hospital, 349 F. Supp. 1078 (1987), California Court of Appeals, http://law.justia.com/cases/california/court-of-appeal/3d/209/1303.html (accessed July 30, 2016); Rivers v. Katz, 67 N.Y.2d 485 (1986), New York Court of Appeals, http://scholar.google.com/scholar_case?case=12167532942286784057&hl=en&as_sdt=6&as_vis=1&oi=scholarr (accessed July 30, 2016). Rogers v. Okin, 738 F. 2d 1 (1984), US Court of Appeals First Circuit, http://openjurist.org/738/f2d/1/rogers-v-okin (accessed July 30, 2016). *Rennie v. Klein*, 653 F.2d 836 (1981) US Court of Appeals Third Circuit, http://openjurist.org/653/f2d/836/rennie-v-klein-m-d-m-d (accessed July 30, 2016). In *Rennie v. Klein*, the court allowed the hearing to be conducted by independent treatment professionals rather than a court. Rogers v. Mills, 457 US 291 was a case on medication over objection of hospitalized non-criminally involved patients that did make it to the Supreme Court. However, the court remanded the case, and the Massachusetts Supreme Court decided it by relying upon state law.

28. Jurasek v. Utah State Hospital, 158 F. 3d 506 (1998), http://openjurist.org/158/f3d/506/jurasek-v-utah-state-hospital (accessed July 30, 2016).

29. Wyatt v. Stickney, 325 F. Supp. 781 US District Court (1971) https://scholar.google.com/scholar_case?case=16580065974523676222 (accessed July 19, 2016).

30. Morton Birnbaum, "The Right to Treatment," *American Bar Association Journal* 46 (1960): 499–504.

31. Rael Jean Isaac and Virginia C. Armat, *Madness in the Streets: How Psychiatry and the Law Abandoned the Mentally Ill* (New York: Free Press, 1990).

32. A procedural issue did reach the Supreme Court in *Lessard v. Schmidt*, but in this section we only address the mental illness–related decision made by the Appeals Court. Lessard v. Schmidt, 349 F. Supp. 1078 (1972), US District Court. E. D. Wisconsin http://www.leagle.com/decision/19721427349FSupp1078_11264 (accessed July 19, 2016).

33. K. J. Brennan, *Kendra's Law: Final Report on the Status of Assisted Outpatient Treatment* (Albany, NY: New York State Office of Mental Health, 2005), appendix 2, http://mentalillnesspolicy.org/kendras-law/research/kendras-law-study-2005.pdf (accessed July 19, 2016). Unpublished revision at http://mentalillnesspolicy.org/kendras-law/kendras-law-constitutional.html (accessed July 20, 2016).

CHAPTER 16: SOLUTIONS

1. John Talbott and Steven Sharfstein, "A Proposal for Future Funding of Chronic and Episodic Mental Illness," *Hospital and Community Psychiatry* 37, no. 11 (November 1986): 1126–30.

2. *An Act to Amend Title XIX of the Social Security Act to Remove the Exclusion from Medical Assistance under the Medicaid Program of Items and Services for Patients in an Institution for Mental Diseases*, H.R. 2757, 113th Cong. (2013), https://www.congress.gov/bill/113th-congress/house-bill/2757/ (accessed July 19, 2016).

3. Pub. L. 89–97, 79 Stat. 286.

4. Mental Illness Policy Org., "SAMHSA Supports Groups That Lobby against Improved Treatment," Mental Illness Policy Org., 2012, http://mentalillnesspolicy.org/samhsa/samhsa-support-antipsychiatry.pdf (accessed July 21, 2016).

5. Mental Illness Policy Org, "How SAMHSA Mental Health Block Grant Guidance and Application Form Encourages States to Not Use Block Grants for the Most Seriously Ill," Mental Illness Policy Org., 2013, http://mentalillnesspolicy.org/samhsa/samhsa-block-grant-problems.pdf (accessed July 21, 2016).

6. Amanda Peters, "Lawyers Who Break the Law: What Congress Can Do to Prevent Mental Health Patient Advocates from Violating Federal Legislation," *Oregon Law Review* 89, no. 1 (2010): 133–74, http://mentalillnesspolicy.org/myths/mental-health-bar.pdf (accessed July 21, 2016).

7. Health Insurance Portability and Accountability Act of 1996, Pub. L. 104-191, US Statutes at Large, August 26, 1996, http://www.gpo.gov/fdsys/pkg/PLAW-104publ191/html/PLAW-104publ191.htm (accessed July 17, 2016); Regulations: US Department of Health and Human Services (HHS), Office for Civil Rights, "HIPAA Administrative Simplification," HHS, March 26, 2013, http://www.hhs.gov/sites/default/files/ocr/privacy/hipaa/administrative/combined/hipaa-simplification-201303.pdf (accessed August 17, 2016).

8. Medicare Prescription Drug, Improvement, and Modernization Act of 2003 (H.R. 1). Pub L. 108-173, US Statutes at Large, December 8, 2003, https://www.congress.gov/bill/108th-congress/house-bill/1 (accessed July 17, 2016). Effect on prices: Thomas R. Oliver, Philip R Lee, and Helene L Lipton, "A Political History of Medicare and Prescription Drug Coverage," *Milbank Quarterly* 82.2 (2004): 283–354, http://www.ncbi.nlm.nih.gov/pmc/articles/PMC2690175/ (accessed July 21, 2016)

9. Thomas R. Insel, "Transforming Diagnosis," NIMH, April 29, 2013, http://www.nimh.nih.gov/about/director/2013/transforming-diagnosis.shtml (accessed July 19, 2016).

10. Some worry that this proposal will make the FDA too dependent on income from those it regulates. Others worry about placing research within a government bureaucracy. Some propose direct funding of the FDA via a pharmaceutical tax.

11. Thomas R. Insel, "P-Hacking," NIMH, November 14, 2014, http://www.nimh.nih.gov/about/director/2014/p-hacking.shtml (accessed July 19, 2016).

12. Richard Nisbett, "The Crusade Against Multiple Regression Analysis: A Conversation with Richard Nisbett," Edge, January 21, 2016, http://edge.org/conversation/richard_nisbett-the-crusade-against-multiple-regression-analysis (accessed July 21, 2016).

13. "Erick H, Turner, "Publication Bias with a Focus on Psychiatry," *CNS Drugs* 27 (May 2013): 457-6, http://www.ohsu.edu/xd/education/schools/school-of-medicine/

departments/clinical-departments/psychiatry/news-events/upload/CNS-Drugs-2013
-Turner.pdf (accessed July 21, 2016).

14. Insel, "P-Hacking."

15. Unlike antipsychiatrists, "neuro-critics" acknowledge serious mental illness exists, but they are appalled by the shoddy research that passes as science. The Coynster, led by James Coyne (@CoyneoftheRealm and coyneoftherealm.com) often takes a look at the faulty math and modeling that works its way into the peer-reviewed press. NeuroSkeptic (@Neuro_Skeptic and neuroskeptic.blogspot.com) covers a broad swath of psychiatry with a skeptical eye and is always interesting. Keith Laws (@Keith_Laws) often covers overstated claims for cognitive treatments. The Neurocritic (http://neurocritic.blogspot .com/) looks at some of the most sensationalistic findings concerning neuroscience and brain imaging.

16. Various scientists on editorial boards, "Trust in Science Would Be Improved by Study Pre-registration," *Guardian*, June 5, 2013, http://www.theguardian.com/science/ blog/2013/jun/05/trust-in-science-study-pre-registration (accessed July 21, 2016).

17. A problem with making data sets publicly available is that it allows one researcher to analyze and sponge off the work of the researcher who collected the data, essentially creating "research parasites."

18. B. A. Nosek, G. Alter, and GC Banks, "Scientific Standards: Promoting An Open Research Culture," *Science* 348 (6242): 1422–25, June 26, 2015, http://www.ncbi .nlm.nih.gov/pubmed/26113702 (accessed July 21, 2016). The actual guidelines are at https://cos.io/top (accessed July 21, 2016).

19. Katherine Burton, L. Bal, Anna Clark, et al., "Preventing the Ends from Justifying the Means: Withholding Results to Address Publication Bias in Peer-Review," *BMC Psychology*, December 1, 2016, http://bmcpsychology.biomedcentral.com/ articles/10.1186/s40359-016-0167-7 (accessed December 10, 2016).

20. On October 20, 2015, the *New York Times* ran a front page article, "Talk Therapy Found to Ease Schizophrenia," purporting that a large multistate study found people who took lower doses of antipsychotics did better than others. It wasn't true. As a result of advocacy by Mental Illness Policy Org., on October 29, the paper ran a begrudging correction, but the original story is still in circulation. They have also run misleading reports on peer support and Open Dialogue.

21. Charles Krauthammer, "How Best to Help the Homeless," *Deseret News* (Salt Lake City, UT), December 25, 1988, http://www.deseretnews.com/article/28130/HOW -BEST-TO-HELP-THE-HOMELESS.html (accessed February 25, 2015).

22. Treatment Advocacy Center, "Model Assisted Treatment Law," Treatment Advocacy Center, 2011, http://www.treatmentadvocacycenter.org/legal-resources/tac-model -law (accessed March 8, 2015).

23. New York State Legislature, NY MHY. LAW § 9.60 : NY Code--Section 9.60: Assisted Outpatient Treatment, 2010 http://codes.lp.findlaw.com/nycode/MHY/B/9/9.60 (accessed July 21, 2016).

24. Many of these policy recommendations were overwhelmingly endorsed by direct vote of the grassroots membership of NAMI in 1995. But subsequent NAMI National boards and staffs have refused to help enact these reforms. National Alliance on Mental Illness, "Involuntary Commitment and Court-Ordered Treatment," NAMI, 1995, http:// www.nami.org/About-NAMI/Policy-Platform/9-Legal-Issues (accessed July 21, 2016).

25. Involuntarily committed (dangerous) patients maintain the right to refuse treatment unless a capacity hearing is held. As a result, individuals are often committed but not allowed treatment.

26. Rael Jean Isaac and DJ Jaffe, "Mental Illness, Public Safety," *New York Times*, December 23, 1995.

27. Steven K. Erickson, Michael J. Vitacco, and Gregory J. Van Rybroek, "Beyond Overt Violence: Wisconsin's Progressive Civil Commitment Statute as a Marker of a New Era in Mental Health Law," *Marquette Law Review* 89 (Winter 2005): 359–405, http://scholarship.law.marquette.edu/cgi/viewcontent.cgi?article=1102&context=mulr (accessed July 19, 2016).

28. Assembly Bill 1194, October 7, 2015, Chaptered 5150.05 Welfare and Institutions Code, http://leginfo.legislature.ca.gov/faces/codes_displaySection.xhtml?lawCode=WIC&sectionNum=5150.05 (accessed August 3, 2016).

29. In the 1990s, when President Clinton tried to create a universal health plan, anti-treatment mental health lawyers tried to insert a sentence along the lines of, "Only services requested by the patient shall be reimbursed." It seemed reasonable, but their motive was to reduce the use of involuntary commitment and treatment for the seriously ill by preventing reimbursement for it.

30. CIT Center, "CIT Center," University of Memphis, http://www.cit.memphis.edu (accessed July 19, 2016). CIT International, "Welcome to CIT International," CIT International, http://citinternational.org (accessed July 19, 2016). NAMI, "Crisis Intervention Teams," NAMI, 2014, http://www.nami.org/Get-Involved/Law-Enforcement-and -Mental-Health/What-Is-CIT/Creating-a-Successful-CIT-Program (accessed July 2, 2016).

31. The Mental Health Courts Program was created by America's Law Enforcement and Mental Health Project, Pub. L. 106-515 (2000), http://www.gpo.gov/fdsys/pkg/PLAW-106publ515/pdf/PLAW-106publ515.pdf (accessed July 21, 2016). Funding also comes through the Mentally Ill Offender Treatment and Crime Reduction Act of 2004, Pub. L. 108-414 (2004) and renewals, http://www.gpo.gov/fdsys/pkg/PLAW -108publ414/pdf/PLAW-108publ414.pdf (accessed July 21, 2016).

32. In a 2014 video interview with the Vera Institute of Justice, Mathew J. D'Emic, the Brooklyn mental health court presiding judge, disclosed that 24 percent of the mentally ill individuals in it have bipolar disorder; 30 percent have major depression; 21 percent have, schizophrenia; 12 percent have schizoaffective disorder; and 13 percent have PTSD. Vera Institute of Justice, "Justice in Transition–NYC: Cops, Courts, and Corrections: Can NYC's Justice System Help Those with Mental Illness?" YouTube video, 1:25:33, posted by VeraInstitute, March 26, 2014, https://www.youtube.com/watch?v=dzFCfJFHLXo (accessed July 19, 2016).

33. Council of State Governments Justice Center, Criminal Justice/Mental Health Consensus Project, Mental Health Courts: A Primer for Policymakers and Practitioners, Prepared for the Bureau of Justice Assistance, DOJ, 2008, http://csgjusticecenter.org/wp -content/uploads/2012/12/mhc-primer.pdf (accessed July 19, 2016).

34. Department of Justice, Bureau of Justice Assistance, "Mental Health Courts Program," Bureau of Justice Assistance, https://www.bja.gov/ProgramDetails. aspx?Program_ID=68 (accessed March 8, 2015). National Center for State Courts, "Mental Health Courts," NCSC, http://www.ncsc.org/Topics/Problem-Solving-Courts/Mental-Health-Courts/Resource-Guide.aspx (accessed July 19, 2016).

35. Kimberly Collins, Gabe Hinkebein, and Staci Schorgl, "The John Hinckley Trial & Its Effect on the Insanity Defense," University of Missouri–Kansas City School of Law, http://law2.umkc.edu/faculty/projects/ftrials/hinckley/hinckleyinsanity.htm (accessed July 29, 2016).

36. Methods for successfully monitoring patients to ensure they take their medications exist. Assisted Outpatient Treatment programs already monitor potentially dangerous mentally ill individuals. In New York, programs monitor those with tuberculosis to see that they don't go off treatment.

37. "New York State District Attorneys Support Hope House," Greenburger Center for Social and Criminal Justice, http://www.greenburgercenter.org/article?ID=101 (accessed August 16, 2016).

38. Almost all psychiatrists receive public funds because Medicare funds most residency programs. Psychiatrists who receive these public funds could also be required to serve the seriously ill. Some argue this will insure fewer enter the profession. But if they won't serve the seriously ill, they should not be publicly funded. There is general agreement that telepsychiatry could help patients in underserved areas. But some fear that insurers in urban areas will replace face-to-face visits with less expensive and less effective phone visits. A useful model might be Washington's Partnership Access Line (PAL), which doesn't serve patients directly. It is a pediatrician to psychiatrist consult line that provides a rapid connection to a psychiatrist for pediatricians serving clients with mental illness.

39. There are many different proven models, from group homes with on-premises case management to scatter site housing with visits from case managers to in-home services for those who live with relatives.

40. Stephen Eide, "Supportive Housing and the Mentally Ill Homeless," Manhattan Institute, September 2016, http://www.manhattan-institute.org/sites/default/files/R-SE-0916.pdf (accessed September 20, 2016).

41. "Clubhouse International," Clubhouse International, http://www.clubhouse-intl.org (accessed July 19, 2016).

CHAPTER 17: THE FUTURE

1. Alluding to HIPAA, President-elect Donald Trump's policy platform noted, "Finally, we need to reform our mental health programs and institutions in this country. Families, without the ability to get the information needed to help those who are ailing, are too often not given the tools to help their loved ones. There are promising reforms being developed in Congress that should receive bi-partisan support." Donald Trump Presidential Campaign, "Healthcare Reform," Donald J. Trump, https://assets.donaldjtrump.com/HCReformPaper.pdf (accessed December 10, 2016).

On reducing violence, his platform said, "Fix our broken mental health system. All of the tragic mass murders that occurred in the past several years have something in common—there were red flags that were ignored. We can't allow that to continue. We must expand treatment programs, and reform the laws to make it easier to take preventive action to save innocent lives. Most people with mental health problems are not violent, but just need help, and these reforms will help everyone." Donald Trump Presidential Campaign, "Constitution and Second Amendment," Donald J. Trump, https://www

.donaldjtrump.com/policies/constitution-and-second-amendment (accessed December 10, 2016).

APPENDIX A: SERIOUS MENTAL ILLNESS DEFINED

1. The definition derives from two steps included in the legislation creating SAMHSA and requiring it to distribute mental health block grants to states proportional to the number of persons with serious mental illness in each state. As the first step, Congress required CMHS to define "serious mental illness in adults." ADAMHA Reorganization Act of 1991, Pub. L. 102-321, Pub. L. 102-321 (1992), pp. 323–442, https://www.gpo.gov/fdsys/pkg/STATUTE-106/pdf/STATUTE-106-Pg323.pdf (accessed July 17, 2016). The second step, after it was defined, was to estimate its prevalence in each state.

2. "[A]dults with a serious mental illness' are persons: (1) age 18 and over and (2) who currently have, or at any time during the past year, had a diagnosable mental, behavioral, or emotional disorder of sufficient duration to meet diagnostic criteria specified within *DSM-IV* or their *ICD-9-CM* equivalent (and subsequent revisions) with the exception of *DSM-IV* 'V' codes, substance use disorders, and developmental disorders which are excluded, unless they co-occur with another diagnosable serious mental illness, and (3) that has resulted in functional impairment, which substantially interferes with or limits one or more major life activities." "[A]dults who would have met functional impairment criteria during the referenced year without the benefit of treatment or other support services are considered to have serious mental illnesses." The same legislation and steps defined "serious emotional disturbance" in children. Center for Mental Health Services (CMHS), *Federal Register* 58, no. 96 (May 1993): 29422, http://www.samhsa.gov/sites/default/files/federal-register-notice-58-96-definitions.pdf (accessed July 22, 2016).

3. When explaining how functional impairment was defined, CMHS stated: "Strict criteria were used, such as reports of extreme deficits in social functioning. . . . A respondent must either have one of the following two profiles: (i) Complete social isolation, defined as having absolutely no social contact of any type—telephone, mail, or in-person—with any family member or friend and having no one in his or her personal life with whom he/she has a confiding personal relationship; or (ii) extreme dysfunction in personal relationships, defined as high conflict and no positive interactions and no possibility of intimacy or confiding with any family member or friend. These persons comprise about 10% of those classified as having SMI." However, in the actual definition included in the *Federal Register*, the criteria were not quite as strict. For example "consistently missing at least one full day of work per month as a direct result of mental health" counts as a qualifying functional impairment.

4. Center for Behavioral Health Statistics and Quality, "Behavioral Health Trends in the United States: Results from the 2014 National Survey on Drug Use and Health," HHS Publication No. SMA 15-4927, NSDUH Series H-50, 2015, http://www.samhsa.gov/data/sites/default/files/NSDUH-FRR1-2014/NSDUH-FRR1-2014.pdf (accessed July 26, 2016).

5. In 2016, in reaction to outside pressure for its failure to focus on serious mental illness, SAMHSA developed a Byzantine policy paper that expanded the definition of serious mental illness far beyond the one created as a result of SAMHSA's establishing

legislation. For example, the paper argued that ADHD, anxiety, mood disorders, and other often mild illnesses are in fact "nested within" or "interchangeable" with the term "serious mental illness." SAMHSA, "Behind the Term: Serious Mental Illness," SAMHSA, 2016, http://www.nrepp.samhsa.gov/Docs/Literatures/Behind_the_Term_Serious%20%20 Mental%20Illness.pdf (accessed December 26, 2016).

6. National Advisory Mental Health Council, "Health Care Reform for Americans with Severe Mental Illnesses: Report of the National Advisory Mental Health Council," *American Journal of Psychiatry* 150, no. 10 (October 1993): 1447–65. Abstract at http:// www.ncbi.nlm.nih.gov/pubmed/8379547 (accessed July 22, 2016).

7. US Senate, "Senate Report 102-397" attached to "HR 5677, HHS Appropriations Bill. ADAMHA Reorganization Act," *Federal Register* (September 10, 1993): 96. The government sometimes uses "severe" versus "serious." From a policy perspective, there is very little difference. After the 1993 report was issued, autism was reclassified as a developmental disability, not a mental illness.

8. Ronald C. Kessler, Wai Tat Chiu, Olga Demler, et al., "Prevalence, Severity, and Comorbidity of 12-Month DSM-IV Disorders in the National Comorbidity Survey Replication," *Archives of General Psychiatry* 6, no. 2 (June 2005): 617–27, http://archpsyc .jamanetwork.com/article.aspx?articleid=208671 (accessed July 22, 2016).

9. American Psychiatric Association, *Diagnostic and Statistical Manual of Mental Disorders: DSM-5* (Washington, DC: American Psychiatric Association, 2013).

10. COLO. REV. STAT. § 27-65-102(9), http://tornado.state.co.us/gov_dir/leg_dir/ olls/2014TitlePrintouts/CRS%20Title%2027%20(2014).pdf (accessed August 17, 2016).

APPENDIX B: STUDIES ON VIOLENCE AND MENTAL ILLNESS

1. John Monahan, "Mental Disorder and Violent Behavior," *American Psychologist* 47, no. 4 (April 1992): 511–21. Abstract at http://psycnet.apa.org/journals/amp/47/4/511/ (accessed July 6, 2016).

2. Thomas Insel, "Keynote Address," video, 30:19, February 26, 2014, http://www .nationalacademies.org/hmd/Activities/Global/ViolenceForum/2014-FEB-26/Day%201/ Welcome%20and%20Morning%20Presentations/4-Insel-Video.aspx (accessed July 25, 2016).

3. Sarah L. Desmarais, Richard A. Van Dorn, Kiersten L. Johnson, et al., "Community Violence Perpetration and Victimization among Adults with Mental Illnesses," *American Journal of Public Health* 104, no. 12 (December 2014): 2342–49. Abstract at http://ajph. aphapublications.org/doi/abs/10.2105/AJPH.2013.301680 (accessed July 25, 2016).

4. K. S. Douglas, L. S. Guy, and S. D. Hart, "Psychosis as a Risk Factor for Violence to Others: A Meta-Analysis," *Psychological Bulletin* 135, no. 5 (September 2009): 679–706. Abstract at http://www.ncbi.nlm.nih.gov/pubmed/19702378 (accessed July 25, 2016).

5. Richard A. Van Dorn, Jan Volavka, and Norman Johnson, "Mental Disorder and Violence: Is There a Relationship beyond Substance Use?" *Social Psychiatry and Psychiatric Epidemiology* 47, no. 3 (March 12, 2012): 487–503. Abstract at http://www.ncbi.nlm.nih .gov/pubmed/21359532 (accessed July 25, 2016).

6. M. Large, G. Smith, and O. Nielssen, "The Relationship between the Rate of Homicide by Those with Schizophrenia and the Overall Homicide Rate," *Schizophrenia*

Research 112, no. 1–3 (July 2009): 123–29. Abstract at http://www.ncbi.nlm.nih.gov/ pubmed/19457644 (accessed July 25, 2016).

7. Seena Fazel, Niklas Langstrom, Anders Hjern, et al., "Schizophrenia, Substance Abuse, and Violent Crime," *Journal of the American Medical Association* 301, no. 19 (May 2009): 2016–23 http://jama.jamanetwork.com/article.aspx?articleid=183929 (accessed July 25, 2016).

8. C. Rodway, S. Flynn, M.S. Rahman et.al, "Patients with Mental Illness as Victims of Homicide: A National Consecutive Case Series," *Lancet* 1, no. 2 (2014): 129–34.

9. Christine C. Joyal, Jean-Luc Dubreucq, Catherine Gendron, et al., "Major Mental Disorders and Violence: A Critical Update," *Current Psychiatry Reviews* 3 (March 2007): 33–50, https://oraprdnt.uqtr.uquebec.ca/pls/public/docs/GSC409/F1512875772 _Article_2007.pdf (accessed July 25, 2016).

10. Louise Arseneault, Terrie E. Moffitt, Avshalom Caspi, et al., "Mental Disorders and Violence in a Total Birth Cohort," *Archives of General Psychiatry* 57, no. 10 (October 2000): 979–86, http://archpsyc.jamanetwork.com/article.aspx?articleid=481658 (accessed July 25, 2016).

11. Seena Fazel, Paul Lichtenstein, Martin Grann, et al., "Bipolar Disorder and Violent Crime," *Archives of General Psychiatry* 67, no. 9 (September 2010): 931–38, http:// archpsyc.jamanetwork.com/article.aspx?articleid=210872 (accessed July 25, 2016).

12. P. J. Taylor, "Psychosis and Violence: Stories, Fears, and Reality," *Canadian Journal of Psychiatry* 53, no. 10 (October 2008): 647–59. Abstract at http://www.ncbi.nlm .nih.gov/pubmed/18940033 (accessed July 25, 2016).

13. Marvin S. Swartz, Jeffrey W. Swanson, and Virginia A. Hiday, "Violence and Severe Mental Illness: The Effects of Substance Abuse and Nonadherence to Medication," *American Journal of Psychiatry* 155, no. 2 (1998): 226–31. Abstract at http://www.ncbi.nlm .nih.gov/pubmed/9464202 (accessed July 25, 2016).

14. Jeffrey W. Swanson, Charles E. Holzer, Vijay K. Ganju, et al., "Violence and Psychiatric Disorder in the Community: Evidence from the Epidemiologic Catchment Area Surveys," *Hospital and Community Psychiatry* 41, no. 7 (July 1990): 761–70. Abstract at http://www.ncbi.nlm.nih.gov/pubmed/2142118 (accessed July 25, 2016).

15. Bruce G. Link, Howard Andrews, and Francis T. Cullen, "The Violent and Illegal Behavior of Mental Patients Reconsidered," *American Sociological Review* 57, no. 3 (June 1992): 275–92. Abstract at http://www.jstor.org/discover/10.2307/2096235?sid=21 105861640113&uid=3739832&uid=2&uid=4&uid=3739256 (accessed July 25, 2016).

16. Seena Fazel and Martin Grann, "Psychiatric Morbidity among Homicide Offenders: A Swedish Population Study," *American Journal of Psychiatry* 161, no. 11 (November 2004): 2129–31. Abstract at http://www.ncbi.nlm.nih.gov/pubmed/15514419 (accessed July 25, 2016). S. Fazel, P. Buxrud, V. Ruchkin, et al., "Homicide in Discharged Patients with Schizophrenia and Other Psychoses: A National Case-Control Study," *Schizophrenia Research* 123, no. 2–3 (November 2010): 263–69. Abstract at http://www .ncbi.nlm.nih.gov/pubmed/20805021 (accessed July 25, 2016).

17. K. G. W. W. Koh, K. P. Gwee, and Y. H. Chan, "Psychiatric Aspects of Homicide in Singapore: A Five-Year Review," *Singapore Medical Journal* 47, no. 4 (2006): 297–304, http://www.sma.org.sg/smj/4704/4704a8.pdf (accessed July 25, 2016).

18. Jason C. Matejkowski, Sara W. Cullen, and Phyllis L. Solomon, "Characteristics of Persons with Severe Mental Illness Who Have Been Incarcerated for Murder," *Journal*

of the American Academy of Psychiatry and the Law 36, no. 1 (March 2008): 74–86, http://www.jaapl.org/content/36/1/74.full (accessed July 25, 2016).

19. David Tuller, "Nurses Step Up Efforts to Protect against Attacks," *New York Times*, July 8, 2008, http://www.nytimes.com/2008/07/08/health/08nurses.html (accessed July 25, 2016).

20. Marilyn Lewis Lanza, Robert Zeiss, and Jill Rierdan, "Violence against Psychiatric Nurses: Sensitive Research as Science and Intervention," *Contemporary Nurse* 21, no. 1 (2006): 71–84. Abstract at http://www.ncbi.nlm.nih.gov/pubmed/16594884 (accessed July 25, 2016).

21. Joy Jacobson, "Violence and Nursing," *American Journal of Nursing* 107, no. 2 (February 2007): 25–26.

22. Lee Romney, "State Mental Hospitals Remain Violent, Despite Gains in Safety," *Los Angeles Times*, October 9, 2013, http://articles.latimes.com/2013/oct/09/local/la-me -mental-hospital-safety-20131010 (accessed July 25, 2016).

23. American Psychiatric Nurses Association, "Workplace Violence (Position Statement)," APNA, 2008, http://www.apna.org/files/public/APNA_Workplace_Violence _Position_Paper.pdf (accessed July 25, 2016).

24. Henry J. Steadman, Edward P. Mulvey, John Monahan, et al., "Violence by People Discharged from Acute Psychiatric Inpatient Facilities and by Others in the Same Neighborhoods," *Archives of General Psychiatry* 55, no. 5 (May 1998): 393–401. Abstract at http://www.ncbi.nlm.nih.gov/pubmed/9596041 (accessed July 25, 2016).

25. E. F. Torrey, Joe Bruce, DJ Jaffe, et al., "Raising Cain: The Role of Serious Mental Illness in Family Homicide," June 2016, http://www.treatmentadvocacycenter.org/storage/documents/raising-cain.pdf (accessed December 24, 2016).

26. Donald M. Steinwachs, Judith D. Kasper, and Elizabeth A. Skinner, "Family Perspectives of Meeting the Needs for Care of Severely Mentally Ill Relatives: A National Survey," final report to the National Alliance for the Mentally Ill, Johns Hopkins University and the University of Maryland, July 1992.

27. John M. Dawson and Patrick A. Langan, Murder in Families (Washington, DC: Bureau of Justice Statistics, DOJ, July 1994) http://www.bjs.gov/content/pub/pdf/mf.pdf (accessed July 25, 2016).

28. Seena Fazel, Johan Zetterqvist, Henrik Larsson, et al., "Antipsychotics, Mood Stabilisers, and Risk of Violent Crime," *Lancet* 384 (September 27, 2014): 1206–14, http://www.thelancet.com/journals/lancet/article/PIIS0140-6736(14)60379-2/fulltext (accessed July 25, 2016).

29. Robert Keers, Simone Ullrich, Bianca L. DeStavola, et al., "Association of Violence with Emergence of Persecutory Delusions in Untreated Schizophrenia," *American Journal of Psychiatry* 171, no. 3 (March 2014): 332–39. Abstract at http://ajp.psychiatry online.org/article.aspx?articleID=1773703 (accessed July 25, 2016).

30. Olav Nielssen and Matthew Large, "Rates of Homicide during the First Episode of Psychosis and after Treatment: A Systematic Review and Meta-Analysis," *Schizophrenia Bulletin* 36, no. 4 (July 2010): 702–12, http://www.ncbi.nlm.nih.gov/pmc/articles/PMC2894594/ (accessed July 25, 2016).

31. Nelly Alia-Klein, Thomas M. O'Rourke, Rita Z. Goldstein, et al., "Insight into Illness and Adherence to Psychotropic Medications Are Separately Associated with Violence Severity in a Forensic Sample," *Aggressive Behavior* 33, no. 1 (2007): 86–96. Abstract

at http://onlinelibrary.wiley.com/doi/10.1002/ab.20170/abstract;jsessionid=A2A18A8D4 A27C220186B855F2C5F87D5.f01t04 (accessed July 25, 2016).

32. Eric Elbogen, Sarah Mustillo, Richard van Dorn, et al., "The Impact of Perceived Need for Treatment on Risk of Arrest and Violence among People with Severe Mental Illness," *Criminal Justice and Behavior* 34, no. 2 (February 2007): 197–210. Abstract at http://cjb.sagepub.com/content/34/2/197 (accessed July 25, 2016).

33. Eric B. Elbogen, Richard A. Van Dorn, Jeffrey W. Swanson, et al., "Treatment Engagement and Violence Risk in Mental Disorders," *British Journal of Psychiatry* 189, no. 4 (September 2006), http://bjp.rcpsych.org/content/189/4/354 (accessed July 25, 2016).

34. J. Swanson, S. Swartz, and M. Estroff, "Violence and Severe Mental Disorder in Clinical and Community Populations: The Effects of Psychotic Symptoms, Comorbidity, and Lack of Treatment," *Psychiatry* 60 (Spring 1997): 1–22. Abstract at http://www.ncbi .nlm.nih.gov/pubmed/9130311 (accessed July 25, 2016).

35. J. Bartels, R.E. Drake, and M.A. Wallach, "Characteristic Hostility in Schizophrenic Outpatients," *Schizophrenia Bulletin* 17, no. 1 (1991): 163–71, http://schizophrenia bulletin.oxfordjournals.org/content/17/1/163.full.pdf (accessed July 25, 2016)

36. L. D. Smith, "Medication Refusal and the Rehospitalized Mentally Ill Inmate," *Hospital and Community Psychiatry* 40 (1999): 491–96. Abstract at https://www.ncjrs.gov/ App/Publications/abstract.aspx?ID=118885 (accessed July 25, 2016).

37. J. A. Yessavage, "Inpatient Violence and the Schizophrenic Patient: An Inverse Correlation between Danger-Related Events and Neuroleptic Levels," *Biological Psychiatry* 17 (1982): 1331–37. Abstract at http://psycnet.apa.org/psycinfo/1983-23962-001 (accessed July 25, 2016).

APPENDIX C: STUDIES CORRELATING ANOSOGNOSIA WITH VIOLENCE

1. Treatment Advocacy Center, "The Anatomical Basis of Anosognosia (Lack of Awareness of Illness)," Treatment Advocacy Center, September 2012, http://www .treatmentadvocacycenter.org/storage/documents/Anosognosia--Anatomical_Basis_- _August_2012.pdf (accessed July 25, 2016).

2. Lisette van der Meer, Annerieke E. de Vos, and Annemarie P. M. Stiekema, "Insight in Schizophrenia: Involvement of Self-Reflection Networks?" *Schizophrenia Bulletin* 39, no. 6 (November 2013): 1288–95. http://www.ncbi.nlm.nih.gov/pmc/articles/ PMC3796073 (accessed July 25, 2016).

3. For a discussion of overstated claims being made for brain imaging, see Sally Satel and Scott O. Lilienfeld, *Brainwashed: The Seductive Appeal of Mindless Neuroscience* (New York: Basic Books, 2013).

4. Xavier Amador, "Anosognosia and Serious Mental Illness," video, 9:01, June 1, 2011, http://ssnsc.blogspot.com/2011/03/anosognosia-1-of-2.html (accessed July 10, 2016).

5. P. F. Buckley, D. R. Hrouda, and L. Friedman, "Insight and Its Relationship to Violent Behavior in Patients with Schizophrenia," *American Journal of Psychiatry* 161, no. 9 (2004): 1712–14. Abstract at http://www.ncbi.nlm.nih.gov/pubmed/15337667 (accessed December 24, 2016).

6. Marvin S. Swartz, Jeffrey W. Swanson, and Virginia A. Hiday, "Violence and

Severe Mental Illness: The Effects of Substance Abuse and Nonadherence to Medication," *American Journal of Psychiatry* 155, no. 2 (1998): 226–31. Abstract at http://www.ncbi.nlm .nih.gov/pubmed/9464202 (accessed July 25, 2016).

7. Nelly Alia-Klein, Thomas M. O'Rourke, Rita Z. Goldstein, et al., "Insight into Illness and Adherence to Psychotropic Medications Are Separately Associated with Violence Severity in a Forensic Sample," *Aggressive Behavior* 33, no. 1 (2007): 86–96. Abstract at http://onlinelibrary.wiley.com/doi/10.1002/ab.20170/abstract;jsessionid=A2A18A8D4 A27C220186B855F2C5F87D5.f01t04 (accessed July 25, 2016).

8. Michelle Grevatt, Brian Thomas-Peter, and Gary Hughes, "Violence, Mental Disorder and Risk Assessment: Can Structured Clinical Assessments Predict the Short-Term Risk of Inpatient Violence?" *Journal of Forensic Psychiatry and Psychology* 15, no. 2 (2004): 278–92. Abstract at http://www.tandfonline.com/doi/ abs/10.1080/1478994032000199095 (accessed July 25, 2016).

9. Arango Celso, Alfredo Calcedo Barba, Teresa González-Salvador, et al., "Violence in Inpatients with Schizophrenia: A Prospective Study," *Schizophrenia Bulletin* 25, no. 3 (1999): 493–503. Abstract at http://www.ncbi.nlm.nih.gov/pubmed/10478784 (accessed July 25, 2016).

10. Strand Susanne, Henrik Belfrage, and Goran Fransson, "Clinical and Risk Management Factors in Risk Prediction of Mentally Disordered Offenders: More Important than Historical Data?" *Legal and Criminological Psychology* 4, no. 1 (1999): 67–76. Abstract at http://onlinelibrary.wiley.com/doi/10.1348/135532599167798/abstract (accessed July 25, 2016)

11. P. Woods, V. Reed, and M. Collin, "The Relationship between Risk and Insight in a High-Security Forensic Setting," *Journal of Psychiatric and Mental Health Nursing* 10, no. 5 (2003): 510–17. Abstract at http://www.ncbi.nlm.nih.gov/pubmed/12956629 (accessed July 25, 2016).

12. S. R. Foley, B. D. Kelly, and M. Clarke, "Incidence and Clinical Correlates of Aggression and Violence at Presentation in Patients with First Episode Psychosis," *Schizophrenia Research* 72, no. 2–3 (2005): 161–68. Abstract at http://www.ncbi.nlm.nih. gov/pubmed/15560961 (accessed July 25, 2016).

INDEX

Pages in **bold** indicate figures and tables.